MUSCLE RELAXANTS

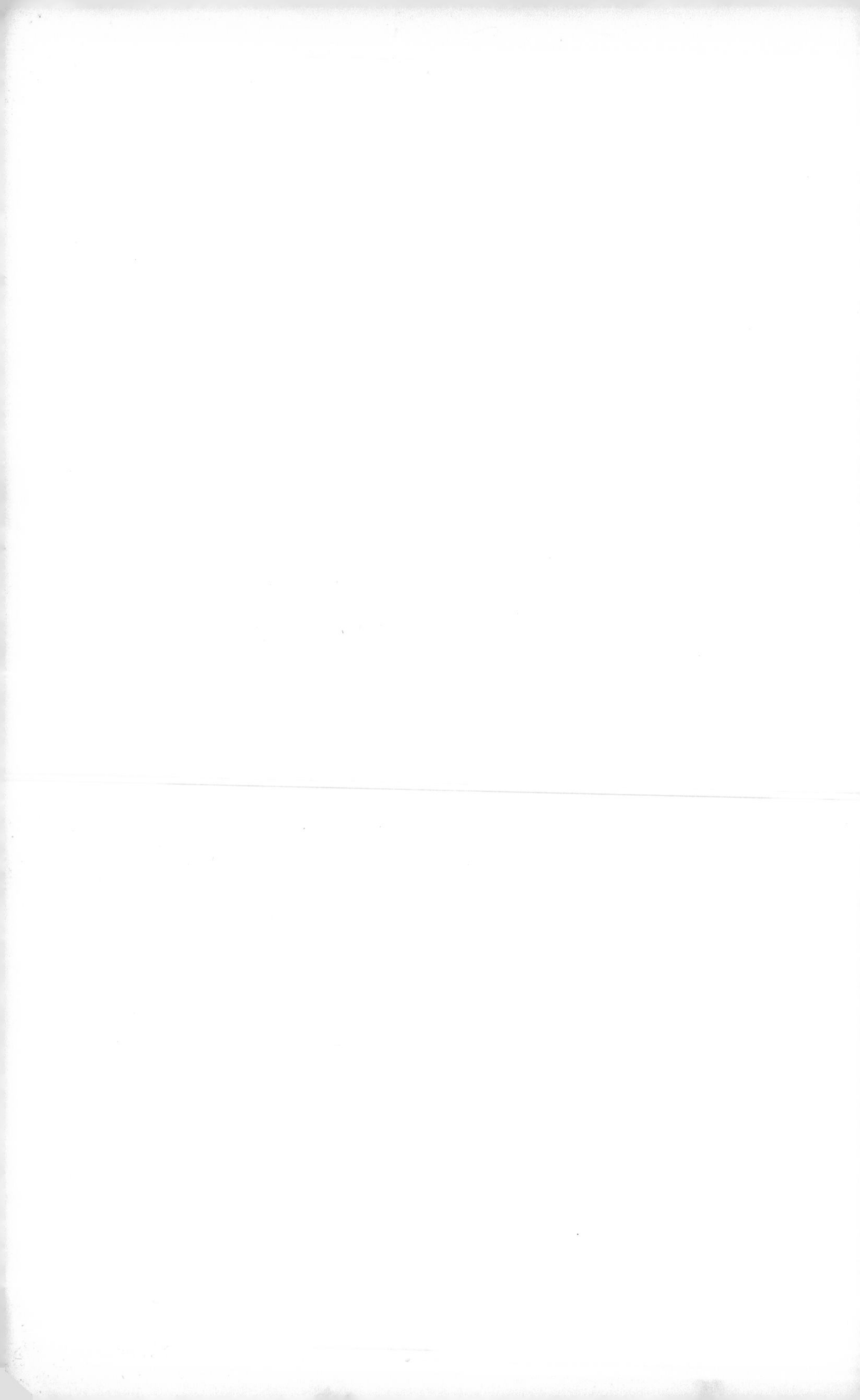

MUSCLE RELAXANTS

Basic and Clinical Aspects

Edited by

Ronald L. Katz, M.D.

Professor and Chairman
Department of Anesthesiology
UCLA School of Medicine
Los Angeles, California

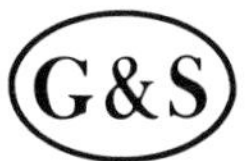

Grune & Stratton
(Harcourt Brace Jovanovich, Publishers)
Orlando San Diego New York London
Toronto Montreal Sydney Tokyo

Muscle Relaxants: Basic and Clinical Aspects is the paperback edition based on December 1984 (Volume III, Number 4) and March 1985 (Volume IV, Number 1) issues of the journal *Seminars in Anesthesia*.

Grune & Stratton, Inc.
Orlando, Florida 32887

Distributed in the United Kingdom by
Grune & Stratton, Ltd.
24/28 Oval Road, London NW 1

Library of Congress Catalog Number 85-081233
International Standard Book Number 0-8089-1784-6
Printed in the United States of America
86 87 88 10 9 8 7 6 5 4 3 2

Contents

Contributors

Sandor Agoston, M.D., Ph.D.
Institute of Anesthesiology
University Hospital
Groningen, THE NETHERLANDS

Hassan H. Ali, M.D.
Department of Anesthesia
Massachusetts General Hospital
Boston, MA

David R. Bevan, M.B., M.R.C.P., F.F.A.R.C.S.
Departments of Anaesthesia
Royal Victoria Hospital and McGill University
Montreal, Quebec, CANADA

W.C. Bowman, B.Pharm., Ph.D., D.Sc., F.P.S., F.R.S.E.
Department of Physiology and Pharmacology
University of Strathclyde
Glasgow, SCOTLAND

Barbara W. Brandom, M.D.
Department of Anesthesiology
Children's Hospital
Pittsburgh, PA

Won W. Choi, M.D.
Department of Anesthesia
University of Iowa Hospitals and Clinics
Iowa City, IA

D. Ryan Cook, M.D.
Department of Anesthesiology
University of Pittsburgh
Pittsburgh, PA

Roy Cronnelly, Ph.D., M.D.
Department of Anesthesia
University of California
San Francisco, CA

Francois Donati, M.D., Ph.D.
Departments of Anaesthesia
Royal Victoria Hospital and McGill University
Montreal, Quebec, CANADA

Nicholas N. Durant, Ph.D.
Department of Anesthesiology
UCLA School of Medicine
Los Angeles, CA

Samir D. Gergis, M.D.
Department of Anesthesia
University of Iowa Hospitals and Clinics
Iowa City, IA

A.J. Gibb, Ph.D.
Department of Physiology and Pharmacology
University of Strathclyde
Glasgow, SCOTLAND

Pim J. Hennis, M.D.
Department of Anesthesia
University of Leiden
Leiden, THE NETHERLANDS

Dieter Langrehr
Institute of Anesthesiology
University Hospital
Groningen, THE NETHERLANDS

Chingmuh Lee, M.D.
Department of Anesthesiology
Harbor/UCLA Medical Center
Torrance, CA

I.G. Marshall, Ph.D.
Department of Physiology and Pharmacology
University of Strathclyde
Glagow, SCOTLAND

Ronald D. Miller, M.D.
Department of Anesthesia
University of California
School of Medicine
San Francisco, CA

Douglas E.F. Newton
Institute of Clinical Pharmacology
University Hospital
Groningen, THE NETHERLANDS

James P. Payne, M.B., F.F.A.R.C.S.
Research Department of Anaesthetics
Royal College of Surgeons of England
London, ENGLAND

Henry Rosenberg, M.D.
Department of Anesthesia
Hahnemann University
Philadelphia, PA

John J. Savarese, M.D.
Department of Anesthesia
Harvard Medical School at Massachusetts
General Hospital
Boston, MA

Ralph P.F. Scott, M.D.
Department of Anesthesia
Harvard Medical School at Massachusetts
General Hospital
Boston, MA

Colin A. Shanks, M.D., Ph.D., F.F.A.R.A.C.S.
Department of Anesthesia
Northwestern University
Chicago, IL

Martin D. Sokoll, M.D.
Department of Anesthesia
University of Iowa Hospital and Clinics
Iowa City, IA

Frank G. Standaert, M.D.
Department of Pharmacology
Georgetown University
Schools of Medicine and Dentistry
Washington, D.C.

Donald R. Stanski, M.D.
Department of Anesthesia
Stanford University
Stanford, California

Robert K. Stoelting, M.D.
Department of Anesthesia
Indiana University School of Medicine
Indianapolis, IN

Jørgen Viby-Mogensen, M.D., Ph.D.
Department of Anaesthesia
Herlev Hospital
Herlev, Ringvej, DENMARK

Frank G. Standaert

1

Donuts and Holes: Molecules and Muscle Relaxants

The site and mechanism of action of neuromuscular blocking drugs have puzzled investigators for over a century. In the early years it was speculated that the fine endings of the nerves to the muscles bore the key spots, but this view changed early in this century when Langley showed that curare antagonized the action of nicotine on denervated muscles and concluded that the sites of action had to be on the muscle. As scientific insight grew, so did knowledge of curare and its receptor, but always there was a search for the single, or at least the principle, site of drug action. In this aspect, laboratory research diverged from clinical experience because those who used the relaxants knew that they were dealing with complicated agents, and it took little reflection to think that there might be more than one site or mechanism of action.

Modern investigations are beginning to bring clinical and laboratory experience together. The experimental work clearly shows that muscle relaxants have several sites and mechanisms of action and that their relative importance can change with changes in dose, activity in a neuromuscular system, disease, and interaction with other drugs. Although it is apparent that the relaxants can have actions on synapses outside the neuromuscular junction, eg, in the heart or ganglia, the neuromuscular junction is the center of interest because it is here that the most desired effects take place and the techniques for experimental investigation are most advanced. Furthermore, although it is well established that drugs have effects on prejunctional receptors in motor nerve endings, the majority of interest follows the lead established by Langley and focuses on the receptors in the membrane of the muscle (Fig 1).

MUSCLE RELAXANTS
ISBN 0-8089-1784-6

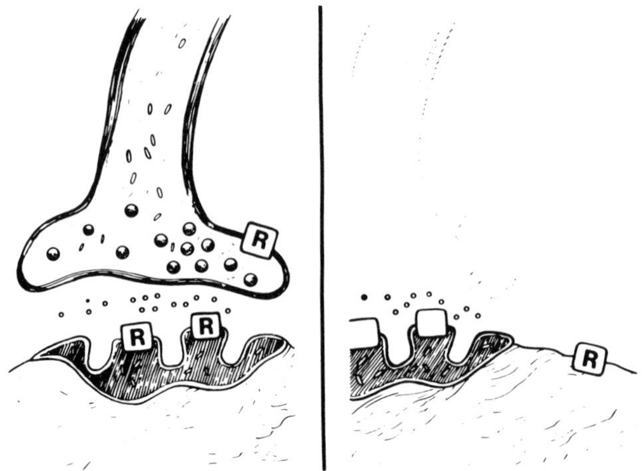

Figure 1. Nicotinic cholinergic receptors (R) on postjunctional folds (bottom left) at the motor endplate of skeletal muscle, on motor nerve endings (top left), and in extrajunctional membrane (right) in immature or denervated skeletal muscle.

JUNCTIONAL AND EXTRAJUNCTIONAL RECEPTORS

Occurrence

Muscles are now known to have at least two distinct receptors that respond to muscle relaxants; the receptors that normally are present in large numbers in the endplate membrane of normal adult junctions and another type that appears throughout the muscle whenever there is deficient stimulation of the muscle by the nerve. The latter, called extrajunctional receptors, are not found in significant numbers in normally active adult muscle, but they become more numerous and contribute to the clinical actions of relaxants, especially to those of succinylcholine, whenever motor nerves are less active than normal,[1] eg, in patients with denervated muscles, burned muscles, or underactive muscles, such as those of individuals with spinal cord injury or a stroke, or even in muscles in limbs immobilized in casts.

Both types of receptors are made in the muscle cell, but apparently by systems that are under different control mechanisms. Extrajunctional receptor synthesis is repressed in the normal adult, but when these receptors are allowed to be made, they are made more rapidly and are destroyed more rapidly (t½ 10 to 30 hours *v* 7 to 14 days) than the receptors in the endplate.[2] Of more practical importance, the extrajunctional receptors are inserted into the membrane all over the muscle instead of being confined to the endplate. Although they are less densely spaced than the latter, they are placed into an area of membrane enormously greater than that of the endplate; hence, pharmacologic effects in response to drug action on them can be significant. Despite differences between them and some pharmacologic characteristics that may have significant consequences when relaxants are used clinically (see following text), the two kinds of receptors are similar and are used interchangeably in many kinds of experiments.

The receptors of the endplate are remarkable in that they seem to have arisen early in evolution; there seems to be little difference between the receptors of human beings, frogs, electric fish, or other organisms.[3-5] This continuity across evolutionary lines greatly facilitates research in this area; while the ultimate object of inquiry may be the receptors of human beings, research is far more readily carried out on lower species or on cells grown in culture. Some of the most valuable creatures have been electric fish of the *Torpedo* family. These fish have such enormous numbers of acetylcholine receptors in their electric organs that it is practical to isolate receptors chemically and to study their morphologic and biochemical properties in the laboratory. It also has been possible to use these receptors and those from higher organisms, including human beings, to study in exquisite detail their physiologic and pharmacologic responses to acetylcholine and related agonists and antagonists.

From studies of isolated receptors and of receptors in situ, it is possible to describe the appearance of receptors, their chemical composition, and even the sequence of nucleic acids that guides their synthesis. It also is possible to measure the electrical activity started by the binding of acetylcholine to a single receptor and to describe the interaction of relaxants and other drugs with receptors.

Electron micrographs of receptors in situ show them to be in the endplate membrane, particularly on the shoulders of the junctional folds, which places them precisely opposite to the acetylcholine release sites in the nerve ending.[6] This area of the membrane is so rich in receptors (10,000 to 20,000/μm^2) that the surface appears to be paved with them.[7] They appear as discrete ring- or rosette-shaped particles, 8 to 9 nm in diameter with a central pit. Both the ring and the pit are believed to be essential for function. The ring is the top view of a cylinder of protein and contains the sites to which acetylcholine and other drugs bind, while the pit is the mouth of a channel in the center of the cylinder through which ions pass across the cell wall. The receptor particles occur in pairs and the pairs are in tidy rows across the surface. Each receptor is believed to operate independently, but there are links between the members of a pair[8] and they may cooperate with each other in some way.

Chemistry

These receptors have been isolated, purified, and analyzed; their structure is known in detail. The key features are sketched in Fig 2. Each receptor is

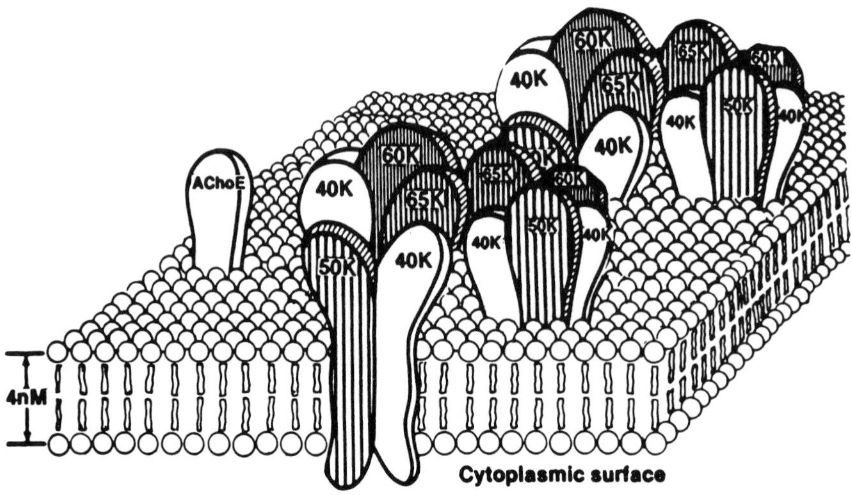

Figure 2. Sketch of postjunctional nicotinic acetylcholine receptors with an acetylcholinesterase (AChoE) molecule nearby.

a protein with a molecular weight of about 250,000 daltons that is made up of five subunits, which are designated alpha, beta, gamma, and delta. There are two alpha units, weighing about 40,000 daltons apiece, and one each of the others, weighing about 50,000, 60,000, and 65,000 daltons, respectively.[9] The receptor complex is approximately 11 nm in length, one half of which protrudes from the extracellular surface of the membrane. The protein passes entirely through the membrane but extends only about 2 nm into the cytoplasm.[10–12]

Each of the five subunits is linear, and the subunits are arranged longitudinally so that the combination is potentially capable of forming a tube or channel[13] that allows cations to flow along the concentration gradient. Sodium and calcium move into the muscle while potassium moves out. This tube is opened when two acetylcholine or other agonist molecules attach to the alpha units, one on each, and cause the subunits to rotate into a new conformation. In the open conformation the channel in the tube is large enough to pass all physiologic cations and even slim organic cations such as decamethonium, but it does not pass either anions or large organic cations.[14] The acetylcholine binding areas on the 40,000-dalton alpha units are the site of competition between cholinergic agonists and antagonists. Both agonists and antagonists are attracted to the site and either may occupy it. When both alpha unit sites are occupied by an agonist, the protein molecule undergoes a conformation change to form a channel through which ions flow (Fig 3). This current depolarizes the adjacent membrane. Both alpha units must be occupied simultaneously by an agonist[15,16]; if only one of them is occupied by an agonist, the

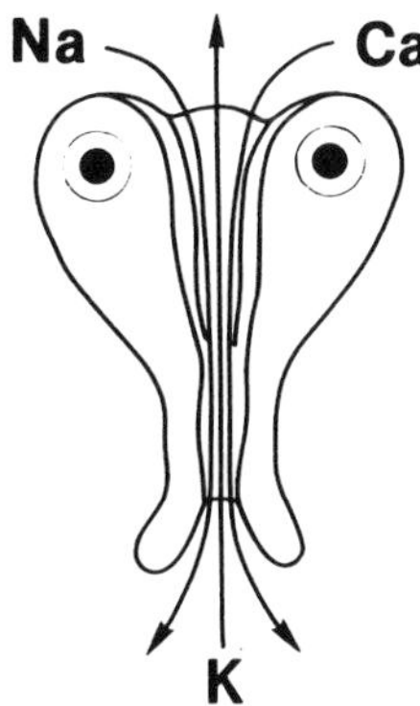

Figure 3. Sketch of the open configuration of the acetylcholine receptor with a molecule of ACh attached to each of the agonist binding sites. (Adapted from Horn and Brodwick.[10])

channel remains closed. This is the basis for the prevention of depolarization by antagonists. Drugs like tubocurarine act because they bind to either or both alpha units and, by doing so, they prevent acetylcholine from binding and opening the channel. This interaction between agonists and antagonists is competitive, and the outcome, transmission or blockade, depends on the relative concentrations and binding characteristics of the drugs involved.

Noncompetitive Drug Actions

The extracellular end of the tube is much larger than the part where the protein crosses the membrane; thus large molecules can enter the tube but not cross it. Drugs that do this can act like plugs in a funnel and prevent or impede the normal flow of ions through the tube, thereby producing a phenomenon called channel blockade. Since channel blockade prevents the flow of physiologic ions, it prevents depolarization of the endplate and can block neuromuscular transmission. Channel blockade is a familiar feature of local anesthetic action on the sodium channels of nerves, yet it is only a recently recognized, but potentially important, feature of drugs that act at the neuromuscular junction. Channel blockade of neuromuscular transmission prevents depolarization, but since the action is not at the acetylcholine site on the alpha subunits, it is not via a competitive antagonism of acetylcholine.[17–20]

Two major types of channel blockade can occur: open channel blockade and closed channel blockade (Fig 4). In the former the drug enters a channel that has been opened by reaction with acetylcholine but cannot penetrate all the way through. When in the channel it impedes the flow of physiologic ions and thus prevents depolarization from occurring. Most of these drugs exhibit two characteristics: (1) they are use dependent, meaning that since they can enter the channel only when it is open, the intensity of their effect depends upon how often the channel is opened, ie; how often the system is used; and (2) they are driven by the electrical interaction between the potential across the

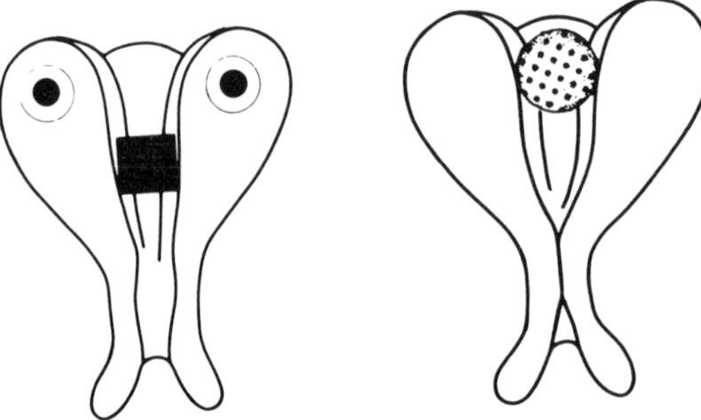

Figure 4. (Left) open channel blockade; (right) closed channel blockade.

membrane and the charge inherent in their molecular structure, which means that only cationic drugs are involved and that the intensity of effect varies with the chemical structure of the molecule. In addition, drugs that penetrate the opened channel may bind temporarily to some point on the wall of the channel, which means that the duration of the blockade also may vary with the molecule.

Closed channel blockade is more difficult to study experimentally so less is known about it, but there are drugs that can react around the mouth of the channel and by their presence prevent physiologic ions from passing through the channel. Since the reaction is around the mouth of the channel, the process can take place whether or not the channel is opened and so is not use dependent. This type of blockade is believed to be part of the pharmacology of, for example, tricyclic antidepressants, piperocaine, naltrexone, and naloxone.[19,21]

Figures 2 and 3 suggest that the receptor molecule is rigid and fixed in shape, but this is not the case. The receptor is made of large flexible macromolecules that are capable of existing in a number of states depending upon the electrical and chemical milieu. Several states of practical importance are illustrated in Fig 5. The three in the top row are the traditional ones that are important to normal receptor function. The resting receptor at the left is free of agonists, so its channel is closed and no ions can flow through to depolarize the membrane. The channel remains closed for an instant after two agonist molecules bind, but then the molecule undergoes the conformation change that results in an active receptor and an open, current passing channel. This is the basis of normal neuromuscular transmission.

The receptors in the bottom row of the figure depict another situation: receptors that bind agonists but that cannot undergo the conformation change that opens the channel. Receptors in these states are termed *densensitized;* ie, they are not sensitive to the channel opening actions of agonists. Desensitized receptors can bind agonists (or antagonists); indeed, they usually bind them with exceptional avidity, but the binding does not result in activation of the receptor or opening of the channel.

Desensitization has practical consequences because, as suggested in Fig 5, normal and desensitized receptors are in equilibrium. One form can change into another, but when receptors are desensitized they are not available to participate in the normal processes of neuromuscular transmission. Since the presence of desensitized receptors means that there cannot be the usual numbers of normal receptors, the production of desensitized receptors weakens the intensity of neuromuscular transmission. If so many receptors are desensitized that there are not enough normal ones remaining to depolarize the motor endplate, neuromuscular transmission will not occur. Even if only some of the receptors are desensitized, the intensity of neuromuscular transmission will be impaired and the system will be more susceptible to blockade by conventional antagonists such as tubocurarine or pancuronium. A significant number of drugs cause or promote desensitization[22–25] (Fig 6), and the phenomenon probably is involved in many of the familiar interactions between relaxants and other drugs used during anesthesia.

Physiology and Pharmacology

Just as we can visualize individual receptors and analyze them biochemically, so can we measure their electrical function. The most direct method is patch clamping,[26] a method in which a glass micropipette is used to probe the membrane surface until a single receptor is encompassed. The tip of the pipette is sealed by the lipid of the membrane, and electronic apparatus is arranged to clamp the membrane potential and to measure the current that flows through the channel of the receptor. The solution in the pipette can contain acetylcholine, tubocurarine, or another drug or mixture of drugs. The arrangement is illustrated in Fig 7.

Figure 8 contains schematized examples of records that are obtained in this way. The top tracing is produced when an agonist, suberyldicholine, an analogue of succinylcholine but more stable than it under experimental conditions, is in the pipette and can react with sites on the receptor. In this situation, randomly occurring descending rectangular pulses are recorded. Each pulse is caused by current flowing across the membrane while two agonist molecules are attached to the receptor, activating it and opening the channel. The pulse stops when one or both agonist molecules detach from the receptor and the channel closes. The current that passes through each channel is minuscule, only a few picoamperes (about 10^7 ions per second), but each neuromuscular junction contains many hundred thousand receptor/channels. The current that flows when many are opened at once, as for example in response to a burst of acetylcholine from the nerve ending, is substantial and can be more than

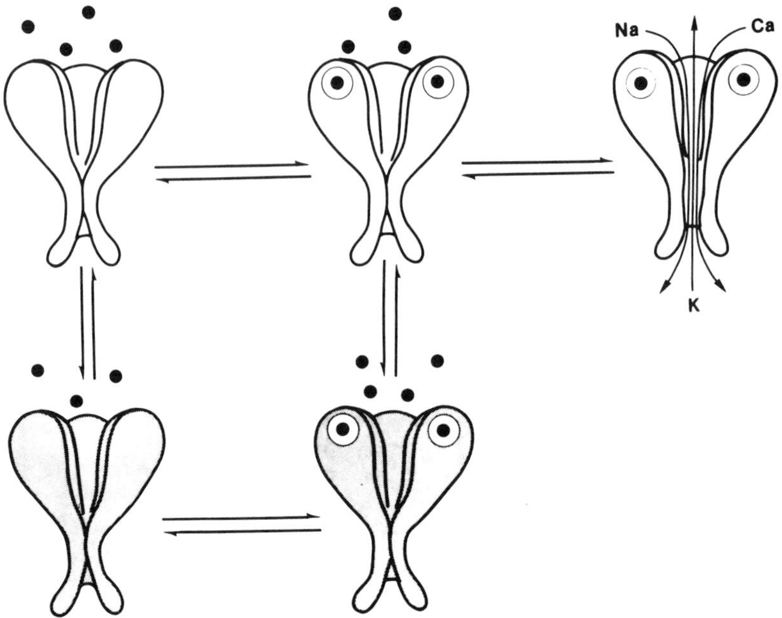

Figure 5. Representations of several receptor conformations. Normal forms are in the top row; desensitized forms are below.

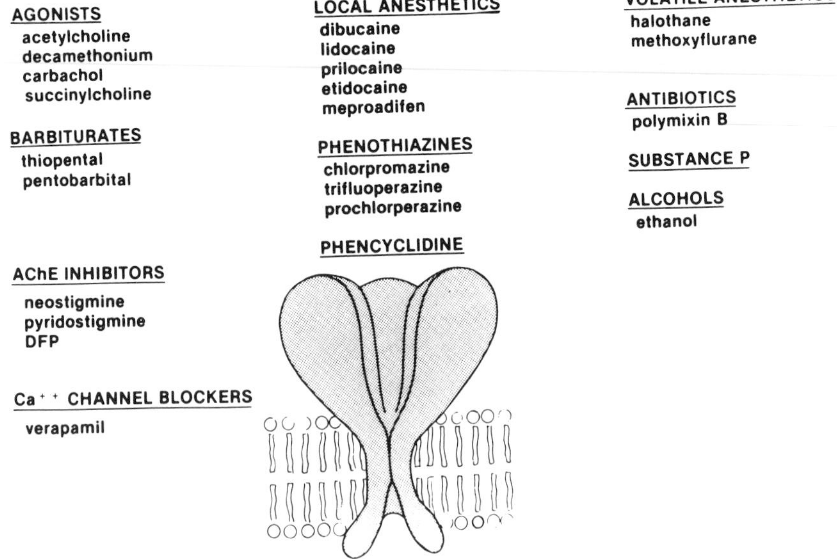

Figure 6. Some drugs that may promote desensitization.

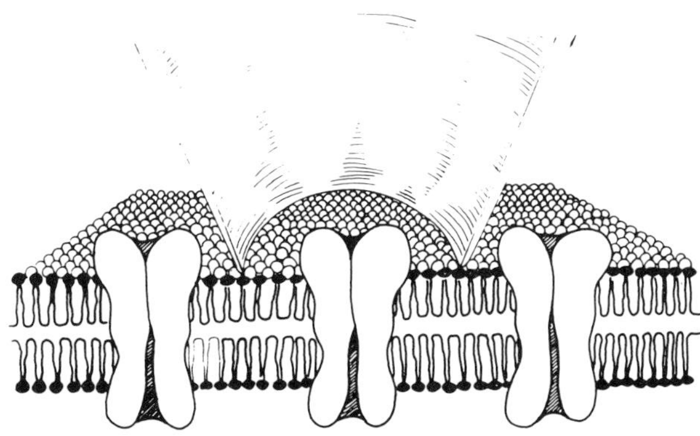

Figure 7. Patch clamp technique for recording current flow through a single acetylcholine receptor.

enough to depolarize the entire region and create the endplate potential that triggers muscle contraction.

Thus, the receptor and its channel make a powerful amplifier, the current carried by two acetylcholine ions is converted into a current carried by tens of thousands of sodium, calcium, and potassium ions. The receptor also is a switch. It is closed and off until acetylcholine is present; then it snaps open and passes current. When acetylcholine leaves, the channel snaps shut and cuts off the current.

The middle tracing (Fig 8) typifies an experiment in which both an agonist (eg, acetylcholine) and tubocurarine are used simultaneously. In this situation, sometimes two agonists attach to the receptor. If this happens, the receptor activates and opens its channel to permit ions to flow and a descending pulse to be recorded. At other times one or two tubocurarine molecules

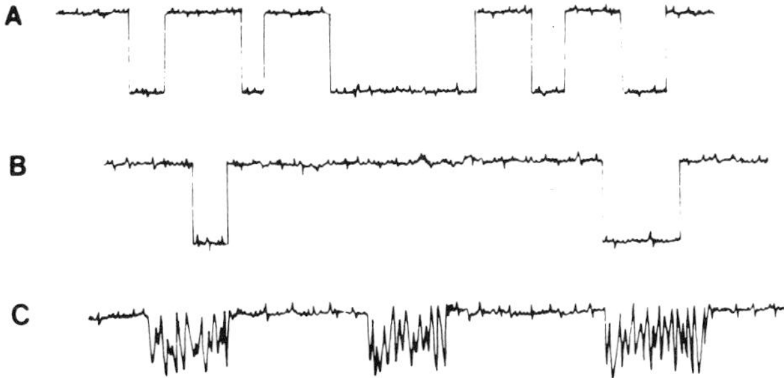

Figure 8. Traces represent patch clamp recordings of ion flow through a single receptor in the presence of an agonist (A), an agonist and tubocurarine (B), and an agonist and a quaternary local anesthetic, QX222 (C). (Adapted from Neher et al.[27])

may attach to the receptor, in which case the receptor is not available to agonists; therefore, the channel stays closed until the tubocurarine leaves. Since the channel is not opened, no current flows and no pulse is recorded. The result is a record of normal-appearing agonist-induced pulses of current, but there are fewer pulses than if tubocurarine was not present.[27] Because current flows through each channel less often, the amount flowing through the endplate at any instant is reduced from normal. This results in a smaller endplate potential and, if carried far enough, a block of transmission. This is a molecular description of the classical competitive interaction between acetylcholine and tubocurarine to reduce neuromuscular transmission.

The bottom tracing (Fig 8) is taken from an experiment in which the pipette contained a mixture of suberyldicholine and QX 222, a derivative of lidocaine. The QX 222 does not compete with an agonist for the receptor, so the channel is open just as often as in the control. However, current does not flow steadily even though the channel remains open.[28] It is thought that this occurs because the QX 222 molecule rapidly and repeatedly hops into and out of the channel. When the molecule is in the channel the flow of physiologic ions is blocked and no current flows, but when the drug is out of the channel the pathway is clear and current flows. This is typical of the channel blocking action of the local anesthetics and other open channel blocking drugs. In practical terms, the channel opens and closes as before, but because of the intermittent block caused by the drug in the channel, the total current per channel opening is less than that of the control. Summed over the entire endplate, this reduces the total endplate current and the endplate potential and so weakens neuromuscular transmission. It also may be noted that since tubocurarine and QX 222 act at different places, receptor site and channel, respectively, the effects of the two can add to reduce current and neuromuscular transmission.

It is now known that channel block is extremely common at neuromuscular junctions; many drugs can and do get into the receptor/channel's mouth and hinder the flow of current.[17–21] Many of these reactions occur with concentrations of drugs used clinically and thus may contribute to the phenomena and drug interactions that are seen in anesthetized patients.

Particularly interesting is the fact that muscle relaxants themselves may cause channel block in addition to acting competitively with acetylcholine on the alpha unit sites.[29] All muscle relaxants are cations and are capable of entering the channel. Even though the drugs may act at both sites, a given drug may prefer to act at one or the other site, ie, there are differences in preferred site of action. In this sense, it takes substantially greater concentrations of pancuronium to affect channels than receptor sites, whereas gallamine acts at both places at all concentrations. Tubocurarine seems to be in between; at low doses, which clinically produce minimal blockage of transmission, the drug is essentially a pure receptor blocker while at high doses, which produce complete or near complete blockade, the drug also affects channels. Decamethonium is particularly interesting because as an agonist it opens channels, but as a cation it enters and blocks them.[30] In fact, as a long slim cation, decamethonium is capable of going all the way through the open channel to enter the muscle cytoplasm.[31]

Figure 9 illustrates some of the classical actions of acetylcholine and muscle relaxants on endplate receptors. The top section depicts a section of membrane exposed to acetylcholine. Some receptors have attracted two molecules of acetylcholine and current flows through the channel, while some channels remain closed because the receptor does not have two molecules of

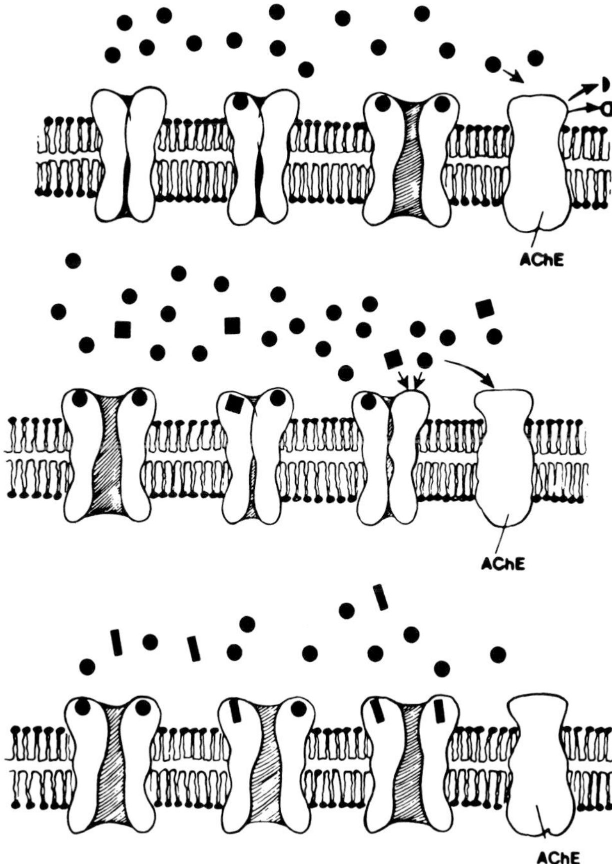

Figure 9. Representation of the classical actions of acetylcholine and muscle relaxants on endplate receptors. Symbols: ● = acetycholine; ◐ = choline; ◐ = acetate; ■ = d-tubocurarine; ▮ = decamethonium.

agonist on it. The sketch also contains a representation of acetylcholinesterase, which may destroy acetylcholine by hydrolyzing it to acetate and choline.

The middle section (Fig 9) depicts a system exposed to a modest concentration of tubocurarine in the junctional cleft. Some receptors attract two acetylcholines and open the channel to depolarize that segment of membrane. Others attract one acetylcholine and one tubocurarine. No current will flow through these channels. The third receptor is particularly interesting because it has acetylcholine on one alpha unit and nothing on the other. What will happen depends upon which of the molecules above it wins the competition for the vacant site. If acetylcholine wins, the channel will open and the membrane will be depolarized. If tubocurarine wins, the channel will stay closed and the membrane will not depolarize. This is where cholinesterase plays a role. Normally the enzyme destroys acetylcholine and removes it from the competition for a receptor, so normally tubocurarine wins the competition and transmission is blocked. If, however, an inhibitor such as pyridostigmine is added, the cholinesterase cannot destroy acetylcholine. This lets the agonist stay in the cleft where its increased concentration tips the competition between acetylcholine and tubocurarine to favor the former. This improves the chances of two acetylcholines binding to a receptor, even though tubocurarine is still in the environment. This is a molecular explanation of how reversing drugs can overcome a neuromuscular block produced by nondepolarizing relaxants.

The third panel (Fig 9) depicts the immediate effects of a modest dose of a depolarizing relaxant, decamethonium. Since it is an agonist, its reaction with receptors is like that of acetylcholine and the membrane is depolarized. Since it is not susceptible to acetylcholinesterase, it is not destroyed and removed from the cleft, so the depolarization persists and leads to neuromuscular blockade.

Figure 10 illustrates the results of exposure to high and prolonged concentrations of muscle relaxants. The top portion represents tubocurarine. In this case there is a much greater concentration of relaxant, and the molecular situation is very different from that depicted previously. The center receptor has two tubocurarines and is closed. The left one is opened by acetylcholine, but a tubocurarine molecule in the channel prevents current from flowing to depolarize the membrane. The right receptor already has one tubocurarine, so it makes no difference whether acetylcholine or tubocurarine binds to the other site; the channel cannot open in either case. When neuromuscular blockade is produced by tubocurarine in doses of this magnitude, inhibiting cholinesterase cannot be expected to be as beneficial as it is against low concentrations of the relaxant.

The bottom portion of the figure depicts some results of exposure to a high concentration of a depolarizing relaxant, decamethonium in this case. Decamethonium and acetylcholine are both agonists, and two molecules of either one, or a combination of the two, can open the channel and depolarize

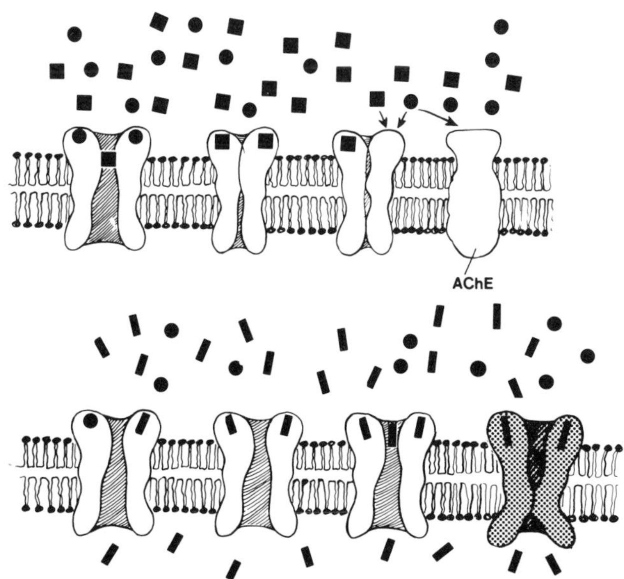

Figure 10. Representations of the effects of exposure to high and prolonged concentrations of muscle relaxants. Symbols: ● = acetylcholine; ■ = d-tubocurarine; ▮ = decamethonium.

the membrane; thus some channels are opened and depolarize the membrane as before. Decamethonium has entered some channels (third receptor from the left). This blocks current flow and prevents depolarization of this membrane segment. Some receptors, like those at the far right, have desensitized in the presence of decamethonium; their channels cannot be opened to carry current. Also, decamethonium is a slim molecule that can pass through opened ion channels; the sketch contains decamethonium molecules that have entered the muscle cytoplasm to cause mischief there. In this situation neuromuscular block is a complex of many things. Some phenomena prevent current flow and thus produce a nondepolarizing blockade, but the total effect consists of depolarizing and nondepolarizing actions, channel effects, receptor desensitization, and intracellular effects. These events are part of phase II block but are not the complete explanation of the syndrome, which at present is not well understood.

PREJUNCTIONAL RECEPTORS

Much less is known about cholinergic receptors in other organs, but the general principles probably apply. Both receptor block and channel block are basic phenomena that can occur whenever a drug and the receptor/channel have characteristics appropriate for an interaction. Some of the most interesting of these drug actions occur at the motor nerve terminal. This structure is known to have cholinergic receptors and it has been postulated that these influence the release of transmitter. In many aspects these postulates are still controversial, but the prejunctional receptors seem to be different from postjunctional ones in their chemical binding characteristics, the nature of the ion channel they control, and their preferential block during high-frequency stimulation.[6,32]

In its action on the prejunctional receptor/channel, tubocurarine seems to block the entry of sodium but not calcium. Accordingly, it interferes with the mobilization of acetylcholine from synthesis sites to release sites rather than interfering with release per se. There may be a specific receptor, a mobilization receptor, that is affected by tubocurarine to slow mobilization and cause failure of transmission at high frequency,[33] or it may be that tubocurarine blocks the flow of sodium needed for the mobilization process by causing block of cholinergic sodium channels in the nerve ending.[6] Practically, the two ideas have the same outcome: prejunctional receptor or receptor/channel blockade diminishes the release of acetylcholine from nerves stimulated at high frequency and this contributes to the weakening of transmission caused by muscle relaxants.

OVERVIEW

Figure 11 offers a framework within which to consider some of these actions of the muscle relaxants. The particular example is tubocurarine and the figure is limited to the neuromuscular junction, but a similar scheme potentially could be drawn for other muscle relaxants and other organs. The figure shows how site and mechanism of action relate to the concentration of the drug and the stimulus imposed on the nerve. At low doses (eg, those that produce minimal blockage of transmission) and at low frequencies (eg, the one shock every few seconds favored by investigators and those monitoring neuromuscular transmission during anesthesia), tubocurarine acts predominantly at the receptor site to compete with acetylcholine. This is the process described for so long by numerous texts.

In more strenuous situations additional things take place. If the dose is increased, the drug enters the ion channel of the endplate to add channel block. This further weakens neuromuscular transmission and diminishes the efficacy of reversing agents. If the rate of nerve stimulation is increased, eg, to tetanizing frequencies, then the nerve is stressed and the capacity to sustain transmitter release is diminished by the prejunctional action of tubocurarine to reduce mobilization. This causes waning of the amount of transmitter released and diminishes the capacity of acetylcholine to compete with the concurrent

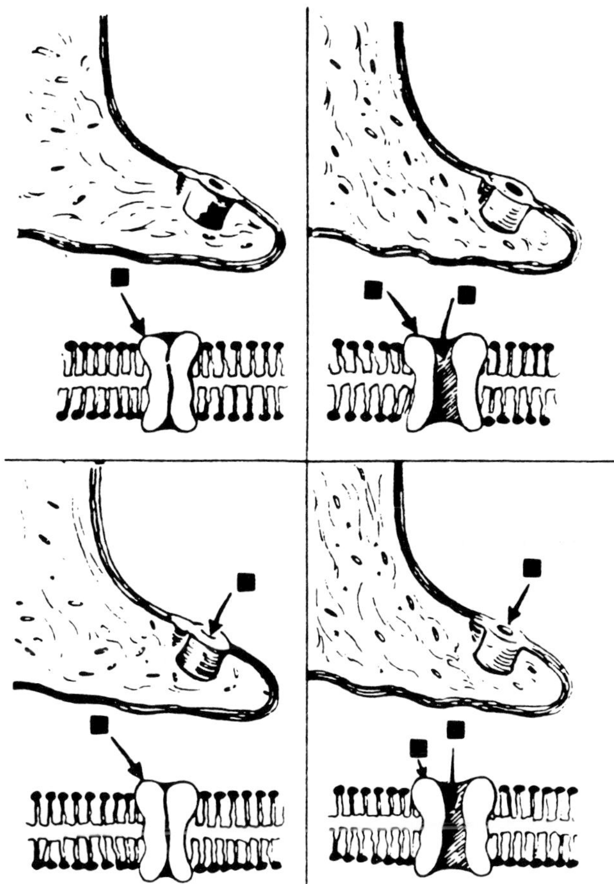

Figure 11. Sketch of some actions of d-tubocurarine at prejunctional and postjunctional receptors of the neuromuscular junction during changes in dose and frequency of stimulation: (upper left) lose dose, low frequency; (upper right) high dose, low frequency; (lower left) low dose, high frequency; (lower right) high dose, high frequency.

actions of tubocurarine at the postjunctional receptor. The sketch at the bottom right summates these events by illustrating a rapidly stimulated junction exposed to a high concentration of tubocurarine. In this situation all mechanisms, prejunctional and postjunctional, are operative and contributing to the blockade of neuromuscular transmission.

Extrajunctional receptors do not participate in the scheme sketched because they are not present in significant number at normal adult neuromuscular junctions. But, as noted previously, they are made rapidly if normal nerve activity to the muscle is not maintained, and they can strongly affect certain clinical uses of the relaxants.

The extrajunctional receptors are very responsive to agonists, such as acetylcholine or succinylcholine, and poorly responsive to antagonists, such as tubocurarine or pancuronium. Since agonists acting on these receptors cause substantial flows of ions across the muscle membrane, they can allow enough potassium to be released to elevate the serum concentration and lead to adverse cardiac affects. Because these receptors are not as strongly affected by nondepolarizing relaxants as are normal receptors, the hyperkalemic effect of succinylcholine may be reduced but not prevented by prior administration of tubocurarine or a related drug. Indeed, the opposite has been observed; tubocurarine can act as an agonist on these receptors; it opens receptor/channels[34] and so causes depolarization and contraction of denervated muscle.[35]

Since extrajunctional receptors are formed rapidly after the slackening of neural influence on muscle and are degraded soon after the neural influence returns, mixtures of normal and extrajunctional receptors are present in many clinical situations and may account for some of the quantitative differences in response to relaxants seen among various clinical states.

The new knowledge of receptors, ion channels, and muscle relaxants seems to complicate things; certainly it was easier to remember when we only thought of a competition between cholinergic agonists and antagonists for receptors in the endplate. However, the newer observations encompass a broader range of sites and mechanisms of action for both agonists and antagonists and in doing so they are more realistic. We intuitively recognize that no drug has only one site or one mechanism of action. We know that the muscle relaxants are not exceptions to this rule, and in recognizing their complexity we begin to bring our theoretical knowledge closer to explaining the variety of things that are seen when these drugs are administered to living human beings.

ACKNOWLEDGMENT

I am deeply indebted to Kitt Booher for her knowledgeable help in assembling and preparing this material for publication.

REFERENCES

1. Tobey RE, Jacobsen PM, Cahle CT, et al: The serum potassium response to muscle relaxants in neural injury. Anesthesiology 37:332–337, 1972
2. Pumplin DW, Fambrough DM: Turnover of acetylcholine receptors in skeletal muscle. Ann Rev Physiol 44:319–335, 1982

3. Gullick WJ, Lindstrom JM: Mapping the binding of monoclonal antibodies to the acetylcholine receptor from *Torpedo californica*. Biochemistry 22:3312–3320, 1983
4. Sargent PB, Hedges BE, Tsavaler L, et al: Structure and transmembrane nature of the acetylcholine receptor in amphibian skeletal muscle as revealed by cross-reacting monoclonal antibodies. J Cell Biol 98:609–618, 1984
5. Raftery MA, Conti-Tronconi BM, Dunn SMJ et al: The nicotinic acetylcholine receptor: Its structure, multiple binding sites, and cation transport properties. Fund Appl Toxicol 4:S34–S51, 1984
6. Standaert F: Release of transmitter at the neuromusclar junction. Br J Anaesth 54:131–145, 1982
7. Heuser JE, Salpeter SR: Organization of acetylcholine receptors in quick-frozen, deep-etched, and rotary-replicated *Torpedo* postsynaptic membrane. J Cell Biol 82:150–174, 1979
8. Karlin A: The anatomy of a receptor. Neurosci Comm 1:111–123, 1983
9. Raftery MA, Hunkapiller MW, Strader CD, et al: Acetylcholine receptor: complex of homologous subunits. Science 208:1454–1457, 1980
10. Horn R, Brodwick MS: Acetylcholine-induced current in perfused rat myoballs. J Gen Physiol 75:297–321, 1980
11. Claudio T, Ballivet M, Patrick J, et al: Nucleotide and deduced amino acid sequence of *Torpedo californica* acetylcholine receptor gamma subunits. Proc Natl Acad Sci USA 80:1111–1115, 1983
12. Stroud RM: Acetylcholine receptor structure. Neurosci Comm 1:124–138, 1983
13. Guy HR; A structural model of the acetylcholine receptor channel based on partition energy and helix packing calculations. Biophys J 45:249–262, 1984
14. Dwyer T, Adams DJ, Hille B: The permeability of the endplate channel to organic cations in frog muscle. J Gen Physiol 75:469–492, 1980
15. Neubig RR, Boyd ND Cohen JB: Conformations of *Torpedo* acetylcholine receptor associated with ion transport and desensitization. Biochemistry 21:3460–3464, 1982
16. Sheridan RE, Lester HA: Functional stoichiometry at the nicotinic receptor. J Gen Physiol 80:499–515, 1982
17. Dreyer F: Acetylcholine receptor. Br J Anaesth 54:115–130, 1982
18. Peper K, Bradley RJ, Dreyer F: The acetycholine receptor at the neuromuscular junction. Physiol Rev 62:1271–1340, 1982
19. Spivak CE, Albuquerque EX: Dynamic properties of the nicotinic acetylcholine receptors ionic channel complex: Activation and blockade, in Hanin I, Goldberg AM (eds): Progress in Cholinergic Biology: Model Cholinergic Synapses. New York, Raven Press, 1982, pp 323–328
20. Lambert JJ, Durant NN, Henderson EG: Drug-induced modification of ionic conductance at the neuromuscular junction. Ann Rev Pharmacol Toxicol 23:505–539, 1983
21. Schofield GG, Witkop B, Warnick JE, et al: Differentiation of the open and closed states of the ionic channels of nicotinic acetylcholine receptors by tricyclic antidepressants. Proc Natl Acad Sci USA 78:5240–5244, 1981
22. Maleque MA, Souccar C, Cohen JB, et al: Meproadifen reaction with the ionic channel of the acetylcholine receptor: Potentiation of agonist-induced desensitization at the frog neuromuscular junction. Mol Pharmacol 22:636–647, 1982
23. Carp JS, Aronstam RS, Witkop B, et al: Electrophysiological and biochemical studies on enhancment of desensitization by phen-othiazine neuroleptics. Proc Natl Acad Sci USA 80:310–314, 1983
24. Brown RD, Taylor P: The influence of antibiotics on agonist occupation and functional states of the nicotinic acetylcholine receptor. Mol Pharmacol 23:8–16, 1983
25. Pascuzzo GJ, Akaike A, Maleque MA, et al: The nature of the interactions of pyridostigmine with the nicotinic receptor-ionic channel complex. Mol Pharmacol 25:92–101, 1984
26. Hamill OP, Marty A, Neher E, et al: Improved patch clamp techniques for high-resolution current recordings from cells and cell-free membrane patches. Pflugers Arch 391:85–100, 1981

27. Neher E, Sakmann B, Steinbach JH: The extracellular patch clamp: A method for resolving currents through individual open channels in biological membranes. Pflugers Arch 375: 219–225, 1978
28. Neher E, Steinbach JH: Local anesthetics transiently block currents through single acetylcholine-receptor channels. J Physiol 277:153–176, 1978
29. Katz B, Miledi R: A re-examination of curare action at the motor endplate. Proc R Soc Lond 211:119–133, 1978
30. Adams PR, Sakmann B: Decamethonium both opens and blocks endplate channels. Proc Natl Acad Sci USA 75:2992–2998, 1978
31. Taylor DB, Creese R, Nedergaard PA, et al: Labelling de-polarizing drugs in normal and denervated muscle. Nature 208:901–902, 1965
32. Standaert F: Sites of action of muscle relaxants. ASA Annual Refresher Course Lectures. Las Vegas, ASA, 1982, pp 226(1–3)
33. Bowman WC: Prejunctional and postjunctional cholinoceptors at the neuromuscular junction. Anesth Analg 59:935–943, 1980
34. Trautmann A: Tubocurarine, a partial agonist for choline receptors. J Neurol Transm 18 (suppl):353–361, 1983
35. McIntyre AR, King RE, Dunn AL: Electrical activity of denervated mammalian skeletal muscle as influenced by *d*-tubocurarine. J Neurophysiol 8:297–301, 1945

Nicholas N. Durant

2

The Physiology of Neuromuscular Transmission

The neuromuscular junction is without doubt the most thoroughly studied synapse of any type, and although some questions remain unanswered, it has become the model of our understanding of synaptic transmission. The neuromuscular junction holds particular importance for anesthetists with regard to peripherally induced muscle relaxation, and so in the present review the physiology of neuromuscular transmission will be addressed from the point of view of both the anesthetist and the fundamentalist.

ANATOMY OF THE NEUROMUSCULAR JUNCTION

A motor nerve enters a muscle, then branches repeatedly depending on the function of that muscle. For example, muscles that perform fine movements are supplied by nerve fibers that innervate relatively few muscle fibers, while muscles that are involved in control of posture are innervated by nerve fibers that may supply many muscle fibers.[1] In the human body, all muscles, with the notable exception of the extraocular muscles of the eye and some muscles of the face and neck, are focally innervated; that is to say that each muscle fiber is served by one or, at the most, three neuromuscular junctions. In muscles in which there is multiple innervation, each muscle fiber may possess many neuromuscular junctions, far more than are found in focally innervated muscle. This muscle type responds to a depolarizing agent with contracture that may, in the case of the eye, raise intraocular pressure. The appearance of the neuromuscular junction in multiply innervated muscle fi-

MUSCLE RELAXANTS
ISBN 0-8089-1784-6

bers lends its name to the type of nerve terminals known as *en grappe* terminations. In contrast, the nerve terminations in focally innervated muscle are flatter and sometimes called *en plaque* terminations.[1]

As the axon forms intimate contact with a single muscle fiber, it looses its myelin sheath and then branches again to form the neuromuscular junction[2] (Fig 1). The nerve terminals themselves lie in synaptic troughs and are capped with Schwann cells (Fig 1), which may serve to mechanically preserve the neuromuscular junction. Although the Schwann cells are responsible for the formation of the nerve myelin sheath, theories as to their function at the mature neuromuscular junction abound and remain unknown for the present.[4] The nerve terminals themselves contain vesicles of the transmitter acetylcholine that line up in "active zones" within the nerve terminal (Fig 2). Also present in the nerve terminal are mitochondria, which make up about 6.6% of the nerve terminal,[5] and cisternae, which are thought to be involved in the "recycling" of the vesicles.[6]

The synaptic cleft, about 50 to 70 nm wide, contains a basement membrane material, which in an electron micrograph shows up as a darker area (Fig 2). The enzyme acetylcholinesterase is also present in the synaptic cleft and is concentrated in the folds. The postjunctional region is immediately recognizable by its folded surface (Fig 3), the mouths of which lie directly opposite the active zones in the nerve terminal shown in Fig 2. It is also in this region that the acetylcholine receptors and their associated ionic channels are located. Thus, the released acetylcholine passes the receptors at the mouths of the folds before being destroyed by the acetylcholinesterase within the folds.

FUNCTION OF THE NEUROMUSCULAR JUNCTION

Neuromuscular transmission starts with the arrival of a nerve action potential at the nerve terminal and concludes with depolarization of the postjunctional membrane. Although the time that elapses between these two events is only a few milliseconds, many different processes take place.

Synthesis of Acetylcholine

The first step is the synthesis of acetylcholine, which takes place within the nerve terminal. Much of the experimental work to determine the stages involved was carried out using the cholinergic nerves of the mammalian CNS; however, this situation is believed to parallel the motor nerve terminal at the neuromuscular junction.[1,7] Acetylcholine is synthesized from choline and acetylcoenzyme A, the latter derived from pyruvate, which in turn is derived from glucose. Choline is present in plasma and consequently in the extracellular fluid surrounding the motor nerve terminal. The source of approxi-

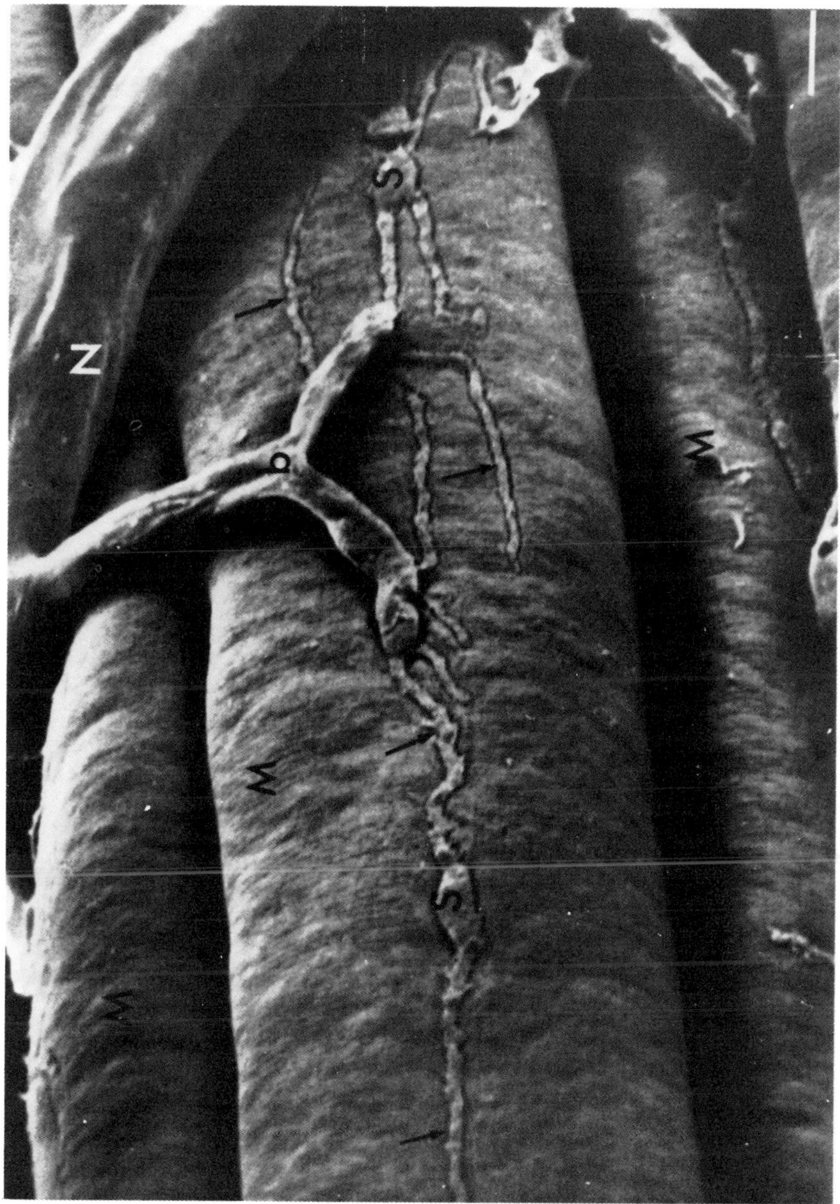

Figure 1. Scanning electron micrograph showing a surface view of the neuromuscular junctions in the sartorius muscle of the frog (*Rana nigromaculata*). The side branch (b) of the motor nerve (N) abruptly narrows into the thin nerve endings (arrows) running along the muscle fiber (M). The cell bodies of Schwann cells (S) are also seen associated within the nerve endings (arrowed). Scale bar: 10 μm. (Reproduced with permission from Desaki and Uehara.[3])

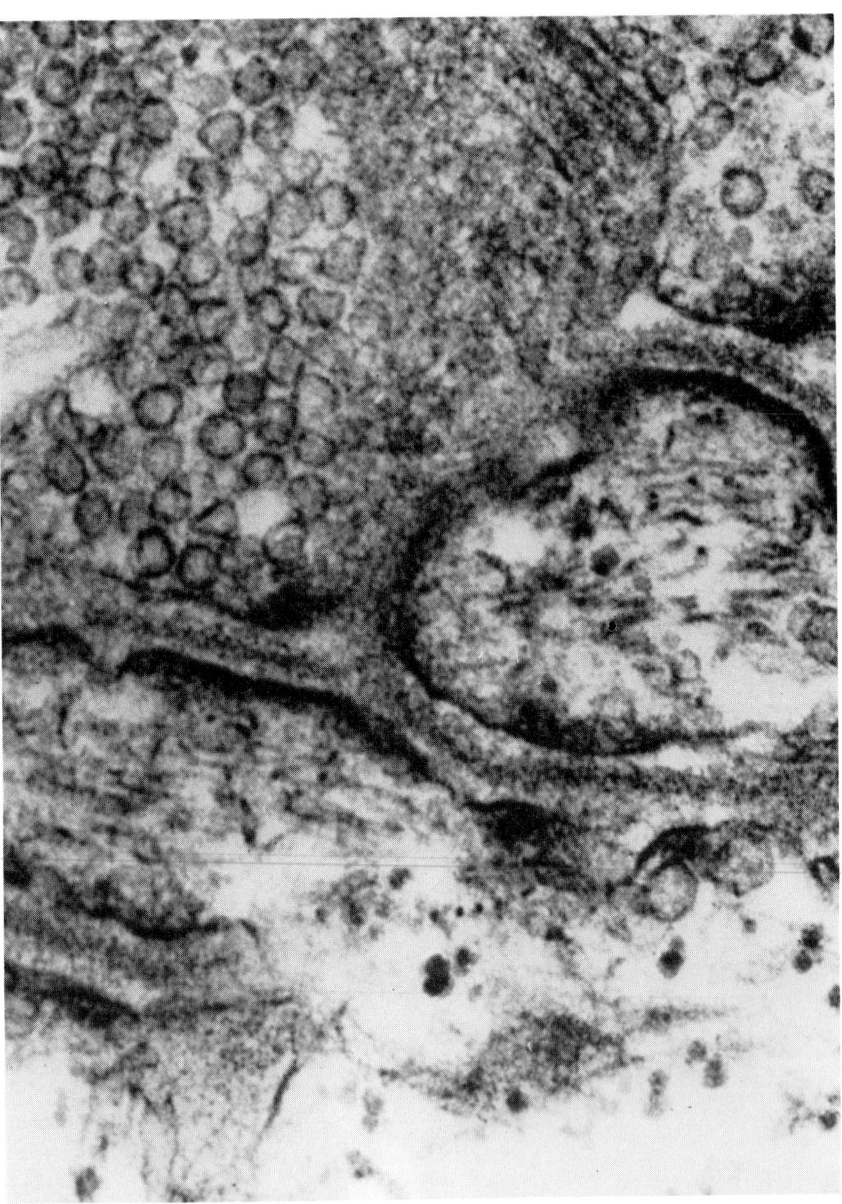

Figure 2. Electron micrograph of the synaptic region of the neuromuscular junction in the cutaneous pectoris muscle of the frog (*Rana pipiens*). The vesicles can be seen within the nerve terminal in the upper part of the micrograph. The active zones of the nerve terminal can be seen at the apex of the projections into the postjunctional folds within the synaptic cleft, and the basement membrane can be clearly seen as the darkened granulation within the synaptic cleft. The postjunctional gutter arcs between the upper left- and right-hand corners of the micrograph also showing the postjunctional folds.

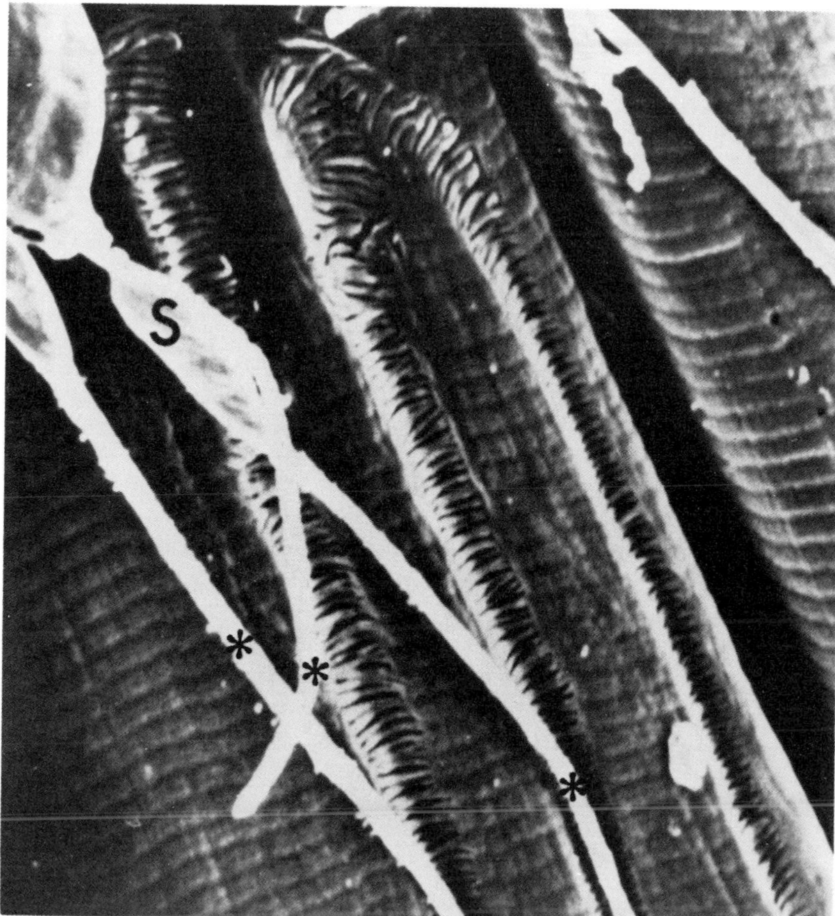

Figure 3. The synaptic gutters and postjunctional folds of the neuromuscular junctions of the sartorius muscle of the frog (*Rana nigromaculata*) after the nerve terminals have been partially detached (asterisks). A Schwann cell (S) is also present on the nerve terminal. Scale bar: 5 μm. (Reproduced with permission from Desaki and Uehara.[3])

mately half of this choline is from the enzymatic destruction of acetylcholine[8,9] (Fig 4). Choline undergoes active transportation into the nerve terminal where it accepts the acetyl group carried by acetylcoenzyme A under the catalytic influence of choline-O-acetyltransferase. The resulting bound acetylcholine is then used to refill the vesicles.[10] The synthesis and breakdown of acetylcholine is shown in Fig 4. Although there are drugs that interfere with the active uptake of choline into the nerve terminal (eg, hemicholinium-3)[11,12] as well as with the incorporation of acetylcholine into vesicles (eg, AH 5183),[13] none of these are clinically used.

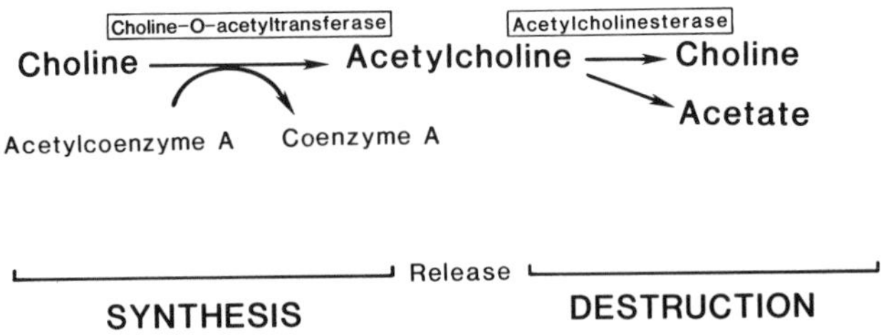

Figure 4. Schematic representation of the synthesis and destruction of acetylcholine within the neuromuscular junction.

Depolarization of the Nerve Terminal

At rest, most living cells maintain an ionic concentration gradient across the cell membrane by means of metabolically driven ion pumps. This results in the potassium ion concentration being about 50 times greater inside the cell and the sodium ion concentration being about 30 times greater outside the cell.[14] Depolarization of the nerve terminal follows the arrival of the nerve action potential and is mainly due to the initial influx of sodium ions through sodium ion channels, which would take the membrane potential from about −90 mV to about +50 mV, the latter being the equilibrium potential for sodium ions. However, at a membrane potential of about 0 mV, potassium ion channels open and the sodium ion channels start to close. In this way, the sodium influx gives rise to a potassium efflux that prevents the membrane potential from going more positive than about +10 mV and then restores the holding potential to −90 mV. Thus, the sodium and potassium ion channels are both sensitive to changes of the membrane potential although at very different potentials.

Calcium is another extremely important ion in the nerve terminal and is, as described later, vital to the release process. Calcium ions enter the nerve terminal during depolarization[15] and are then rapidly sequestered by the sarcoplasmic reticulum[16,17] and the mitochondria.[5] The calcium ions are removed from the nerve terminal by a Na/Ca antiporter or by adenosine triphosphate (ATPase).[18,19]

THE THEORY OF QUANTAL RELEASE

The first clues to the process of release were provided by the observations of small (approximately 0.5 mV) spontaneous (1 to 3 Hz) depolarizations of the endplate recorded using intracellular electrodes placed in the endplate region of isolated frog skeletal muscle.[20] The small endplate potentials, known as miniature endplate potentials (MEPP) do not result in any muscle movement. If the nerve is stimulated and a microelectrode can be kept in the endplate region of the muscle fiber during the resulting twitch response, then a voltage recording similar to that shown in Fig 5A will be seen. However, if the microelectrode is moved away from the endplate region, the initial depolarization or shoulder is lost[20] (Fig 5B). Thus, the endplate potential is only seen at the endplate and must reach a threshold of about −50 mV to trigger a muscle action potential. Several groups of workers have demonstrated quite clearly that if the magnesium concentration in the solution surrounding the muscle is raised and the calcium concentration lowered, then the nerve-muscle preparation becomes paralyzed due to the fact that the initial depolarization recorded at the endplate, otherwise known as the endplate potential (EPP), in response to nerve stimulation becomes smaller[21–24] and does not reach threshold amplitude. These EPPs possess very similar rise and decay times to the MEPPs[4,22] and are also in ratio to the amplitude of the MEPPs. If several EPPs are recorded in the presence of a low-calcium and high-magnesium Ringer solution, then their amplitude varies considerably, but they are still in ratio to the mean MEPP amplitude.[21] The observations of Del Castillo and Engbaek[21] and of Del Castillo and Katz[23] led to the quantal theory of acetylcholine release, which describes a MEPP as being the single unit, packet, or quanta of trans-

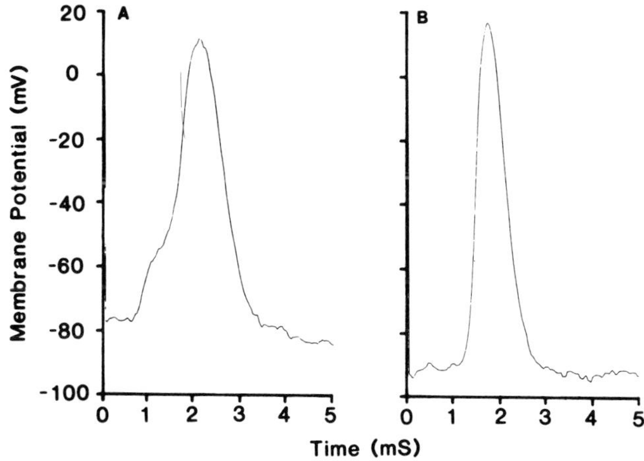

Figure 5. (A) Intracellular voltage recordings made using a microelectrode in the endplate region of the cutaneous pectoris muscle of the frog (*Rana pipiens*) during a single nerve stimulation that elicits an endplate potential and muscle action potential. The endplate potential comprises the initial shoulder of the muscle action potential. (B) An intracellular recording made from the same muscle preparation as in Fig 5A except the intracellular electrode was distant from the endplate, and no shoulder or endplate potential is seen.

mitter. The EPP recorded in the presence of low calcium and high magnesium is simply composed of a low number of these quanta.[22,25] This theory is illustrated in Fig 6. Examination of the smallest EPP and the MEPP in Figs 6A and 6B, respectively, reveals their peak amplitudes to be in the approximate ratio of 5:1; thus, the number of quanta (quantal content) that make up the smallest EPP is about 5. Similarly, the two larger EPPs have quantal contents of about 8 and 10. It should be stressed that this is an oversimplification since such factors as the nonlinear summation of EPPs[26] must also be taken into account.

When the quantal content is low (less than 10), as it usually is in a low-calcium and high-magnesium bathing solution, the statistical properties of the EPPs can be analyzed.[25] Such analyses suggest that the quantal content of an EPP equals the product of the size of the available pool of quanta and the probability of release[22] (Fig 7). In these circumstances, the quantal content of the EPP is reduced, the size of the available pool is unaffected, and thus the probability of release will be markedly decreased.[26]

The Role of Calcium

Calcium is essential to the exocytotic release process; without this ion no transmitter release will occur, although the nerve terminal will still depolar-

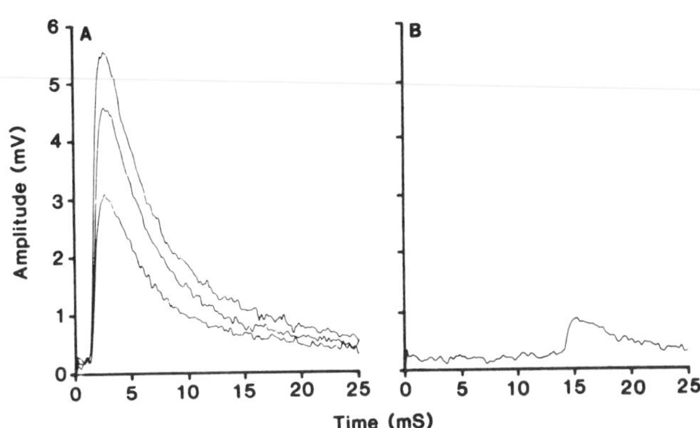

Figure 6. (A) Intracellular recordings made using the same method as described in Fig 5A except the concentration of calcium chloride was lowered from 2 μmol/L to 0.9 μmol/L, and the concentration of magnesium sulphate was 10 μmol/L. Under these conditions the amplitude of the endplate potential is reduced. Three superimposed endplate potentials are shown. (B) A recording made from the same endplate as in Fig 6A in the absence of nerve stimulation, showing a spontaneous miniature endplate potential.

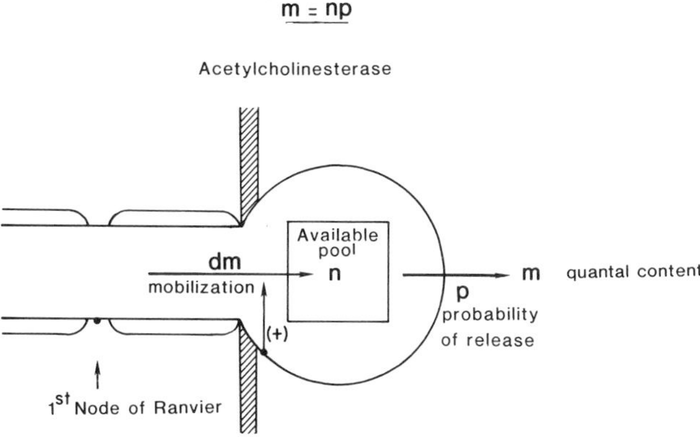

Figure 7. Schematic representation of the theoretical parameters of quantal release at the neuromuscular junction; the availability of quanta (n), the probability of release (p), the quantal content (m), and the mobilization rate (dm). The possible sites of action of acetylcholine on the nerve terminal are also indicated (●).

ize.[4] Calcium ions enter the nerve terminal during depolarization along with the sodium ions,[27] and it has been suggested that specific binding sites for calcium ions exist within the nerve terminal.[28] Calcium and magnesium ions may be considered to have an antagonistic action toward each other in their effect on release.[24,25] It is this depressant effect of magnesium that results in its interaction with neuromuscular blocking agents when magnesium is administered to treat pre-eclampsia and eclamptic toxemia.[29] Some of the antibiotics depress acetylcholine release in a manner similar to magnesium (eg, polymyxin B),[30] and although calcium is not effective in reversing neuromuscular block produced by a mixture of d-tubocurarine and polymyxin B, it is effective in reversing the block produced by some other antibiotics and d-tubocurarine.[29]

The number of acetylcholine molecules in a single quantum has been estimated to be between 6,000 and 10,000[31,32] and the usual number of quanta released from a single nerve terminal in response to a single nerve stimulus is thought to be 200 to 400 at untreated amphibian[33] and mammalian neuromuscular junctions.[34]

The aminopyridines have been investigated for their clinical potential as reversal agents,[35,36] and this group of drugs block potassium conductance, which results in a prolonged nerve terminal action potential and a consequently greater influx of calcium ions.[27,37,38] Experimentally, EPP quantal contents exceeding 10,000 have been estimated in the presence of 3,4-diaminopyridine.[33]

The Present Status of the Quantal Release Theory

It was about the same time as the quantal theory of transmitter release was proposed that vesicles were demonstrated to be present in the nerve terminal,[39] which led to the natural conclusion that a vesicle and a quanta of transmitter were one and the same.[26] However, it should be brought to the attention of the reader that there is evidence for two other types of acetylcholine release at the neuromuscular junction. The first type is nonquantal in nature and consists of leakage of acetycholine from the motor nerve terminal; this leakage is large and not affected by nerve terminal depolarization.[40] The second type, more recently proposed, is quantal in nature and not dependent on extracellular calcium.[41] Furthermore, it should be noted that acetylcholine can also be synthesized and released from nonneural cells such as the Schwann cells.[42]

The nonevoked nonquantal release of acetylcholine is considered by some to be an obstacle to the vesicle hypothesis. Other obstacles include the observations that (1) 50% of the acetylcholine in the nerve terminal is not in vesicles but is in the cytosol; (2) vesicles that can be isolated do not contain recently synthesized acetylcholine; and (3) stimulation does cause the release of recently synthesized acetylcholine.

Marchbanks[43] discusses these points and suggests the acetylcholine may be released through pores or channels in the nerve terminal; however, it should be pointed out that this hypothesis also arouses vigorous discussion.[44,45] Other complicating factors include the observation of MEPPs that are smaller in size than the quantal unit[46–48]; these events are commonly known as sub-MEPPs. Kriebel et al[49] postulated that the sub-MEPPs are the basic quantal unit and that MEPPs are multiples of these; however, the statistical evidence for such a hypothesis is poor. Another type of MEPP that has been observed following a variety of treatments including 3,4-diaminopyridine,[38] high-frequency nerve stimulation,[50] lanthanum ions,[51] vinblastine,[52] and 4-aminoquinoline[53] is the "giant" MEPP. Molgó and Thesleff[53] suggest that the giant MEPPs produced by 4-aminoquinoline arise from release sites outside the active zones, and this is the second type of release listed previously.[41]

The aforementioned alternative points of view are presented in order to demonstrate that the vesicle hypothesis is not universally accepted. The status of this hypothesis is examined further by MacIntosh.[7] It should be pointed out that strong evidence for release of vesicular acetylcholine by exocytosis has been recently demonstrated.[54,55] Also, pharmacologically induced massive release of acetylcholine induced by the venom from black widow spider (*Latrodectus mactans*) produces swelling of the nerve terminal.[56] This would not be seen unless the vesicles become a part of the presynaptic membrane.

Once exocytosis has occurred, the vesicles are then thought to be recycled by invaginating at sites distant from the active zones, coalescing with the cisternae in the nerve terminal, filling with acetylcholine, and forming new vesicles ready for release.[6]

Mobilization of Transmitter

Mobilization of transmitter is a factor that can also affect transmitter release if release is high. Mobilization is the rate at which the available pool of transmitter refills (Fig 7), and the effect of acetylcholine antagonists such as the nondepolarizing neuromuscular blocking agents has led to the suggestion that mobilization is increased by released acetylcholine in a positive feedback loop that is intercepted by antagonists.[1,57,58] Further evidence for this action of released acetylcholine is supplied by the fact that cholinergic agonists such as decamethonium appear to increase mobilization.[59] The fade of tetanic tension and train-of-four produced by nondepolarizing neuromuscular blocking agents is postulated to be due to their prejunctional effect on mobilization of transmitter.[1,58]

The reader is referred to recent reviews by Standaert[60] and by Bowman et al[61] for further reading on the release process at the neuromuscular junction.

POSTJUNCTIONAL EVENTS

Following release of acetylcholine from the nerve terminal and diffusion across the synaptic cleft, acetylcholine interacts with the endplate to produce depolarization. If the release of the acetylcholine is quantal in nature, a MEPP or an EPP may be recorded if a microelectrode is in the endplate region. In order for the molecules of acetylcholine to produce a depolarization, a change in the ionic permeability of the endplate must occur. This is achieved via the acetylcholine-activated ionic channel, a protein with the appearance of a rosette made up of five or six protein subunits.[62] The receptor density at the endplate region is estimated to be between 10,000 and 30,000 μm^{-2}.[63–65] The receptor channel complex is roughly cylindrical in shape, with a length of 11 nm and a diameter of 8.5 to 9.0 nm,[66–68] and is inserted through the membrane and distributed asymmetrically, projecting 5.5 nm from the membrane surface on the synaptic side and 1.5 nm on the cytoplasmic side.[67,68] This knowledge of the structure of the acetylcholine receptor-channel complex is derived from studies on the receptors in the membrane of the electric organ of the *Torpedo,* which are believed to be biochemically similar to those in mammalian endplates.[69]

Two agonist molecules must bind to the receptor before it will undergo the conformational change necessary to allow ionic flow.[70,71] Unlike the voltage-sensitive sodium and potassium ion channels in the nerve terminal, the ion channels in the endplate region are chemically sensitive and, when open,

Figure 8. A family of endplate currents recorded from the untreated transected cutaneous pectoris muscle of the frog (*Rana pipiens*). The endplate currents are superimposed and were recorded at membrane holding potentials of (in descending order) −40, −60, −80, −100, −120, and −140 mV. The rate of decay of the endplate currents becomes faster at less negative membrane holding potentials, reflecting the shorter lifetime of the acetylcholine-activated ionic channels of the endplate. (Reproduced with permission from Durant and Horn.[75])

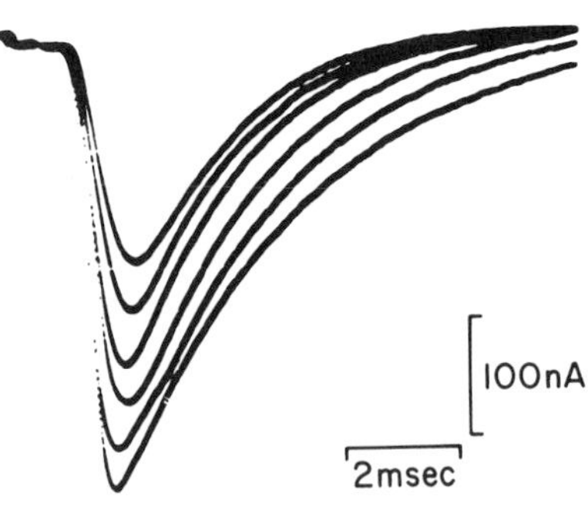

cannot discriminate between sodium and potassium ions, which flow inward and outward, respectively, at a membrane potential of −90 mV.[72] This ionic flow makes the endplate region become more positive, the extent of this depolarization being dependent on the number of channels that open and therefore the amount of acetylcholine present. The acetylcholine-activated ionic channels remain open for an exponentially distributed period of time that is dependent upon the membrane potential.[73] Ionic conductance can be measured at the endplate by recording the endplate currents (EPC) using the voltage clamp technique,[72] and the exponential decay of the EPCs is an indirect estimate of channel lifetime. Shortening of EPC decay rates, and consequently the channel lifetime, occurs as the membrane potential is made more positive (Fig 8). Single acetylcholine-activated ionic channels can be recorded, and computer-assisted summation of these single-channel events will produce a hypothetical miniature EPC.[74]

Channel lifetime is also affected by drugs,[75] including the nondepolarizing neuromuscular blocking agents,[76] and the effect of gallamine on EPCs is shown in Fig 9. This muscle relaxant, besides blocking the acetylcholine receptors, also blocks the conductance of the open channel, although only for a relatively short period of time at −90 mV, such that it leaves the channel during the time the EPC is still being recorded and acetylcholine-activated channels become conductive again, giving rise to the biphasic EPC decay at −90 mV shown in Fig 9.[77] A biphasic decay is not seen at more positive potentials due to the shorter channel lifetime and a voltage-dependent action of gallamine. The properties of the acetylcholine-activated channel are covered in further detail elsewhere.[78]

How important is blockade of the acetylcholine-activated ionic channel by drugs that are clinically used? In the case of the nondepolarizing neuromuscular blocking agents, this effect does not make a large contribution to neuromuscular blockade. It has been estimated with d-tubocurarine that only 1% of the channels in the endplate are blocked during a train of nerve stimuli,[79]

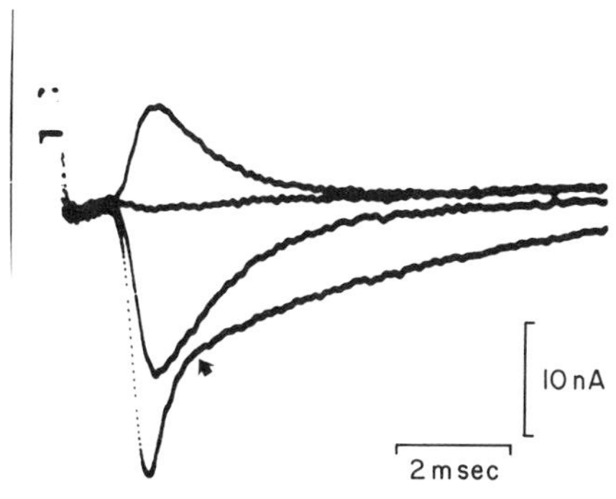

Figure 9. A family of endplate currents recorded under the same experimental conditions as described in Fig 8, except 10 μmol/L gallamine is present in the bathing solution. The membrane holding potentials are (in descending order) 30, 0, −30, and −90 mV. Compared with the control in Fig 8, the amplitudes of the endplate currents are reduced and the endplate current decay at −90 mV is biphasic due to the gallamine. The point at which the endplate current decay becomes biphasic is indicated by the arrow.

mainly due to the low number of receptor-channel complexes that will still open in response to released acetylcholine because of the receptor blockade produced by the drug. The same situation does not apply to other agents that do not produce acetylcholine receptor blockade such as ketamine, which is an extremely potent agent in producing blockade of open acetylcholine-activated channels but does not block acetylcholine receptors.[80,81] Many other agents (eg, the inhalation anesthetics) do affect ionic conductance of the endplate and these may interact with the nondepolarizing neuromuscular blocking agents.

The EPP will, if large enough, trigger voltage-sensitive sodium channels in the muscle membrane area adjacent to the endplate region, to open and initiate a muscle action potential that is propagated away from the endplate region, and excitation-contraction coupling of the muscle fiber rapidly follows. Whether the EPP potential reaches the threshold of approximately −50 mV will determine whether a muscle action potental is triggered (Fig 5). This part of the process of neuromuscular transmission is open to manipulation by peripherally acting muscle relaxants and anticholinesterase drugs.

The Margin of Safety

As discussed, the nondepolarizing neuromuscular blocking agents block primarily the receptors; however, many receptors have to be blocked before a diminution of response is observed. This is known as the margin of safety of neuromuscular transmission[82,83] and describes the fraction of available receptors that must be blocked before depression of the muscle response is observed. The most sensitive indicator is the train of stimuli applied at 100 Hz, and in this situation approximately half of the receptors must be blocked before a decrease in tetanic tension is observed. The margin of safety was estimated by Paton and Waud[82] to lie between 4 and 12 in anesthetized cats, using a nerve stimulation frequency of 0.1 Hz. It should also be pointed out that the margin of safety of neuromuscular transmission can also be significantly affected by agents that decrease the release of acetylcholine, eg, magnesium ions.

The Action of Neuromuscular Blocking Agents and Anticholinesterases

The action of the nondepolarizing agents at the neuromuscular junction is almost entirely confined to the acetylcholine receptors of the endplate (see preceding text), where they competitively bind and prevent released acetylcholine from causing sufficient depolarization (EPP) to trigger a muscle action potential. Since this action is competitive, a lowered synaptic concentration of the antagonist will cause dissociation and recovery. Similarly, recovery will ensue if the synaptic concentration of acetylcholine is raised, thus displacing the antagonist by the law of mass action. Such is the case with the anticholinesterases, which will prevent the destruction of released acetylcholine by acetylcholinesterase (Fig 4) and lead to the reversal of nondepolarizing neuromuscular block. These drugs will also permit the access of released acetylcholine to the 1st node of Ranvier,[1,84] which will cause antidromic firing, although only when the frequency of nerve stimulation is less than 2 Hz.[1]

The depolarizing agent succinylcholine may initially depolarize the nerve terminal, thereby causing fasiculations; however, it also will rapidly depolarize the endplate region and take it to a more positive potential above the threshold for muscle action potential initiation.[85] Clinically, this type of neuromuscular blockade is termed phase I block, and with time this may progress to phase II block, which is more akin to nondepolarizing neuromuscular block and may be reversed by anticholinesterases.[85] Prolonged exposure in vitro of the endplate to succinylcholine results in desensitization of the endplate region[86]; however it is not possible to make the conclusion that phase II block with succinylcholine is due to desensitization. The modes of action of the neuromuscular block produced in vitro by d-tubocurarine, succinylcholine, and magnesium are summarized in Fig 10.

Physiologic Factors That Affect Neuromuscular Transmission

Neuromuscular transmission may be different in certain situations, which will have a bearing on the clinical use of muscle relaxants. For example, newborns exhibit an inability to maintain a tetanus applied at a frequency of nerve stimulation of 100 Hz until approximately 2 to 3 months of age.[87,88] An in vitro study using the phrenic nerve-hemidiaphragm of the rat also suggests that the safety factor is reduced at the immature neuromuscular junction.[89] Other factors beyond the scope of this review such as pharmaco-

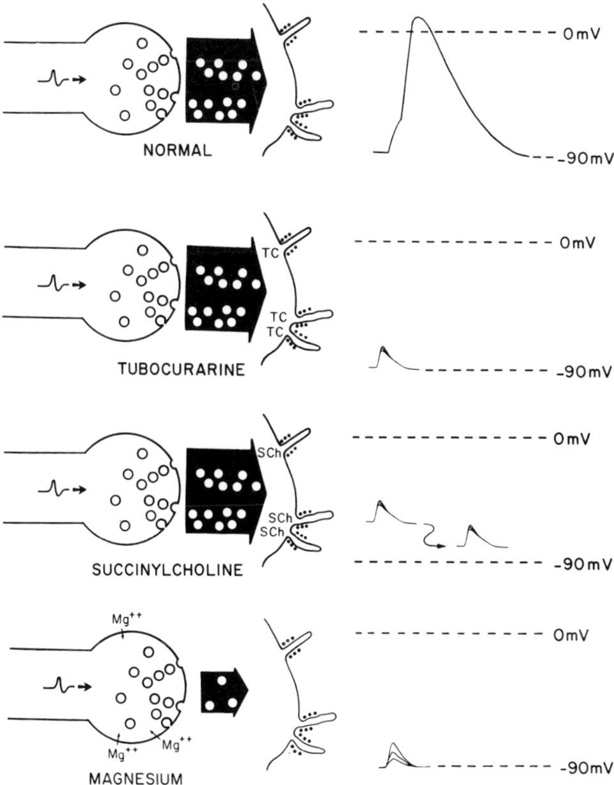

Figure 10. Diagrammatic representation of the actions in vitro of d-tubocurarine, succinylcholine, and magnesium compared with control. The nerve terminal, release of quanta, and the endplate are shown in the left-hand half of the illustration, and the corresponding theoretical intracellular endplate voltage recordings are shown on the right. The endplate potentials shown in the presence of magnesium are similar to the actual recordings shown in Fig 6A.

kinetics also play a role in the sensitivity of infants to neuromuscular blocking agents.[90]

Myasthenia gravis is characterized by muscle weakness and exquisite sensitivity to nondepolarizing agents and resistance to depolarizing agents.[29] The patient behaves as if already partially curarized, and it appears that myasthenic lgG binds to receptors,[91] while release of acetylcholine is apparently normal.[92]

In contrast to myasthenia gravis, in the Eaton-Lamberet syndrome release of acetylcholine is impaired,[93] but the symptoms (generalized muscle weakness and fatiguability) are superficially similar to myasthenia gravis. Due to its ability to increase the release of acetylcholine, 4-aminopyridine has been found to produce some improvement.[94–97] Some success has also been achieved using the synthetic *Veratrum* alkaloid germine monoacetate to treat myasthenia gravis.[98] This alkaloid acts primarily by causing repetitive firing of the axon and the muscle fiber in response to a single stimulus.[99]

ACKNOWLEDGMENT

The secretarial assistance of R. Antonucci and the illustrative expertise of N. Nguyen are most gratefully acknowledged. I would also like to thank Dr B. Bloor and D. Tinnion for reading the manuscript and offering their constructive criticism.

REFERENCES

1. Bowman WC: Pharmacology of Neuromuscular Function. Bristol, England, Wright, 1980
2. McMahan UJ, Spitzer NC, Peper K: Visual identification of nerve terminals in living isolated skeletal muscle. Proc R Soc Lond 181:421–430, 1972
3. Desaki J, Uehara Y: The overall morphology of neuromuscular junctions as revealed by scanning electron microscopy. J Neurocytol 10:101–110, 1981
4. Katz B: Nerve, Muscle and Synapse. New York, McGraw-Hill, 1966
5. Alnaes E, Rahamimoff R: On the role of mitochondria in transmitter release from motor nerve terminals. J Physiol 248:285–306, 1975
6. Heuser JE, Reese TS: Evidence for recycling of synaptic vesicle membrane during transmitter release at the frog neuromuscular junction. J Cell Biol 57:315–344, 1973
7. MacIntosh FC: The present status of the vesicle hypothesis. Adv Behav Biol 24:297–322, 1977
8. Collier B, Katz HS: Acetylcholine synthesis from recaptured choline by a sympathetic ganglion. J Physiol 238:639–655, 1974
9. Potter LT: Synthesis, storage and release of ^{14}C acetylcholine in isolated rat diaphragm muscle. J Physiol 206:145–166, 1970
10. Hubbard JI: Microphysiology of vertebrate neuromuscular transmission. Physiol Rev 53:674–723, 1973
11. Elmqvist D, Quastel DMJ: Presynaptic action of hemicholinium at the neuromuscular junction. J Physiol 177:463–482, 1965
12. Jones SF, Kwanbunbumpen S: The effects of nerve stimulation and hemicholinium on synaptic vesicles at the mammalian neuromuscular junction. J Physiol 207:31–50, 1970
13. Marshall IG: Studies on the blocking action of 2-(4-phenyl piperidino)-cyclohexanol (AH5183). Br J Pharmacol 38:503–516, 1970
14. Cookson JC, Paton WDM: Mechanisms of neuromuscular block. Anaesthesia 24:395–416, 1969
15. Miyamoto MD: The actions of cholinergic drugs on motor nerve terminals. Physiol Rev 29:221–247, 1978
16. Blaustein MP, Ratzlaff RW, Kendrick NK: The regulation of intracellular calcium in presynaptic nerve terminals. Ann NY Acad Sci 307:195–211, 1978
17. Blaustein MP, McGraw CF, Somlyo AV, et al: How is cytoplasmic calcium concentration controlled in nerve terminals? J Physiol 76:459–470, 1980
18. Baker PF: The regulation of intracellular calcium in giant axons of *Loligo* and *Myxicola*. Ann NY Acad Sci 307:250–268, 1978
19. Rahamimoff R, Lev-Tov A, Meiri H: Primary and secondary regulation of quantal transmitter release: Calcium and sodium. J Exp Biol 89:5–18, 1980

20. Fatt P, Katz B: Some observations on biological noise. Nature 166:597–598, 1950
21. Del Castillo J, Engbaek L: The nature of the neuromuscular block produced by magnesium. J Physiol 124:370–384, 1954
22. Del Castillo J, Katz B: The effect of magnesium on the activity of motor nerve endings. J Physiol 124:553–559, 1954
23. Del Castillo J, Katz B: Quantal components of the end-plate potential. J Physiol 124:560–573, 1954
24. Hubbard JI, Jones SF, Landau EM: On the mechanism by which calcium and magnesium affect the release of transmitter by nerve impulses. J Physiol 196:75–86, 1968
25. Del Castillo J, Katz B: Statistical factors involved in neuromuscular facilitation and depression. J Physiol 124:574–585, 1954
26. Martin AR: Quantal nature of synaptic transmission. Physiol Rev 46:51–66, 1966
27. Molgó J, Thesleff S: Electrotonic properties of motor nerve terminals. Acta Physiol Scand 114:271–275, 1982
28. Silinsky EM: On the calcium receptor that mediates depolarization-secretion coupling at cholinergic motor nerve terminals. Br J Pharmacol 73:413–429, 1981
29. Miller RD, Savarese JJ: Pharmacology of muscle relaxants, their antagonists, and monitoring of neuromuscular function, in Miller R (ed): Anesthesia, chap 17. New York, Churchill-Livingstone, 1981, pp 487–538
30. Durant NN, Lambert JJ: The action of polymyxin B at the frog neuromuscular junction. Br J Pharmacol 72:41–47, 1981
31. Kuffler SW, Yoshikami D: The number of transmitter molecules in a quantum: An estimate from iontophoretic application of acetylcholine at the neuromuscular synapse. J Physiol 251:465–482, 1975
32. Bierkamper GG, Goldberg AM: Release of acetylcholine from the isolated perfused diaphragm, in Hanin I, Goldberg AM (eds): Progress in Cholinergic Biology. New York, Raven Press 1982, pp 113–136
33. Katz B, Miledi R: Estimates of quantal content during ‘chemical potentiation’ of transmitter release. Proc R Soc Lond 205:369–378, 1979
34. Hubbard JI, Wilson DF: Neuromuscular transmission in a mammalian preparation in the absence of blocking drugs and the effect of D-tubocurarine. J Physiol 228:307–325, 1973
35. Stoyanov E, Vulchev P, Shturbova M, et al: Clinical electromyomechanographic and electromyographic studies in decurarization with Pymadine. Anaesth Resus Inten Therap 4:139–142, 1976
36. Thesleff S: Aminopyridines and synaptic transmission. Neuroscience 5:1413–1419, 1980
37. Durant NN, Marshall IG: The effects of 3,4-diaminopyridine on spontaneous and evoked transmitter release at the frog neuromuscular junction. J Physiol 280:21P, 1978
38. Durant NN, Marshall IG: The effects of 3,4-diaminopyridine on acetylcholine release at the frog neuromuscular junction. Eur J Pharmacol 67:201–208, 1980
39. Robertson JD: The ultrastructure of a reptilian myoneural junction. J Biophys Biochem Cytol 2:381–393, 1956
40. Katz B, Miledi R: Transmitter leakage from motor nerve endings. Proc R Soc Lond 196:59–72, 1977
41. Thesleff S, Molgó J: A new type of transmitter release at the neuromuscular junction. Neuroscience 9:1–8, 1983
42. Ito K, Miledi R: The effect of calcium-ionophores on acetylcholine release from Schwann cells. Proc R Soc Lond 196:51–58, 1977
43. Marchbanks RM: Role of storage vesicles in synaptic transmission. Symp Soc Exp Biol 33:251–276, 1979
44. Whittaker VP: The vesicular hypothesis. Trends in Neuroscience 2:55–56, 1979
45. Marchbanks RM: In reply to Dr Whittaker. Trends in Neuroscience 2:56, 1979

46. Kriebel ME, Gross CE: Multimodal distribution of frog miniature endplate potentials in adult, denervated, and tadpole leg muscle. J Gen Physiol 64:85–103, 1974
47. Dennis MJ, Miledi R: Characteristics of transmitter release at regenerating frog neuromuscular junctions. J Physiol 239:571–594, 1974
48. Bevan S: Sub-miniature end-plate potentials at untreated frog neuromuscular junctions. J Physiol 258:145–155, 1976
49. Kriebel ME, Llados F, Matteson DR: Spontaneous subminiature end-plate potentials in mouse diaphragm muscle: Evidence for synchronous release. J Physiol 262:553–581, 1976
50. Heuser JE: A possible origin of the 'giant' spontaneous potentials that occur after prolonged transmitter release at frog neuromuscular junctions. J Physiol 239:106P–107P, 1974
51. Heuser J, Miledi R: Effect of lanthanum ions on function and structure of frog neuromuscular junctions. Proc R Soc Lond 179:247–260, 1971
52. Pécot-Dechavassine M: Action of vinblastine on the spontaneous release of acetylcholine at the frog neuromuscular junction. J Physiol 261:31–48, 1976
53. Molgó J, Thesleff S: 4-Aminoquinoline-induced 'giant' miniature endplate potentials at mammalian neuromuscular junctions. Proc R Soc Lond 214:229–247, 1982
54. Pécot-Dechavassine M: Synaptic vesicle openings captured by cooling and related to transmitter release at the frog neuromuscular junction. Biol Cell 48:43–50, 1982
55. Heuser JE, Reese TS, Dennis MJ, et al: Synaptic vesicle exocytosis captured by quick-freezing and correlated with quantal transmitter release. J Cell Biol 71:275–300, 1979
56. Ceccarelli B, Grohovaz F, Hurlbut WP, et al: Freeze-fracture studies of frog neuromuscular junctions during intense release of neurotransmitter. I. Effects of black widow spider venom and Ca^{2+}-free solutions on the structure of the active zone. J Cell Biol 81:163–177, 1979
57. Bowman WC, Webb SN: Tetanic fade during partial transmission failure produced by non-depolarizing neuromuscular blocking drugs in the cat. Clin Exp Pharmacol Physiol 3:545–555, 1976
58. Bowman WC: Prejunctional and postjunctional cholinoceptors at the neuromuscular junction. Anesth Analg 59:935–943, 1980
59. Blaber LC: The prejunctional action of some non-depolarizing blocking drugs. Br J Pharmacol 47:109–116, 1973
60. Standaert FG: Release of transmitter at the neuromuscular junction. Br J Anaesth 54:131–145, 1982
61. Bowman WC, Marshall IG, Gibb AJ: Is there feedback control of transmitter release at the neuromuscular junction? Semin Anesth 3:275–283, 1984
62. Heuser JE, Salpeter SR: Organisation of acetylcholine receptors in quick-frozen, deep-etched, and rotary-replicated *Torpedo* postsynaptic membrane. J Cell Biol 82:150–173, 1979
63. Matthews-Bellinger J, Salpeter MM: Distribution of acetylcholine receptors at frog neuromuscular junctions with a discussion of some physiological implications. J Physiol 279:197–213, 1978
64. Land BR, Salpeter EE, Salpeter MM: Acetylcholine receptor site density affects the rising phase of miniature endplate currents. Proc Natl Acad Sci USA 77:3736–3740, 1980
65. Fertuck HC, Salpeter MM: Quantitation of junctional and extrajunctional acetylcholine receptors by electron microscope autoradiography after ^{125}I-α-bungarotoxin binding at mouse neuromuscular junctions. J Cell Biol 69:144–158, 1976
66. Raftery MA, Changeux J-P: The nicotinic acetylcholine receptor (AChR). Neurosci Res Program Bull 20:277–301, 1982
67. Ross MJ, Klymkowski MW, Agard DA, et al: Structural studies of a membrane-bound acetylcholine receptor from *Torpedo californica.* J Mol Biol 116:635–659, 1977
68. Kistler J, Stroud RM, Klymkowsky MW, et al: Structure and function of an acetylcholine receptor. Biophys J 37:371–383, 1982
69. Lindstrom J, Walter B, Einarson B: Immunochemical similarities between subunits of acetyl-

choline receptors from *Torpedo, Electrophorus*, and mammalian muscle. Biochemistry 18:4470–4480, 1979

70. Trautmann A, Feltz A: Open time of channels activated by binding of two distinct agonists. Nature 286:291–293, 1980
71. Feltz A, Trautmann A: Densitization at the frog neuromuscular junction: a biphasic process. J Physiol 322:257–272, 1982
72. Takeuchi A, Takeuchi N: On the permeability of end-plate membrane during the action of transmitter. J Physiol 154:52–67, 1960
73. Magleby KL, Stevens CF: The effect of voltage on the time course of end-plate currents. J Physiol 223:151–171, 1972
74. Neher E, Steinbach JH: Local anaesthetics transiently block currents through single acetylcholine-receptor channels. J Physiol 277:153–176, 1978
75. Lambert JJ, Durant NN, Henderson EG: Drug-induced modification of ionic conductance at the neuromuscular junction. Ann Rev Pharmacol Toxicol 23:505–539, 1983
76. Durant NN, Horn R: ORG 6368: A nondepolarizing neuromuscular blocking agent with a novel effect on end-plate conductance. J Pharmacol Exp Ther 228:567–572, 1984
77. Colquhoun D, Sheridan RE: The modes of action of gallamine. Proc R Soc Lond 211:181–203, 1981
78. Standaert FG: Donuts and holes: Molecules and muscle relaxants. Semin Anesth 3:251–261, 1984
79. Magleby KL, Pallotta BS, Terrar DA: The effect of (+)-tubocurarine on neuromuscular transmission during repetitive stimulation in the rat, mouse, and frog. J Physiol 312:97–113, 1981
80. Volle RL, Alkadhi KA, Branisteanu DD, et al: Ketamine and ditran block endplate ion conductance and [^{3}H]phencyclidine binding to electric organ membrane. J Pharmacol Exp Ther 221:570–576, 1982
81. Aronstam RS, Narayanan L, Wenger DA: Ketamine inhibition of ligand binding to cholinergic receptors and ion channels. Eur J Pharmacol 78:367–370, 1982
82. Paton WDM, Waud DR: The margin of safety of neuromuscular transmission. J Physiol 191:59–90, 1967
83. Waud BE, Waud DR: The relation between the response to "train-of-four" stimulation and receptor occlusion during competitive neuromuscular block. Anesthesiology 37:413–416, 1972
84. Webb SN, Bowman WC: The role of pre- and post-junctional cholinoceptors in the action of neostigmine at the neuromuscular junction. Clin Exp Pharmacol Physiol 1:123–134, 1974
85. Durant NN, Katz RL: Suxamethonium. Br J Anaesth 54:195–208, 1982
86. Katz B, Thesleff S: A study of 'desensitization' produced by acetylcholine at the motor end-plate. J Physiol 138:63–80, 1957
87. Goudsouzian NG: Maturation of neuromuscular transmission in the infant. Br J Anaesth 52:205–214, 1980
88. Crumrine RS, Yodlowski EH: Assessment of neuromuscular function in infants. Anesthesiology 54:29–32, 1981
89. Kelly SS, Roberts DV: The effect of age on the safety factor in neuromuscular transmission in the isolated diaphragm of the rat. Br J Anaesth 49:217–222, 1977
90. Fisher DM, Miller RD: Neuromuscular effects of vecuronium (ORG NC 45) in infants and children during N_2O halothane anesthesia. Anesthesiology 58:519–523, 1983
91. Pennefather P, Quastel DMJ: The effects of myasthenic IgG on miniature endplate currents in mouse diaphragm. Life Sci 27:2047–2054, 1980
92. Cull-Candy SG, Miledi R, Trautmann A: End-plate currents and acetylcholine noise at normal and myasthenic human end-plates. J Physiol 287:247–265, 1979
93. Swift TR: Disorders of neuromuscular transmission other than myasthenia gravis. Muscle Nerve 4:334–353, 1981

94. Lundh H, Nilsson O, Rosén I: 4-Aminopyridine — A new drug tested in the treatment of Eaton-Lambert syndrome. J Neurol Neurosurg Psychiatry 40:1109–1112, 1977
95. Agoston S, van Weerden T, Westra P, et al: Effects of 4-aminopyridine in Eaton-Lambert syndrome. Br J Anaesth 50: 583–585, 1978
96. Sanders DB, Kim YI, Howard JF, et al: Eaton-Lambert syndrome: A clinical and electrophysiological study of a patient treated with 4-aminopyridine. J Neurol Neurosurg Psychiatry 43:978–985, 1980
97. Thesleff S: Aminopyridines and synaptic transmission. Neuroscience 5:1413–1419, 1980
98. Flacke W: Treatment of myasthenia gravis. N Engl J Med 288:27–31, 1973
99. Higashi H, Yonemura K, Shimoji K: Antagonism of neuromuscular blocks by germine monoacetate. Anesthesiology 38:145–152, 1973

W.C. Bowman
I.G. Marshall
A.J. Gibb

3

Is There Feedback Control of Transmitter Release at the Neuromuscular Junction?

There is no serious opposition to the established concept that neuromuscular transmission is brought about by the release of acetylcholine from the nerve endings by nerve impulses, and that the released acetylcholine then acts on postjunctional endplate cholinoceptors to bring about the permeability change that gives rise to the endplate potential, and hence to a propagated action potential, followed by the series of events that results in contraction. Nor is there argument about the view that neuromuscular blocking drugs such as tubocurarine impair neuromuscular transmission by reversibly blocking the postjunctional cholinoceptors. Vigorous controversy does arise, however, over whether the postjunctional cholinoceptor blocking action of tubocurarine and similarly acting drugs is their only important contributory action, or whether a prejunctional action on the nerve endings also comes into play. Furthermore, even among those who accept that tubocurarine exerts a prejunctional action, there are relatively few who would go so far as to agree that its prejunctional action arises from the blockade of a population of nerve terminal cholinoceptors that play an important role in the transmission process under appropriate circumstances. We believe (and have done so for a long time) that tubocurarine, and most related drugs, act both prejunctionally and postjunctionally and that the main prejunctional action constitutes blockade of a population of nicotinic autoreceptors that are normally activated by the transmitter and that serve to mediate mobilization of reserve transmitter to the

MUSCLE RELAXANTS
ISBN 0-8089-1784-6

readily releasable situation within the terminal axoplasm. The physiologic importance of the postulated prejunctional autoreceptors is that they function in a positive feedback control system, activated by the transmitter itself, that serves to maintain the availability of acetylcholine when the demand for it is high, ie, when there is a heavy traffic of nerve impulses. The concept is illustrated in Fig 1. Our earlier views are expressed in several review articles,[1–7] but the idea that tubocurarine owes part of its neuromuscular blocking effect to an action on the nerve endings is not new. It was eloquently put forward by Lilleheil and Naess in 1961[8] and later by others.[9–11] Miyamoto[12] has reviewed the earlier literature on the subject.

TETANIC FADE AND TRAIN-OF-FOUR FADE

Most of the discussion about a possible prejunctional action of tubocurarine has centered around its ability to produce fade of responses at frequencies of stimulation above the very low ones (eg, 0.1 Hz) often used experimentally, ie, its ability to produce the familiar tetanic fade and train-of-four fade. The electrical counterpart of the mechanical phenomenon called tetanic fade is the so-called rundown of the endplate potentials within a high-frequency train (Fig 2). Hutter[13] showed in 1952 that during partial curarization, contraction of the cat's tibialis anterior muscle produced by close arterially injected

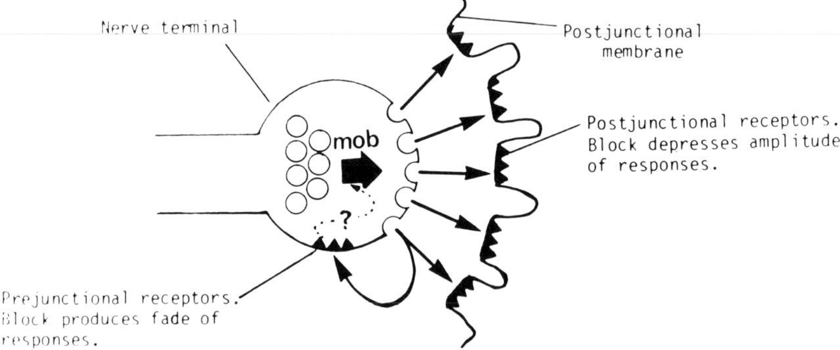

Figure 1. Diagrammatic representation of the proposed actions of released acetylcholine on prejunctional and postjunctional nicotinic cholinoceptors. Mobilization should be taken to include all those processes that serve to place acetylcholine in a readily releasable situation between nerve impulses, and not merely the movement of vesicles toward the terminal membrane as suggested by the diagram. The question mark near the prejunctional receptors is intended to indicate that any second messenger involved is unknown. It should be noted that the prejunctional receptors are not those that mediate antidromic repetitive firing in motor nerves under some circumstances.

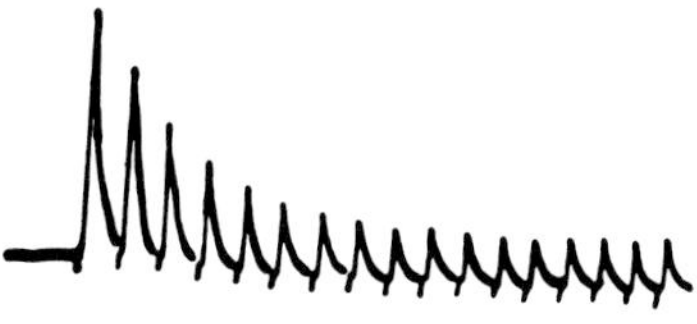

Figure 2. Endplate potentials recorded extracellularly from an isolated diaphragm preparation of the rat in response to stimulation of the phrenic nerve at a frequency of 180 Hz in the presence of tubocurarine. The so-called early tetanic rundown, which is the electrical counterpart of tetanic fade, is clearly evident (Reproduced with permission from Liley.[30])

acetylcholine was not depressed more during tetanic fade than it was before or after. In a similar kind of experiment 10 years later, Otsuka et al[14] showed on an isolated frog muscle that the endplate potential produced by microionophoretic application of acetylcholine was not smaller at the time of maximal tetanic rundown of neurally evoked endplate potentials than it was later, after a rest, when rundown was no longer present. These observations of Hutter[13] and of Otsuka et al[14] show that although sensitivity to acetylcholine is of course depressed by tubocurarine, it is not depressed to an increasing extent during tetanic fade or tetanic rundown. If there is no progressive diminution in acetylcholine sensitivity, then, as the authors concluded, these fade phenomena must be the result of a diminishing output of acetylcholine from the motor nerve endings. It was assumed that tubocurarine had merely unmasked a spontaneously occurring event. That is, it was supposed that acetylcholine output per impulse normally fell progressively during the early part of a tetanus, but such was the safety factor in the transmission process that no tetanic fade was evident unless tubocurarine was present to raise the threshold for transmission (ie, to abolish the safety factor). It should be noted that, at that time, techniques were not available to record trains of endplate potentials except in the presence of tubocurarine (or some other means of impairing transmission) to prevent dislodging or breaking the microelectrode. Therefore, it was not possible to record trains of endplate potentials that could serve as proper predrug controls.

If it could be shown that tetanic rundown of endplate responses was absent or less marked in the absence of tubocurarine than in its presence, then the implication would be that tubocurarine actually caused the effect. And since evidence has been provided that the effect arises from a progressively diminishing acetylcholine output, the inference would be that tubocurarine causes a progressive diminution of acetylcholine output during high-frequency stimulation and that this contributes to tetanic fade. Hubbard et al[9] and Blaber[11] attempted to study the problem by recording endplate potentials from isolated muscle fibers that had been cut on either side of the endplate, whereas Galindo[10] achieved similar ends by stretching the isolated muscle fibers. These procedures cause sufficient depolarization of the fiber membranes to prevent action potential generation and contraction, so that endplate potential trains can be recorded in the absence of tubocurarine. Under these conditions, rundown is virtually absent in the control trains, but it appears, along with an overall depression of amplitude, as soon as tubocurarine is present. The authors concluded that tubocurarine was causing the rundown, rather than merely unmasking it. However, these results have been criticized on the grounds that the procedures themselves (cutting, stretching) cause a pronounced, depolarization, possibly to near the equilibrium potential, so that the control trains of endplate potentials might not be able to reach the full magnitude commensurate with the amount of acetylcholine released. Consequently, rundown, which might have been present but invisible in the controls, so the critics held, only became evident when overall amplitude was depressed by tubocurarine.

Bowman and Webb[1,2] then returned to the less esoteric method of simply recording twitch and tetanic tension in the anaesthetized cat, but using a range of acetylcholine antagonists. They argued that if tension depression and tetanic fade are a consequence of one and the same mechanism, the fade being merely an unmasking of a spontaneously occurring event, then the two effects should hold a constant relationship with one another regardless of which drugs are used, or of the route of administration (if only one drug is used). They found that this was not so and therefore concluded that the two effects—peak tension depression and fade—are consequences of two different actions of the drugs, even though during tetanic contractions the latter must reinforce the former. Lee et al[15] supported this view by showing that, in the anaesthetized cat, α-bungarotoxin, which is known to be a powerful and virtually irreversible blocker of postjunctional motor endplate cholinoceptors, greatly depressed the amplitude of contractions but produced no tetanic fade or train-of-four fade. Clearly, fade is not merely a consequence of unmasking, by blocking postjunctional acetylcholine receptors, a spontaneously occurring event. We have confirmed in vitro the result of Lee et al[15] using another snake toxin, erabutoxin b, which is also a powerful ligand for the postjunctional acetylcholine receptors. Figure 3 illustrates the extremes of the lack of correlation between the two effects that it is possible to demonstrate with acetylcholine antagonists. Thus, hexamethonium produced complete tetanic fade in a concentration that was too small to depress the twitches, whereas erabutoxin b produced no detectable fade even when there was pronounced tension depression. The clinically used neuromuscular blocking drugs produce effects that lie between these extremes, and when studied under the equilibrium conditions that pertain in vitro, it is difficult to demonstrate any clear-cut differences between them. However, they do behave differently in vivo. For a given degree of block, tetanic fade is more pronounced with tubocurarine, for example, than with pancuronium or vecuronium,[2,16] and in any case, fade is slower to develop than is peak tension depression.

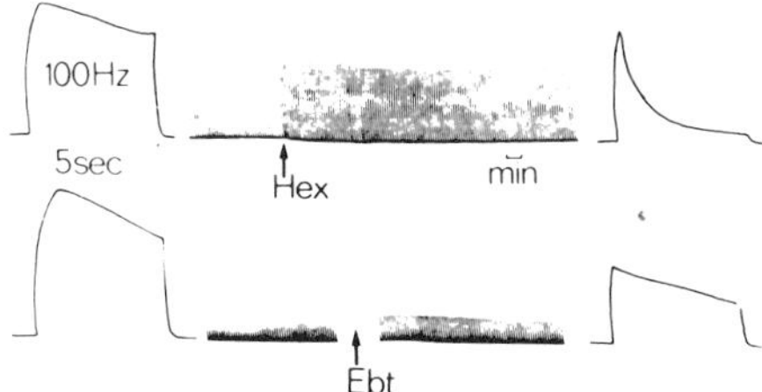

Figure 3. Isolated phrenic nerve hemidiaphragm preparations of the rat. The top and bottom traces are from different experiments. Twitches were evoked by stimulating the motor nerve at a frequency of 0.1 Hz, and tetani (100 Hz for 5 seconds) were interposed. The tetani were recorded on faster moving paper and the gain for the tetani was halved. At Hex, 150 μg/mL hexamethonium was added to the bath. This dose was too small to depress the twitches but produced marked tetanic fade in the subsequent tetanus. At Ebt, 0.32 μg/mL of erabutoxin b was added to the bath. The twitches were slowly depressed by more than 50%. Tetanic tension was also depressed, but tetanic fade was no greater than that occurring in the control tetani at the start of the experiments.

RUNDOWN OF ENDPLATE CURRENTS

In 1979, Glavinović[17] showed beyond reasonable doubt that the rundown of endplate responses that occurs in the presence of tubocurarine is not merely the result of unmasking a spontaneously occurring event. He made use of the technique of voltage clamp and recorded trains of neurally evoked endplate currents in cut rat diaphragm fibers. The voltage clamp technique is referred to again later in the text. Suffice to say at this point that the technique allows endplate responses to be recorded in the absence of tubocurarine and that there is no danger of complications arising through depolarization because the purpose of the clamp is to hold the membrane potential constant and, therefore, to prevent that effect. Glavinović found that in the absence of tubocurarine there was little or no rundown. Rundown was in fact an effect of tubocurarine.

If it is agreed that fade and rundown are not simply consequences of unmasking a spontaneously occurring event but that they are actually produced by tubocurarine and related drugs through a separate action, then that action must be to reduce transmitter output during high-frequency stimulation if the early results of Hutter[13] and of Otsuka et al[14] are accepted. There is, however, a great reluctance among many pharmacologists to accept that tubocurarine might act on the nerve endings to impair transmitter release. This reluctance probably stems from early observations by Dale et al,[18] who failed to detect by bioassay any effect of tubocurarine on the release of acetylcholine evoked by nerve stimulation in the muscle of the tongue perfused with a physiologic salt solution. However, anyone who has attempted a similar procedure (as we have) will be aware of the wide margin of error inherent in this type of experiment. Furthermore, in order to collect acetylcholine it is necessary to inhibit cholinesterase, yet anticholinesterase drugs act to prevent the very effects (ie, tetanic fade, train-of-four fade) that are being analyzed. Additionally, it is now known that there is a considerable spontaneous release of acetylcholine that is nonquantal in nature, perhaps up to 100 times as much as that giving rise to the miniature endplate potentials.[19] This large spontaneous release will of course be included in that collected in the perfusate, and it may well be that any falloff in evoked release during the initial part of a tetanus would be too small to be detected by relatively crude bioassay methods in the face of a constant background of spontaneous release.

Those who accept that fade of tetanic tension or of train-of-four is a separate phenomenon from tension depression, yet who cannot accept a prejunctional origin of the fade effect, have recruited the concept of use-dependent postjunctional ion channel occlusion in order to explain it.[20] Such an explanation, however, necessarily ignores the finding of Hutter[13] and of Otsuka et al[14] that tubocurarine-induced fade is associated with a diminished acetylcholine release. Furthermore, Magleby et al[21] have shown that tubocurarine-induced rundown of trains of endplate currents is independent of the membrane potential in voltage-clamped muscle fibers. This result constitutes good evidence that ion channel occlusion is not involved, because ion channel occlusion by cations, when it occurs, is strongly dependent upon membrane potential.

We have conducted a further electrophysiologic analysis, and we believe the results overwhelmingly point to a prejunctional origin of the fade effects of tubocurarine and related drugs. The philosophy of our approach is illustrated by Fig 4. We have used the voltage-clamped isolated cut diaphragm muscle fibers of the rat. In a voltage clamp experiment, two microelectrodes are inserted into the muscle fiber. One microelectrode continually monitors the voltage across the membrane and the other passes current into the fiber. The voltage-recording electrode is connected through a feedback amplifier to the current-passing electrode, and the arrangement is such that current will be instantly passed to maintain (ie, clamp) the voltage at any level preset by the experimenter. We chose to clamp the voltage at or near the resting membrane potential. Thus, any tendency for acetylcholine to depolarize the endplate membrane by opening the receptor-linked ion channels is immediately detected by the one (voltage-recording) and counteracted by the other (current-passing) microelectrode. The current passed by the current-passing electrode is exactly equal to the ionic current flow caused by acetylcholine. Hence,

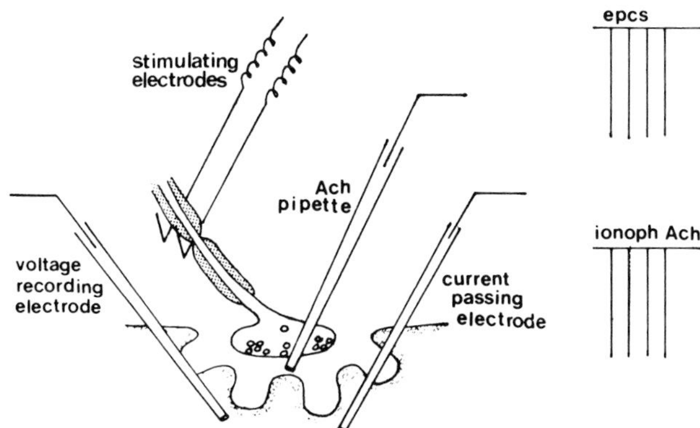

Figure 4. Diagrammatic representation of the voltage-clamped cut muscle fiber preparation. Abbreviations: Ach = acetylcholine; epcs = endplate currents. See text for further explanation.

measurement of the current passed by the current-passing electrode is an accurate reflection of the amount of acetylcholine released to interact with its postjunctional receptors. It is important to realize that in this type of arrangement there is no problem of a safety factor or of any ceiling to the effect of acetylcholine that might mask some of its activity. The amount of current that flows is in fact a direct measure of the amount of acetylcholine that interacts with its receptors and, therefore, of the amount of acetylcholine released to evoke transmission.

Acetylcholine was applied to the motor endplate receptors in two ways to evoke trains of endplate currents: (1) by stimulating the motor nerve and (2) by releasing it ionophoretically in jets from a micropipette. We have assumed that an action of a drug that is evident regardless of the manner in which the endplate currents are evoked must be exerted postjunctionally. On the other hand, a drug action that is evident when the nerve is stimulated at a given frequency, but not when jets of acetylcholine are released from a micropipette at the same frequency, must be exerted on the nerve. Many of the results with this preparation have been reported in detail by Gibb and Marshall.[22] Results with tubocurarine are illustrated in Fig 5. Tubocurarine depressed the amplitudes of brief trains of endplate currents (50 Hz) whether they were evoked by nerve stimulation or by ionophoretic application of acetylcholine, and so we conclude that amplitude depression is the result of postjunctional receptor block. Some rundown in the early part of each train was usually evident in the control neurally evoked trains before tubocurarine was added, but this was greatly enhanced in the presence of tubocurarine, as Glavinović[17] had also shown. However, there was uniform depression, with no sign of progressive rundown, when jets of acetylcholine were applied ionophoretically. We there-

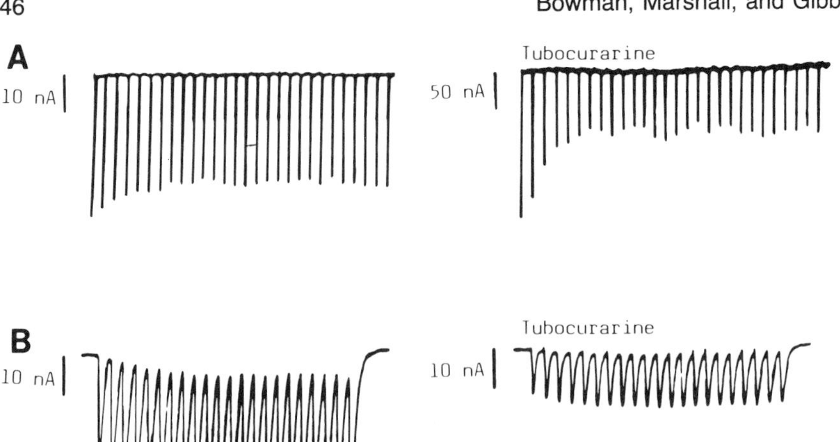

Figure 5. (A) Trains of endplate currents (50 Hz) evoked by stimulating the nerve and recorded in the absence (left) and in the presence (right) of tubocurarine (0.5×10^{-6} mol/L). The gain was increased fivefold in the presence of tubocurarine so that the height of the initial response approximately matched that of the control. (B) Trains of jets of acetylcholine recorded in the absence (left) and in the presence (right) of tubocurarine (0.25×10^{-6} mol/L). Tubocurarine produced a uniform depression of amplitude but there was no rundown, which is therefore deduced to be the result of an action on the nerve. Temperature was 37 °C, and membrane potential was −60 mV.

fore conclude that rundown with tubocurarine (the electrical counterpart of fade) is the result of an action on the nerve and so cannot be a consequence of postjunctional ion channel occlusion. Despite some quantitative differences, essentially similar results were obtained with other clinically used neuromuscular blocking drugs such as atracurium, pancuronium, and vecuronium. (For results with vecuronium, see Bowman et al.[6]) However, erabutoxin b, in accordance with the absence of tetanic fade in its presence (Fig 3), produced a uniform depression of the amplitude of the responses in a train whether the responses were evoked by nerve stimulation or by ionophoretic application. There was no sign of rundown, indicating that erabutoxin b acts only postjunctionally. This is in agreement with the report by Jones and Salpeter[23] that the similarly acting toxin, α-bungarotoxin, does not bind to motor nerve endings.

ION CHANNEL OCCLUSION

Trimetaphan (a ganglion-blocking drug) produces ion channel occlusion in the high concentrations necessary to affect the neuromuscular junction.[24] This drug produced both amplitude depression and rundown of trains of endplate currents whether they were evoked by nerve stimulation or by microionophoresis of acetylcholine (Fig 6). In accordance with its ion channel occluding effect, its ability to produce rundown was enhanced when the membrane was clamped at higher potentials.

EFFECT OF ACETYLCHOLINE

The fact that those drugs used in this study that produce the postulated prejunctional effect are acetylcholine antagonists does not prove that their prejunctional action is a consequence of this effect; that is, it cannot be taken as proof of the existence of prejunctional acetylcholine receptors. In order to postulate the existence of a specific receptor, it should be demonstrated that specific antagonists and the corresponding agonists have mutually opposing effects. Blaber[25] provided evidence that low concentrations of decamethonium, which in this context can be regarded as possessing acetylcholine-like action, increased the mobilization of transmitter in the nerve endings of the

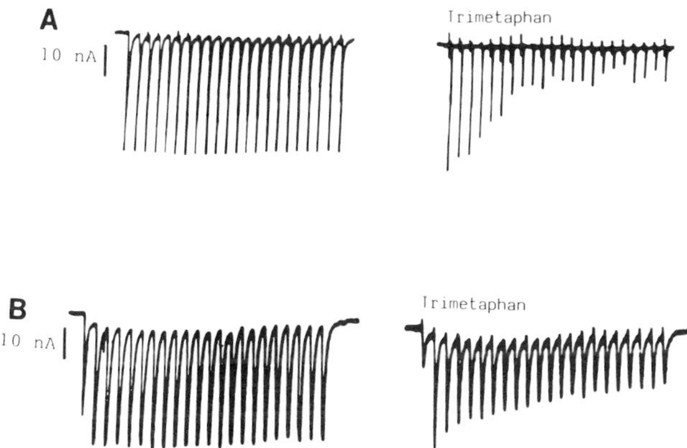

Figure 6. This figure shows experiments similar to those illustrated in Fig 5 except that trimetaphan (A) 10^{-4} mol/L and (B) 2.5×10^{-5} mol/L was added instead of tubocurarine. With these concentrations of trimetaphan there was little depression of amplitude of the initial responses, but rundown was evident in both A and B, indicating that it was mainly the result of a postjunctional use-dependent action (ie, ion channel occlusion). A and B are from different experiments and therefore not too much importance can be attached to the fact that rundown in A is more marked than in B. Nevertheless, we gained the impression from many experiments that there are both prejunctional and postjunctional components of action with trimetaphan.

isolated tenuissimus muscle of the cat, and that this action was blocked by tubocurarine. (This action of decamethonium is of course separate from its neuromuscular blocking action, which occurs with higher concentrations.)

In the experiment illustrated in Fig 7, depression and rundown of neurally evoked endplate current trains in the rat diaphragm were produced by tubocurarine added to the bath. Then, in the continued presence of tubocurarine, acetylcholine was applied to the endplate region by microionophoresis. The acetylcholine caused a further depression of peak amplitude probably because of desensitization of some receptors, and so we increased the gain on the recording. However, the important result is that the rundown produced by tubocurarine was largely overcome by the acetylcholine. We therefore feel

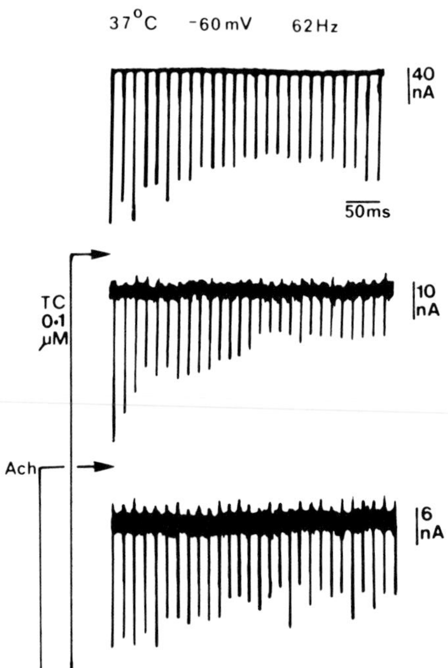

Figure 7. Trains of endplate currents (62 Hz) were evoked by stimulating the nerve. The top record is in the absence of tubocurarine, and the middle and bottom records are in the presence of tubocurarine (10^{-7} mol/L). Acetylcholine was applied microionophoretically during the train in the bottom record. The gain was adjusted so that the first epc in each train was approximately the same size (temperature 37 °C; membrane potential −60 mV). The rundown produced by tubocurarine (middle) was reduced in extent by acetylcholine (bottom) to little more than that in the control (top).

justified in proposing that the rundown produced by tubocurarine is a consequence of its blocking acetylcholine receptors, which for the reasons already given, we believe to be located on the nerve endings. We admit that the prevention of rundown by acetylcholine was not always as pronounced as that illustrated in Fig 7, although it was a statistically significant effect when recordings were made at 37 °C. We are inclined to the view that the reason for the variation in our results with acetylcholine lies in the method of administration. The acetylcholine pipette (Fig 4) was positioned in the neuromuscular junction by locating the point at which it gave the sharpest endplate current when acetylcholine was released from it. This point is thus the best position for stimulating postjunctional receptors, but it is unlikely to be optimal for acting on prejunctional receptors, and this may be why our success varied.

The electrophysiologic results described previously were obtained with trains of pulses of 50 to 70 Hz, but we have obtained similar results with train-of-four stimulation, and some of these have been described elsewhere.[6] Indeed, we have reason to suppose that the prejunctional receptors come in to play at frequencies of stimulation as low as 1 Hz.

CONCLUSION

Since tubocurarine and related drugs produce rundown or fade of responses evoked by nerve stimulation apparently by blocking prejunctional acetylcholine receptors, we conclude that these receptors must normally be activated by the transmitter and that they mediate a positive feedback control mechanism as described at the beginning of this article and illustrated in Fig 1.

Waud and Waud[26] have repeatedly emphasized that in the presence of nondepolarizing blocking drugs, the safety margin in transmission is substantially diminished at higher stimulation frequencies. When train-of-four stimulation was used, we noted that train-of-four fade was more pronounced in the mechanical responses than in the endplate currents.[6] The implication, therefore, is that the loss of safety factor arises from two effects of nondepolarizing neuromuscular blocking drugs: (1) block of postjunctional receptors, an effect that is independent of stimulation frequency, and (2) block of prejunctional receptors resulting in an initial progressive diminution of acetylcholine release, which greatly exaggerates the consequences of postjunctional receptor block. Block of prejunctional receptors increases in importance with increase in frequency.

Figure 8 is more complicated than Fig 1 in that it includes an additional population of prejunctional nicotinic receptors (RN rep) and a population of prejunctional muscarinic receptors (RM). Riker[27] has done much to further our understanding of these additional nicotinic receptors (RN rep), although even now there is controversy as to their existence.[28] In any case, these

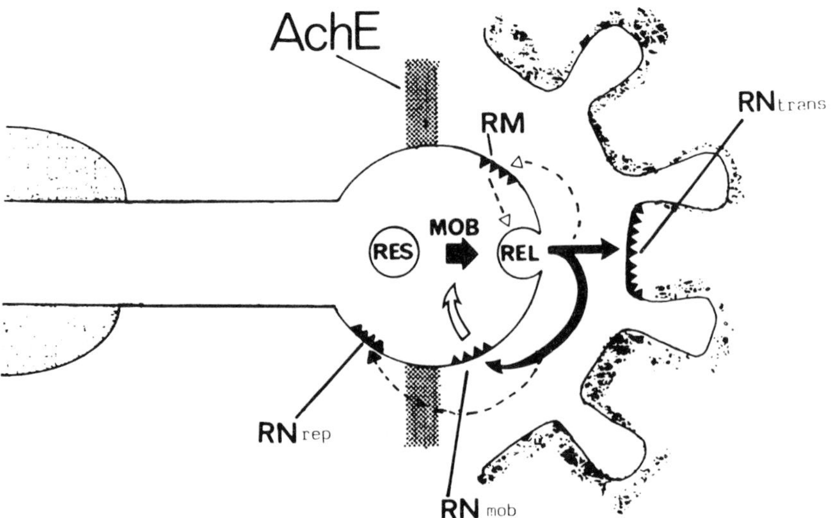

Figure 8. Vesicular acetylcholine is depicted as existing in two main stores in the nerve ending, a readily releasable store (REL) and a reserve store (RES). The former is replenished by the latter through the process of mobilization (MOB), which is postulated to be stimulated by transmitter acetylcholine acting on prejunctional nicotinic autoreceptors (RN mob). Block of these receptors produces the various fade phenomena. A separate population of prejunctional nicotinic receptors (RN rep) is postulated to mediate terminal depolarization, which can either act as a generator potential for antidromic repetitive firing or block conduction depending on the extent of the depolarization. A third group of prejunctional cholinoceptors (RM), which are muscarinic in nature, is depicted. These may mediate inhibition of transmitter release under certain circumstances. The postjunctional receptors (RN trans) are those mediating transmission.

particular receptors probably have only pharmacologic rather than physiologic relevance, being responsible for the production of repetitive firing in nerve by anticholinesterase drugs and cholinomimetics. These receptors are thought to be stimulated by the transmitter only when junctional acetylcholinesterase is inhibited. That component of the acetylcholinesterase that is known to be associated with the nerve ending (represented by AchE in Fig 8) may function to protect the RN rep receptors from being stimulated by the transmitter. Repetitive firing in the nerve has no obvious relevance to the normal physiologic transmission process, and so we regard these particular receptors as a red herring in relation to any consideration of normal neuromuscular transmission. The existence of prejunctional muscarinic receptors is also controversial, although the results of Abbs and Joseph[29] seem difficult to explain on other grounds. They propose that prejunctional muscarinic receptors are inhibitory in nature, and more recent experiments (personal communication with D. Joseph) suggest that they function only during low rates of stimulation. It is possible that blockade of these muscarinic receptors by those neuromuscular blocking drugs that possess atropine-like action (eg, gallamine) accounts for the reports that under certain circumstances (eg, low-frequency stimulation) these drugs may initially cause a small increase in acetylcholine release.

There is accumulating evidence that presynaptic autoreceptors play modulatory roles in the transmission mechanisms (both positive and negative) at many central synapses and at neuroeffector junctions in the autonomic nervous system. We propose that the neuromuscular junction is not different in this respect, and that the most important prejunctional modulation occurs via the nicotinic receptors labeled RN mob in Fig 8. It may be worth considering whether the various fade phenomena characteristic of myasthenia gravis could be the result of blockade of these prejunctional receptors by the continually circulating antibodies to the postjunctional acetylcholine receptors.

REFERENCES

1. Bowman WC, Webb SN: Acetylcholine and anticholinesterase drugs, in Cheymol J (ed): International Encyclopedia of Pharmacology and Therapeutics. Oxford, Pergamon Press, 1972, pp 427–502
2. Bowman WC, Webb SN: Tetanic fade during partial transmission failure produced by non-depolarizing neuromuscular blocking drugs in the cat. Clin Exp Pharmacol Physiol 3:545–555, 1976
3. Bowman WC: Prejunctional and postjunctional cholinoceptors at the neuromuscular junction. Anesth Analg 59:935–943, 1980
4. Bowman WC: Pharmacology of Neuromuscular Function. Bristol, England, John Wright & Son, 1980, pp 93–97
5. Bowman WC, Marshall IG: Die Rolle prä-und postsynaptischer cholinergische Rezeptoren bei der neuromuskulären Übertragung und deren Beeinflussbarkeit durch Muskelrelaxantien, in Buzello W (Hrsg): Muskelrelaxantien. Stuttgart, George Thieme, 1981, pp 34–48
6. Bowman WC, Gibb AJ, Marshall IG: Prejunctional and postjunctional effects of vecuronium, in Agoston S, Bowman WC, Miller RD, et al (eds): Clinical Experiences with Norcuron. Amsterdam, Elsevier, 1983, pp 26–32
7. Bowman WC, Harvey AL, Gibb AJ, et al: Prejunctional actions of cholinoceptor agonists and antagonists and of anticholinesterase drugs, in Kharkevich DA (ed): Handbook of Experimental Pharmacology. Berlin, Springer-Verlag (in press)
8. Lilleheil G, Naess K: A presynaptic effect of d-tubocurarine in the neuromuscular junction. Acta Physiol Scand 52:120–136, 1961
9. Hubbard JI, Wilson DF, Miyamoto M: Reduction of transmitter release by d-tubocurarine. Nature 223:531–533, 1969
10. Galindo A: The role of prejunctional effects in myoneural transmission. Anesthesiology 36:598–608, 1972
11. Blaber LC: The prejunctional actions of some non-depolarizing blocking drugs. Br J Pharmacol 47:109–116, 1973
12. Miyamoto MD: The actions of cholinergic drugs on motor nerve terminals. Pharmacol Rev 29:221–247, 1978

13. Hutter OF: Post-tetanic restoration of neuromuscular transmission blocked by d-tubocurarine. J Physiol Lond 118: 216–227, 1952
14. Otsuka M, Endo M, Nonomura Y: Presynaptic nature of neuromuscular depression. Jap J Pharmacol 12:573–584, 1962
15. Lee C, Chen D, Katz RL: Characteristics of nondepolarizing neuromuscular block I. Postjunctional block by alpha-bungarotoxin. Can Anaesth Soc J 24:212–219, 1977
16. Williams NE, Webb SN, Calvey TN: Differential effects of myoneural blocking drugs on neuromuscular transmission. Br J Anaesth 52:1111–1115
17. Glavinović MI: Presynaptic action of curare. J Physiol 290:499–506, 1979
18. Dale HH, Feldberg W, Vogt M: Release of acetylcholine at voluntary motor nerve endings. J Physiol 86:353–380, 1936
19. Katz B, Miledi R: Transmitter leakage from motor nerve endings. Proc R Soc Lond 196:59–72, 1977
20. Dreyer F: Acetylcholine receptor. Br J Anaesth 54:115–130, 1982
21. Magleby KL, Pallotta BS, Terrar DA: The effect of (+)-tubocurarine on neuromuscular transmission during repetitive stimulation in the rat, mouse and frog. J Physiol 312:97–113, 1981
22. Gibb AJ, Marshall IG: Pre- and postjunctional effects of tubocurarine and other nicotinic antagonists during repetitive stimulation in the rat. J Physiol 351:275–297, 1984
23. Jones SW, Salpeter MM: Absence of $[^{125}I]\alpha$-bungarotoxin binding to motor nerve terminals of frog, lizard and mouse muscle. J Neurosci 3:326–331, 1983
24. Gibb AJ, Marshall IG: The effects of trimetaphan on tetanic fade and on endplate ion channels at the rat neuromuscular junction. Br J Pharmacol 76:187P, 1982
25. Blaber LC: The effect of facilitatory concentrations of decamethonium on the storage and release of transmitter at the neuromuscular junction of the cat. J Pharmacol Exp Ther 175:664–672, 1970
26. Waud BE, Waud DR: Physiology and pharmacology of neuromuscular blocking agents, in Katz RL (ed): Muscle Relaxants. New York, American Elsevier, 1975, pp 1–58
27. Riker WF: Prejunctional effects of neuromuscular blocking and facilitatory drugs, in Katz RL (ed): Muscle Relaxants. New York, American Elsevier, 1975, pp 60–102
28. Hohlfeld R, Sterz R, Peper K: Prejunctional effects of anticholinesterase drugs at the endplate mediated by presynaptic acetylcholine receptors or by postsynaptic potassium efflux. Pflugers Arch 391:213–218, 1981
29. Abbs ET, Joseph DN: The effects of atropine and oxotremorine on acetylcholine release in rat phrenic nerve-diaphragm preparations. Br J Pharmacol 73:481–483, 1981
30. Liley AW: The quantal components of the mammalian endplate potential. J Physiol 133:571–587, 1956

Hassan H. Ali

4

Monitoring of Neuromuscular Function

It is generally acknowledged that the response to neuromuscular blocking drugs is unpredictable in the population at large. This is more so in several physiologic and pathologic conditions directly or indirectly involving the neuromuscular junction. Monitoring of neuromuscular function provides valuable information to the anesthesiologist. The acquisition of relevant data contributes to a more predictable and rational approach to the use of muscle relaxants, and hence to better patient care.

CLINICAL MONITORING OF NEUROMUSCULAR FUNCTION

Early attempts to assess residual neuromuscular block in humans were based on observation of clinical signs such as the ability to open the eyes, protrude the tongue, swallow, as well as hand-grip strength and head lift. Some anesthetists measured certain respiratory variables such as tidal volume, vital capacity, and inspiratory force to indicate the presence or absence of any residual weakness secondary to neuromuscular block.[1] However, measurement of voluntary movement cannot be carried out in unconscious patients, and during anesthesia, both tidal volume and inspiratory force measurements may be depressed by the central actions of analgesics and anesthetics rather than by peripherally acting neuromuscular blocking agents. The assumption that relaxants are responsible for respiratory depression at the end of anesthesia can only be ascertained when impairment of neuromuscular function is demonstrated. The only reliable method of monitoring neuromuscular func-

MUSCLE RELAXANTS
ISBN 0-8089-1784-6

tion is stimulation of an accessible peripheral motor nerve and measurement of the evoked response of the skeletal muscle innervated by that nerve. In contrast to voluntary movement, evoked responses do not require the cooperation of the patient. Furthermore, supramaximal nerve stimuli can be used to ensure full activation of all nerve and muscle fibers.

METHODS OF MEASUREMENT OF EVOKED RESPONSES

Measurement of the force of muscle contraction or electrical activity resulting from indirect stimulation of the motor nerve is primarily an index of the number of muscle fibers that have been activated. The response of the muscle to indirect supramaximal stimulation applied to the motor nerve may be measured in two ways.

Evoked Tension Measurement (Mechanomyography)

Adduction of the thumb is most commonly chosen for mechanical twitch measurement because the adductor pollicis brevis is normally the only muscle supplied by the ulnar nerve to effect thumb adduction.[2] Consequently, the human ulnar nerve-adductor pollicis approaches the precision of an experimental nerve-muscle preparation. Recording evoked plantar flexion of the big toe in response to posterior tibial nerve stimulation or dorsiflexion of the foot to peroneal nerve stimulation has also been employed.[3]

It is important to realize that the evoked tension measures the contractile responses of the whole muscle. In contrast, the evoked compound action potential provides a measure of the electrical activity only in those fibers that are near enough to the recording electrodes.[4] Appropriate conditions are required to allow a valid and reliable interpretation of tension measurement. These conditions include the capacity of the force transducer used, the initial tension of the muscle, and the direction of movement of the muscle in relation to the transducer.[5]

Evoked Electrical Activity (Electromyography)

The evoked electromyography (EMG) provides a more versatile method than evoked tension. The EMG can be measured in response to ulnar nerve stimulation from the adductor pollicis brevis (thenar EMG),[6] the abductor digiti quanti (hypothenar EMG),[6] or the first dorsal interosseous muscle of the hand.[7] Undoubtedly, employing the evoked EMG avoids problems with transducer fixation, orientation, and overload.[5] If the surface or needle electrodes are correctly placed on the motor point of the muscle studied, a number of biphasic motor unit action potentials are recorded as a single large summated compound action potential. The latter represents the activity of only a limited number of muscle fibers, and this explains some of the reported discrepancies between the evoked EMG and tension responses, since different things are being measured.[6] The potentials picked up by the electrodes are usually small in amplitude. Consequently, they must be amplified to a level that can be conveniently studied. Measuring the evoked EMG is still not widely available for routine clinical monitoring of neuromuscular function because of the cost involved in recording high-speed events.

Modern computer technology has made it possible to develop a compact, fully automated solid-state electronic storage system.[8] In this device, the EMG wave is dissected by an analog-to-digital converter and stored in an electronic memory. Read-out of the memory through digital-to-analog converter at a much slower rate allows the reconstructed wave to be recorded on a slower recorder. The EMG amplitude can subsequently be measured in a manner similar to the measurement of mechanical twitch responses.

Several computerized evoked EMG analyzers are now commercially available in addition to the already available evoked muscle tension analyzers. The former can process the raw EMG signal in response to train-of-four stimuli (T_4) that are generated from a built-in constant current stimulator utilizing surface electrodes. The computer searches for the supramaximal stimulus and establishes the control response. Further, it computes the ratio of the height of the first response of the train to the height of the control response (ie, single twitch response) and the ratio of the fourth response to the first response in the train (T_4 ratio). When the fourth response is no longer detectable (75% block), the number of the remaining responses can be displayed. Work is in progress to correlate the EMG response measured by this method with the tension response evoked in the same muscle and measured with the conventional technique.[1] Both criteria for clinical relaxation and recovery are assessed as well and correlated with data of evoked responses obtained using both methods.

PATTERN OF NERVE STIMULATION AND ITS CLINICAL RELEVANCE

As indicated earlier, the ulnar nerve is most commonly used either at the wrist or elbow to elicit evoked tension or electrical response of the adductor of the thumb. Other peripherally accessible motor nerves that can be utilized to evoke muscle activity are (1) the posterior tibial nerve behind the medial malleolus (plantar flexion of the foot), (2) the lateral popliteal nerve, lateral to the neck of the fibula (dorsiflexion of the foot), or (3) the facial nerve. The point of stimulation of the latter nerve should be localized to the area close to the tragus of the ear as the nerve emerges from the stylomastoid foramen to pass through the parotid gland and anterior to the external carotid artery. This is important to avoid direct stimulation of the closely interdigitated facial muscles (eg, the orbicularis occuli and adjoining muscles).

The evoked muscle response depends on the pattern of nerve stimulation, which may be one of the following: (1) single twitch, (2) tetanic, (3) post-tetanic single twitch, or (4) train-of-four.

Single Twitch Stimulation

Proper stimulus characteristics should be defined.[9]

Stimulus wave form. An inappropriate wave form can result in repetitive nerve firing and a tetanic-like response. Ideally, it should be a rectangular pulse.

Duration. The pulse duration should be as short as possible, around 0.2 ms. If the duration is greater than the refractory period of the nerve, a second action potential will be triggered by the falling phase of the stimulating pulse. Furthermore, excessively long pulse may directly stimulate the muscle.

Stimulus intensity. This should be supramaximal to ensure recruitment of all nerve fibers and consequent activation of all muscle fibers.

Stimulus frequency. This is important because changing the frequency of stimulation would change the effective dose of a nondepolarizing relaxant necessary to achieve a certain point on the dose-response curve.[10]

The single twitch is useful as an approach to the comparative study of neuromuscular blocking drugs. A control response is obtained, and the percentage change from control establishes the onset of action and potency of the drug. The duration of action is indicated by the time required for recovery of the evoked twitch response to control level. The 25% to 75% recovery time defines the recovery rate or recovery index. The latter can be used to compare different relaxants. Stimulus frequency of the single twitch plays a significant role in the interpretation of evoked responses. Changing the stimulus frequency, eg, from 0.1 Hz (one stimulus every 10 seconds) to 1.0 Hz (one stimulus every second) can decrease the ED_{95} for d-tubocurarine (the effective dose for 95% twitch suppression of thumb adduction) by a factor of 3 or more[10] (Fig 1). In other words, the ED_{95} of d-tubocurarine at 0.1 Hz is approximately 0.5 mg/kg compared with 0.16 mg/kg at 1.0 Hz. The onset time and the duration of action of the relaxant accordingly appear to differ when the stimulation frequency is varied. The ED_{95} of d-tubocurarine at 0.1 Hz seems to be more clinically relevant, since this level of twitch inhibition consistently corresponds with degrees of relaxation sufficient for smooth tracheal intubation and adequate surgical relaxation.

The control level of the twitch response will not be available unless

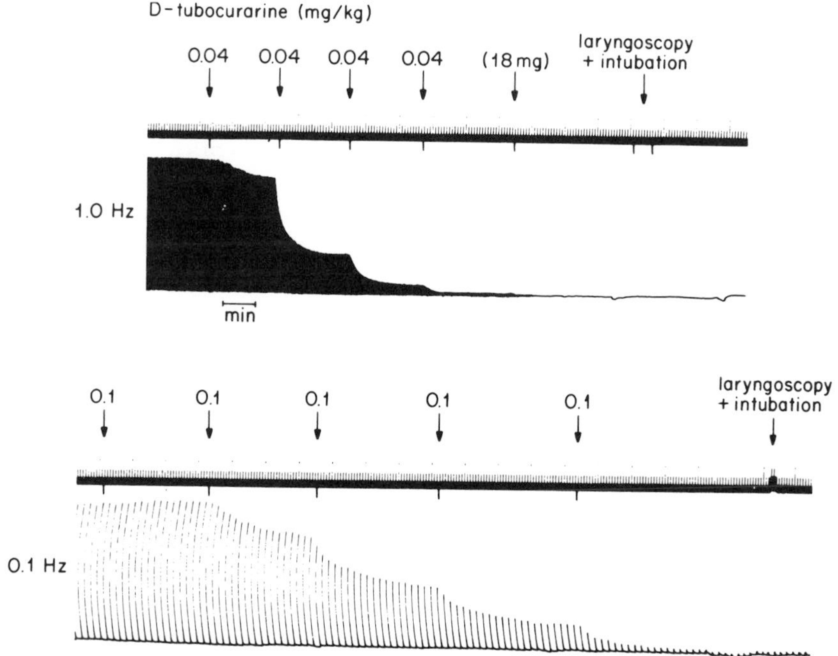

Figure 1. A d-tubocurarine incremental dose response at two stimulus frequencies. The upper panel shows evoked thumb adduction in response to ulnar nerve stimulation at a frequency of 1.0 Hz. Note that the twitch was suppressed to 95% of control after the fourth dose of 0.04 mg/kg (total: 0.16 mg/kg). Laryngoscopy was impossible at this degree of block. An extra 0.3 mg/kg (18.0 mg) was required for adequate laryngoscopy and intubation. The lower panel shows the same as above, except the frequency of stimulation was changed to 0.1 Hz. The effective dose required to achieve 95% suppression of the twitch was 0.5 mg/kg of d-tubocurarine. This level of block appeared to be adequate for laryngoscopy and intubation. Stimulating the nerve too rapidly (more often than once every 5 to 7 seconds) will give a false sense of clinically significant block.

monitoring is performed routinely and a control response is obtained. However, single twitch stimuli are helpful at anytime to decide whether postoperative apnea is peripheral or central in origin. It is also valuable in monitoring the administration of succinylcholine drip. Intermittent train-of-four stimulation is extremely helpful to detect the onset and development of phase II block.[11,12]

Tetanic Stimulation

The endplate potential is more than adequate to trigger a propagated response over a wide range of frequencies of stimulation, hence the response to tetanic stimulation is sustained at high frequencies during normal neuromuscular transmission, despite the decrement in acetylcholine (Ach) release.

When the margin of safety is decreased by disease of the myoneural junction (eg, myasthenia gravis) or the use of curare-like drugs, then the decrease in Ach output that is either induced by the nondepolarizing relaxant during high-frequency stimulation (prejunctional effect) or by repetitive nerve stimulation will be manifested as fade or nonsustained response. High-frequency tetanic stimulation of 100 or 200 Hz has been advocated to test for residual curarization by demonstration of fade.[13] It has been shown, however, that the tension developed during maximal voluntary effort is comparable to the tension evoked by a 50-Hz (50 stimuli per second) tetanus.[2] This indicates that a higher frequency is neither necessary nor physiologic. In addition, high-frequency stimulation increases the duration of the refractory period, and it is possible that part of the fade seen is secondary to decreased ability of the muscle to respond rapidly rather than to receptor blockade.[9] Moreover, fade has been observed during the use of potent inhalation anesthetics and in the absence of neuromuscular blocking drugs.[14–16] Consequently, at best it is difficult to interpret the response to tetanic stimulation. Application of tetanic stimulation at 50 Hz for 5 seconds has been suggested to detect intense nondepolarizing neuromuscular blockade in the absence of the response to a single or train-of-four nerve stimulation.[17] The posttetanic twitch appeared, on average, 36 minutes before the first response to train-of-four (T_4) during anesthesia in which pancuronium (0.1 mg/kg) was administered for tracheal intubation. There was a good correlation between the number of posttetanic twitches (posttetanic count) and the return of the first response of T_4.[17]

Posttetanic Single Twitch Stimulation

Posttetanic single twitch stimulation refers to the repeated single twitch 5 to 10 seconds after cessation of tetanic stimulation at the pretetanic single twitch frequency (Fig 2). Posttetanic potentiation (PTP) during partial curarization can be explained by increased mobilization and enhanced synthesis of acetylcholine during and after tetanic stimulation. Mechanical PTP can be demonstrated in the absence of neuromuscular block. This is in contrast to measurement of evoked EMG posttetanic response.[6,9] The mechanical posttetanic potentiation may be explained by a change in the contractile response of the muscle induced by tetanic stimulation. Since this phenomenon does not appear during evoked EMG, the presence of evoked electromyographic PTP will indicate the presence of residual nondepolarizing neuromuscular block.[6,9]

Train-of-Four Stimulation*

The ability to estimate quantitatively the degree of neuromuscular block without the need for a control response is desirable and definitely advanta-

---

**Two stimuli per second for 2 seconds.*

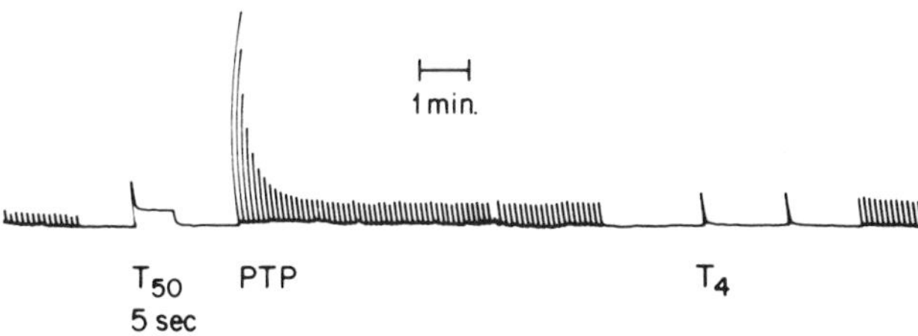

Figure 2. This figure shows (1) pretetanic single twitch response at a frequency of 0.15 Hz, (2) tetanic fade at a frequency of 50 Hz for 5 seconds, and (3) PTP of the single twitch at 0.15 Hz during partial d-tubocurarine block in a patient during N_2O-O_2-narcotic anesthesia.

geous. This seems to be accomplished by a method utilizing trains-of-four (T_4) stimuli at a frequency of 2 Hz (two stimuli per second).[18] Each train is repeated once every 10 to 12 seconds when necessary. The ratio of the amplitude of the fourth to the first evoked response in the same train appeared to provide a convenient method for assessment of neuromuscular transmission. This ratio correlates well with a simple clinical test commonly used for evaluating recovery from neuromuscular block (ie, sustained head lift). Nerve trunks contain both afferent and efferent nerve fibers, and high-frequency stimulation may evoke a powerful sensory input as well as stimulate motor fibers. Thus, T_4 stimulation causes significantly less discomfort to the conscious patient than does tetanic stimulation at 30 Hz or more. Additionally, T_4 stimulation may be as sensitive, and is often more so, than tetanic stimulation (50 Hz for 5 seconds)[19] (Figs 3 and 4). Unlike tetanic stimulation, it does not affect the subsequent pattern of recovery from neuromuscular block. In addition to its use in monitoring nondepolarizing neuromuscular block, T_4 has proven of great clinical value in detecting and following the changing pattern of succinylcholine (Sch) block (ie, from phase I to phase II block)[11,12] (Figs 5 and 6).

The train-of-four can be utilized to assess the dose of a nondepolarizing relaxant required to achieve a certain degree of block, without the need for transducing the evoked response[20] (Fig 7). Thus, the movement of thumb in response to T_4 applied to the ulnar nerve is simply observed or felt by the anesthetist. During the onset of neuromuscular block, the fourth response in the train is eliminated at approximately 75% depression of the first twitch. The third and fourth twitches are abolished at 80% suppression of the first twitch, while in addition, the second twitch becomes undetectable at about 90% block of the first twitch. Thus, for clinical purposes, merely counting the number of twitches in the T_4 response may make it possible to quantify the extent of block and the dose of nondepolarizing relaxant required to achieve a certain

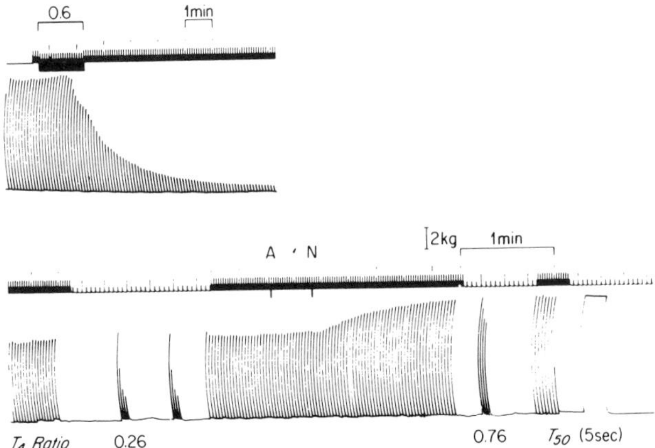

Figure 3. The upper panel shows evoked thumb adduction to ulnar nerve stimulation at 0.15 Hz before and after d-tubocurarine 0.6 mg/kg. The lower panel shows the single twitch recovered spontaneously to 75% of control height and a train-of-four (T_4) ratio of only 0.26, 150 minutes after the injection of curare. Atropine and neostigmine were administered at A and N, respectively. The single twitch recovered to control height in four minutes, and one minute later T_4 ratio increased to 0.76. At T_{50} for 5 seconds, tetanus at 50 Hz was fully sustained.

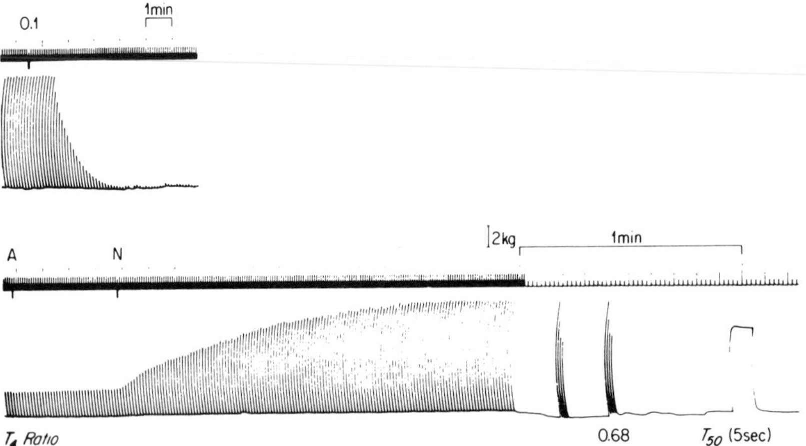

Figure 4. The upper panel is similar to that of Fig 3, showing the response to pancuronium 0.1 mg/kg. In the lower panel, single twitch recovered spontaneously to 20% of control height 90 minutes after pancuronium administration. After reversal with atropine and neostigmine at A and N, respectively, the single twitch recovered to control height in ten minutes. The T_4 ratio was 0.68 15 minutes after reversal, while tetanus at 50 Hz for 5 seconds was fully sustained.

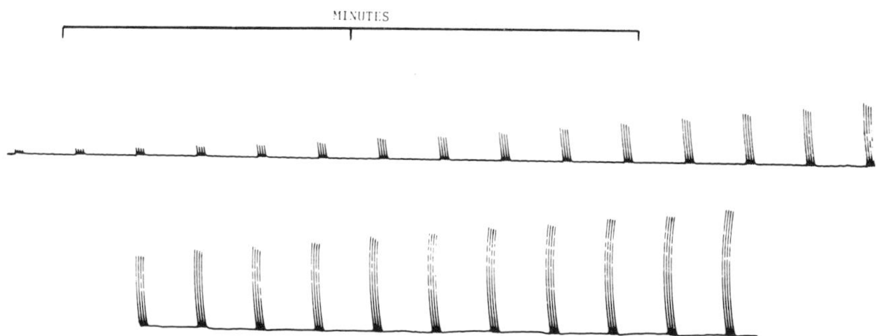

Figure 5. Both panels show spontaneous recovery of thumb adduction in response to T_4 stimulation at 2 Hz, repeated once every 10 seconds. This recovery followed the administration of succinylcholine 1.0 mg/kg, resulting in complete ablation of the twitches for eight minutes in a patient anesthetized with thiopental-N_2O-O_2-narcotic. Note that the four responses recovered equally without fade at any degree of block.

degree of muscle relaxation, ie, a clinically relevant range of neuromuscular block (75% to 95% block).

The degree of neuromuscular blockade ranging from 95% to 75% twitch inhibition (ie, 5% to 25% twitch height) is generally accepted to define satisfactory clinical relaxation. This is true for nitrous narcotic anesthesia. With potent inhalation agents (halothane, enflurane, isoflurane) which produce muscle relaxation by central mechanisms other than neuromuscular block (although they may in addition have peripheral neuromuscular effects), lesser degrees of twitch depression are needed to provide adequate clinical relaxation. At 25% twitch recovery (three detectable responses to train-of-four stimulation), a small supplemental dose of the nondepolarizing relaxant may be indicated to provide approximately 90% block (one response to T_4) if clinical relaxation is to be maintained. This may be important especially with the new relaxants atracurium and vecuronium. The incremental doses of the latter two drugs needed to suppress the twitch height from 25% to 5% are 80 and 20 μg/kg, respectively. Alternatively, continuous relaxation to approximately 90% block employing either of the two drugs and utilizing T_4 monitoring can be achieved by constant drug infusion. The rate of the latter is about 6 μg/kg/min for atracurium and 1.0 to 2.0 μg/kg/min for vecuronium.

It is important to realize that direct stimulation of the long flexor of the fingers in the forearm may cause difficulty and confusion. This can be avoided if monitoring of the evoked response is restricted to adduction of the thumb in response to T_4 ulnar nerve stimulation.[6] If the little finger or the other three fingers are observed, pure indirect responses cannot be guaranteed. A component of direct stimulation would lead to underestimation of the degree of neuromuscular block and unnecessary overdosage with nondepolarizing re-

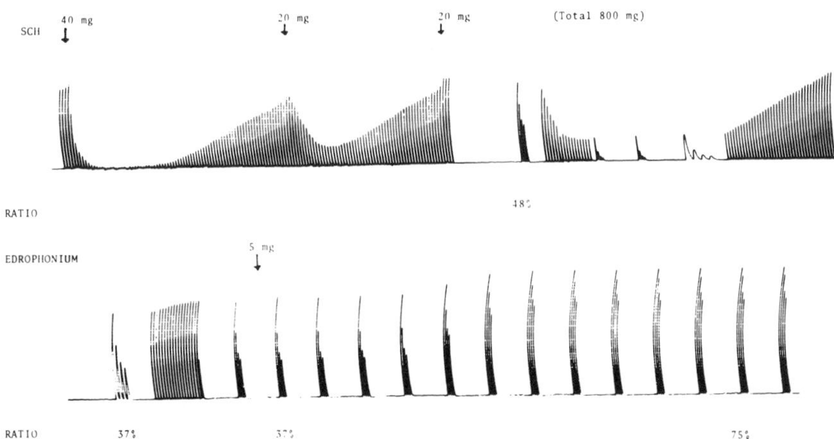

Figure 6. The tracing is from the same patient as in Fig 5, where relaxation was maintained with Sch infusion following the recovery from the initial dose. The patient received 10.0 mg/kg in two hours. In the upper panel, the response to T_4 after three increments of Sch following discontinuation of the infusion is shown. Note the development of fade, which is more manifest during the recovery from each dose (recorder speed 10 mm/min). The lower panel is a continuation of the tracing from the upper panel, showing a T_4 with a ratio of 0.37. Two minutes later, T_4 ratio persisted at 0.37 despite the continued recovery of the four responses. At the arrow, edrophonium 5.0 mg was injected intravenously resulting in progressive recovery of the T_4 responses, and the ratio increased from 0.37 to 0.75 in two minutes.

laxants. The same consideration holds true if when using the facial nerve the stimulating electrodes are applied close to the orbicularis occuli muscle, because direct stimulation of the latter is inevitable. Hence, the stimulating electrodes should be placed close to the tragus of the ear as indicated earlier.

FACTORS ALTERING NEUROMUSCULAR FUNCTION AND THE RESPONSE TO MUSCLE RELAXANTS

Knowledge of the interaction between neuromuscular blocking drugs and inhalation anesthetics, adjuvants, and preoperative medication is quite valuable. Some physiologic or pathologic conditions such as hypothermia, electrolyte imbalance, pH changes, enzymatic abnormalities (eg, atypical plasma cholinesterase), hepatic and/or renal insufficiency, and neuromuscular diseases are other examples where abnormal response to muscle relaxants can be anticipated. This emphasizes the importance of monitoring neuromuscular function. The information obtained would be extremely helpful for dosage

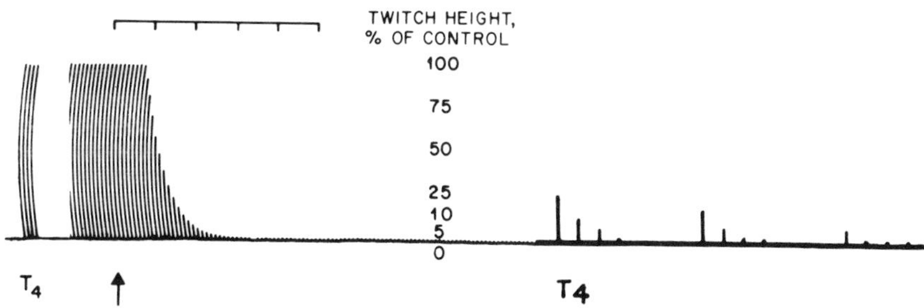

Figure 7. This figure shows the train-of-four count. (Read from left to right.) Control T_4, control single twitch response at 0.15 Hz. At the arrow, pancuronium 0.1 mg/kg was given, resulting in 99% twitch inhibition. The vertical numbers represent estimates of percent twitch height. At T_4, a diagram superimposed on the tracing demonstrates three levels of block of the first twitch of T_4: three responses = 75% block; two responses = 80% block; and one response = 90% block. See text for further details.

adjustment of relaxants and safer conduct of anesthesia. There are numerous examples of the value of monitoring neuromuscular function on one hand, and the unpredictability of the response to muscle relaxants on the other. For the purpose of space limitations, only the following two case reports will be briefly outlined.

Case 1

A 62-year-old female patient weighing 60 kg was admitted to the hospital for total abdominal hysterectomy. She had a previous history of difficulty breathing that required postoperative ventilation in another hospital several years prior to this admission. No further details could be obtained, and the possibility of abnormal response to Sch was raised. Figure 8 demonstrates a recording of evoked thumb adduction to percutaneous ulnar nerve stimulation at the wrist at a frequency of 0.15 Hz (approximately one stimulus every 7 seconds) with intermittent train-of-four stimuli. In the upper panel is the control twitch height before the administration of Sch. A test dose of Sch 0.05 mg/kg (3.0 mg) was given at the mark. This dose resulted in complete ablation of the twitch in four minutes and provided excellent conditions for endotracheal intubation. Recovery to 25% was 16 minutes. Note the response to train-of-four (T_4) showed minimal fade. At 50% twitch recovery, another increment of Sch 0.05 mg/kg resulted in disappearance of the twitch for 14 minutes (second panel). A third similar increment that was administered at 75% twitch height resulted in ablation of the twitch for another 14 minutes and additional 20 minutes for complete recovery of the twitch to control. In the lowermost panel, we see that a fourth increment of 0.05 mg/kg Sch did not completely abolish the twitch as the first increment. This required 28 minutes for com-

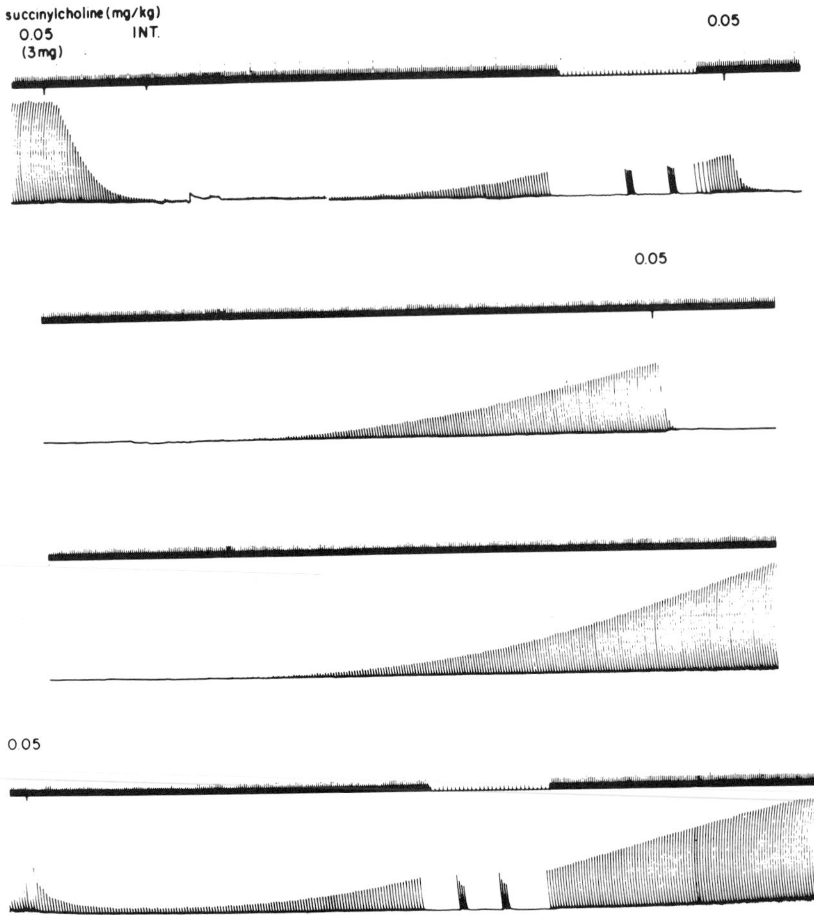

Figure 8. Sensitivity to succinylcholine in a patient homozygous for the atypical or dibucaine-resistant plasma cholinesterase enzyme under N_2O-O_2-narcotic anesthesia. See text for further details.

plete recovery at which time the patient was extubated. Note that the response to T_4 shows more fade, indicating an early development of phase II block. A total of 12.0 mg of Sch was given over two hours. Dibucaine number and esterase activity indicated that this patient is homozygous for the atypical or dibucaine-resistant enzyme. The case emphasizes the importance of monitoring the response of a test dose of Sch that may substitute for the aforementioned biochemical studies, which were once suggested to be a routine workup for patients about to receive Sch. Simple clinical monitoring is cheaper, the results are obtained faster, and lab error is less likely.

Case 2

Figure 9 shows evoked thumb adduction in response to train-of-four stimuli from a 50-year-old 50-kg female secretary who had a 20-year history of myasthenia gravis. She was given a daily dose of 360 mg of pyridostigmine and 20 mg of prednisone. The control T_4 showed slight fade. A test dose of d-tubocurarine 0.05 mg/kg (2.5 mg) produced approximately 98% depression of the first response of T_4. The 50% recovery time in this patient was approxi-

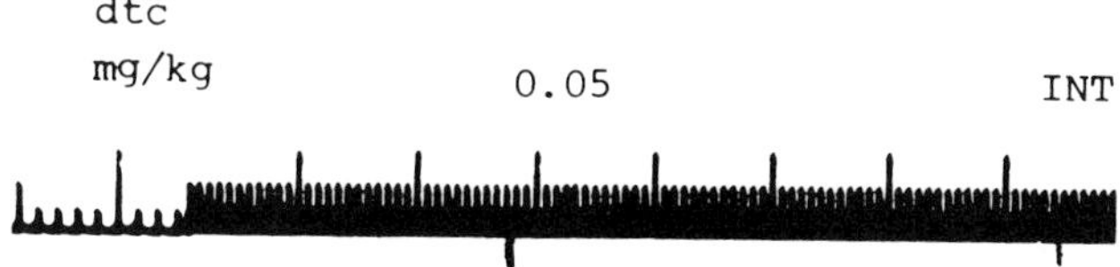

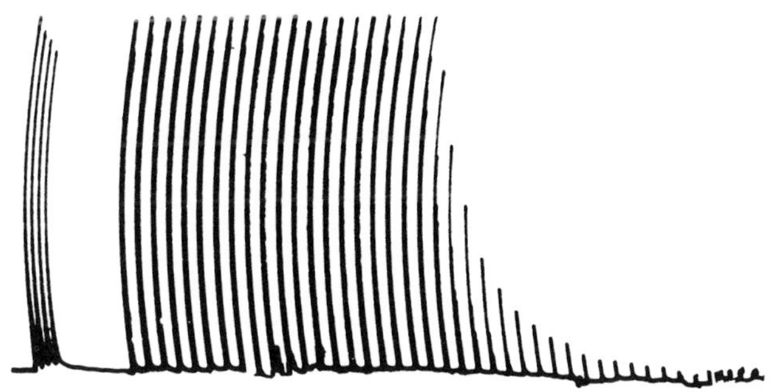

Figure 9. Evoked thumb adduction in response to train-of-four (T_4) ulnar nerve stimulation in a 50-kg myasthenic patient. Control T_4 response showing moderate fade 4th/1st = 0.85. At the mark, d-tubocurarine 0.05 mg/kg (2.5 mg) was administered under N_2O-O_2-fentanyl anesthesia. Note that the first twitch of T_4 became 98% depressed in four minutes and the patient could be easily intubated at the mark (INT). Time scale = one minute between each two high spikes. See text for further details.

mately two hours. In contrast, we had another myasthenic patient with a full-blown clinical picture and controlled with a daily dose of 900 mg of pyridostigmine and 60 mg of prednisone who required a total dose of 0.3 mg/kg of d-tubocurarine (30 mg) to achieve 95% twitch depression. The latter recovered completely in two hours during a thymectomy procedure. This patient had at this time a T_4 ratio of 75% and a fully sustained tetanus at 50 Hz for 5 seconds with excellent respiratory mechanics. We would not have predicted or known this information without monitoring neuromuscular function (unpublished data).

CORRELATION OF EVOKED RESPONSES WITH CLINICAL CRITERIA FOR ADEQUATE RECOVERY

It has been shown that after the recovery of the single twitch (at 0.15 Hz) to control height and sustained response to tetanic stimulation at 50 Hz for 5 seconds, the T_4 still shows variable degrees of fade, denoting that the latter parameter is more sensitive than either the single twitch or the tetanus at 50 Hz for 5 seconds.[19,*]

The ratio of the amplitude of the fourth to the first response of T_4 correlates well with clinical criteria employed for assessment of recovery from neuromuscular block. With a ratio above 60%, patients were able to sustain head lift for 3 seconds or more.[9] In conscious unmedicated volunteers, at a similar ratio of T_4, the changes in the measured respiratory variable (ie, tidal volume, vital capacity, inspiratory force, and peak expiratory flow rate) were negligible compared with control.[21] This is because the lowest measured values were well above the clinically acceptable limits. A ratio above 75% was found to correlate with signs of adequate clinical recovery from d-tubocurarine following awakening from N_2O-O_2-narcotic anesthesia.[22,23] These clinical signs included the ability of the patient, in response to command, to open the eyes widely, cough effectively, protrude the tongue, sustain head lift for at least 5 seconds, generate a vital capacity of at least 15 to 20 mL/kg, generate an inspiratory force of 20 to 25 cm H_2O negative pressure,[24] and exhibit sustained response to tetanic stimulation at 30 to 50 Hz for 5 seconds. Finally, after reviewing the literature and abstracts submitted to scientific meetings in the last several years, it is clear that the train-of-four has enjoyed significant popularity as a research tool for the quantitative analysis of neuromuscular blocking drugs.

**Editor's note: This point is still a controversial matter, with some experts feeling that tetanic stimulation may be more sensitive under some circumstances.*

SUMMARY

Clinical monitoring of neuromuscular function can be accomplished by either measuring the evoked mechanical or EMG response of a skeletal muscle via an accessible motor nerve. The pattern of motor nerve stimulation varies from supramaximal single repeated stimuli at a specified frequency to tetanic stimulation, posttetanic single stimuli at the pretetanic frequency, and train-of-four stimuli at 2 Hz.

The response to relaxants is unpredictable in the population at large and more so in pathologic states. This makes monitoring of the muscle response to motor nerve stimulation extremely valuable and helpful. The train-of-four technique of measurement has proved to be valuable not only as a reliable clinical tool to measure the response to relaxants and monitoring recovery, but also as a research tool for studies of old and new neuromuscular blocking drugs. Evoked responses and clinical criteria for adequate recovery from muscle relaxants should complement each other. The more criteria fulfilled, the better and safer the conclusion that the patient has recovered from clinical neuromuscular blockade.

REFERENCES

1. Ali HH, Savarese JJ: Monitoring of neuromuscular function. Anesthesiology 45:216, 1976
2. Merton PA: Voluntary strength and fatigue. J Physiol 123:553, 1954
3. Kaplan R, Ali HH: Unpublished data, 1980
4. Ali HH: Mechanomyography and electromyography, in Buzello W, (ed): Muscle Relaxation. New York, Georg Thieme Verlag Stuttgart, 1981, pp 82–88
5. Gissen AJ: Standardized technique for transmission studies. Anesthesiology 39:567, 1973 (letter)
6. Katz RL: Electromyographic and mechanical effects of suxamethyonium and tubocurarine on twitch, tetanic and post-tetanic responses. Br J Anaesth 45:849, 1973
7. Ali HH, Utting JE, Gray TC: Quantitative assessment of residual antidepolarizing block (Part I). Br J Anaesth 43:473, 1971
8. Lee C, Katz RL, Lee ASJ, et al: A new instrument for continuous recording of the evoked compound electromyogram in the clinical setting. Anesth Analg 56:260, 1977
9. Epstein RA, Epstein RM: The electromyographic and the mechanical response of indirectly stimulated muscle in anesthetized man following curarization. Anesthesiology 38:212, 1973
10. Ali HH, Savarese JJ: Stimulus frequency and the dose response to d-tubocurarine in man. Anesthesiology 52:35, 1980
11. Lee C, Katz RL: Dose relationships of phase II, tachyphylaxis and train-of-four fade in suxamethonium-induced dual neuromuscular block in man. Br J Anaesth 47:841, 1975
12. Ramsey FM, Lebowitz PW, Savarese JJ, et al: Clinical characteristics of long-term succinylcholine neuromuscular blockade during balanced anesthesia. Anesth Analg 59:110, 1980
13. Gissen AJ, Katz RL: Twitch, tetanus and post-tetanic potentiation as indices of nerve-muscle block in man. Anesthesiology 30:481, 1969
14. Cohen PJ, Heisterkamp CV, Skovsted P: The effect of general anesthesia on the response to tetanic stimulus in man. Br J Anaesth 42:543, 1970

15. Miller RD, Eger El II, Way WL, et al: Comparative neuromuscular effects of forane and halothane alone and in combination with d-tubocurarine in man. Anesthesiology 35:38, 1971
16. Stanec A, Heyduk J, Stanec D, et al: Tetanic fade and post-tetanic tension in the absence of neuromuscular block in anesthetized man. Anesth Analg 57:102, 1978
17. Viby-Mogensen J, Howardy-Hansen P, Chraemer-Jorgensen B, et al: Post-tetanic count (PTC). A new method of evaluating an intense nondepolarizing neuromuscular blockade. Anesthesiology 55:458, 1981
18. Ali HH, Utting JE, Gray TC: Stimulus frequency in the detection of neuromuscular block in humans. Br J Anaesth 42:967, 1970
19. Ali HH, Savarese JJ, Lebowitz PW, et al: Twitch, tetanus and train-of-four as indices of recovery from nondepolarizing neuromuscular blockade. Anesthesiology 54:294, 1981
20. Lee C: Train-of-four quantitation of competitive neuromuscular block. Anesth Analg 54:649, 1975
21. Ali HH, Wilson RS, Savarese JJ, et al: The effect of tubocurarine on indirectly elicited train-of-four muscle response and respiratory measurements in humans. Br J Anaesth 47:570, 1975
22. Ali HH, Kitz RJ: Evaluation of recovery from nondepolarizing neuromuscular block, using a digital neuromuscular transmission analyser: Preliminary report. Anesth Analg 52:740, 1973
23. Brand JB, Cullen DJ, Wilson NE, et al: Spontaneous recovery from non-depolarizing neuromuscular blockade: Correlation between clinical and evoked responses. Anesth Analg 56:55, 1977
24. Pontoppidan H, Geffin B, Lowenstein E: Acute Respiratory Failure in the Adult. Boston, Little, Brown, 1973, p 60

Chingmuh Lee

5

Succinylcholine: Its Past, Present, and Future

Succinylcholine is one of the most important, popular, and controversial drugs in modern anesthesia practice. At this juncture of enthusiastic anticipation of the new relaxants, atracurium and vecuronium, one finds it interesting and enlightening to review the past of succinylcholine, to examine its present, and to make projections regarding its future.

THE BEGINNING OF BASIC AND CLINICAL NEUROMUSCULAR PHARMACOLOGY

It is difficult to understand why some land plants contain neuromuscular poisons. Except for the possible bad taste, the poisons do not serve any conceivable purposes toward the survival of the plants. These poisons are harmless when ingested by animals, and the plants have no mechanisms of injecting these poisons into animals. It is even more difficult to conceive how South American Indians discovered curare compounds and how natives from Zaire discovered steroidal arrow poisons.

The discovery of America was soon followed by the excitement about the arrow poisons of the Amazonian Indians. Poets, scientists, explorers, and politicians mentioned in the early legends include such famous figures as Raleigh, von Humbolt, and Magendie, who received samples of the poisons from Napoleon III.

It was Claude Bernard whose classic experiments with the arrow poisons in the 19th century laid the foundation of modern concepts of neuromuscular junction, neuromuscular transmission, and neuromuscular pharmacology. Al-

MUSCLE RELAXANTS
ISBN 0-8089-1784-6

though Läwen first described the use of curarine on humans as an adjunct to anesthesia in 1912, his report (in German) was ignored. The report of Griffith and Johnson of Canada in 1942 was generally credited for the introduction of neuromuscular relaxants into modern anesthesia.[1] For a historical account of discoveries of peripherally acting muscle relaxants in general, see Bowman.[2]

DISCOVERY OF SUCCINYLCHOLINE

Hunt and de Taveau (1906) described succinylcholine as "similar to that of the valeryl compound" and showed that the physiologic action of valeryl-choline was to slow the heart and, more often than not, to raise BP.[3] It is said that in their study concerning primarily the cardiovascular effects of these compounds, Hunt and de Taveau did their experiments on curarized animals and missed out on the neuromuscular effects of succinylcholine. The neuromuscular effects of succinylcholine were not discovered until 1949 (Table 1).

CLINICAL DEBUT OF SUCCINYLCHOLINE

Ever since the introduction of curare into clinical anesthesia, the search for better neuromuscular relaxants never ceased. Curare opened a new page in the history of modern anesthesia. However, it did not take long for its disadvantages to be recognized. Beecher and Todd, in an authoritative report published in 1954, submitted that curare increased surgical mortality.[4] However, the conclusion of the famous Harvard study was soon modified. The apparent increase in mortality might have resulted from increased acceptance of ever sicker patients to surgery. Safe relaxation made safe light anesthesia possible, which in turn also made development of new surgical techniques possible.

Soon after the discovery of its neuromuscular effects, succinylcholine was introduced into clinical use in Europe in 1951 by Brüke et al and in the United States in 1952 by Foldes et al, then of Pittsburgh.[5] The Foldes et al

Table 1
Early History of Succinylcholine

1906	Hunt and de Taveau, cardiovascular effects in curarized cats
1949	Bovet et al, neuromuscular effect
1949	Phillips, neuromuscular effect
1951	Brüke et al, clinical use in Europe
1952	Foldes et al, clinical use in USA

Table 2
Types of Operations*

Operation	No. of Cases	Percentage
Gastric	43	21.3
Gall bladder	57	28.2
Other upper abdomen	38	18.8
Large bowel	20	9.9
Appendectomy	8	4.0
Intra-abdominal gynecologic procedure	36	17.8

*Data taken from Foldes et al.[5]

report proved to be a magnificent classic, although some of the original conclusions have since been revised. Table 2 lists the types and numbers of surgical operations described in the Foldes et al paper. An extensive variety of abdominal surgeries were performed under primarily succinylcholine-thiopental anesthesia. The anesthetic and relaxant doses are shown in Table 3. The dose ranges of succinylcholine and thiopental were great.

The single most important advantage of succinylcholine, instantaneous changes in the degree of muscular relaxation, was recognized on its debut:

> Compared to other muscle relaxants used in anesthesiology, succinylcholine possesses several advantages, the outstanding one, in our experience, being its easy controllability, which permitted almost *instantaneous changes* in the degree of muscular relaxation. With succinylcholine, both the increasing and the decreasing of muscular relaxation took *less than a minute* [italics added].[5]

This superior advantage of succinylcholine remains unchallenged to date, more than 32 years later.

Table 3
Succinylcholine Diiodide and Thiopental Doses*

	Range	Average
Duration of anesthesia	35–363 min	126 min
Initial dose of succinylcholine diiodide	10–50 mg	29.2 mg
Total dose of succinylcholine diiodide	66–1830 mg	597 mg
Dose of succinylcholine diiodide/min	1.1–9.2 mg	4.0 mg
Initial dose of thiopental sodium	250–1000 mg	560 mg
Total dose of thiopental sodium	540–3500 mg	1432 mg
Dose of pentothal sodium/min	2.3–34.8 mg	13.1 mg

*Data taken from Foldes et al.[5]

It is of interest that Foldes et al used "less than a minute" as criterion for rapid action. This criterion remains generally accepted in 1984. Other generally accepted criteria for the ideal muscle relaxant were also clearly stated in the Foldes report:

> It is generally accepted that the ideal muscle relaxant should have *specificity* and *rapid onset* of action, *readily controllable* intensity, wide *margin* between muscular relaxation and respiratory arrest and *rapid and complete recovery* after the cessation of its administration [italics added].[5]

The "wide margin" criterion was important in clinical practice until the liberal use of controlled respiration prevailed in anesthesia practice. The so-called respiratory sparing advantage of any relaxant has since been de-emphasized, and succinylcholine is no longer described as respiratory sparing.

Disadvantages of succinylcholine were not readily recognizable in the initial clinical experience. Most of the serious complications of succinylcholine were unheard of in the history of medicine and are *unique* to succinylcholine. Regarding the usual side effects common to most neuromuscular relaxants such as cardiovascular and autonomic effects, succinylcholine is indeed rather benign. At the time of its introduction, succinylcholine "approximated most closely the definition of the ideal muscle relaxant."[5] Of all the complications of succinylcholine, the unexpected prolongation of duration of action occurring in some patients was the first to be recognized. All other complications took years of clinical use to recognize. It appears as though complications occurring 1 in 1,000 took 1 year to recognize, while complications occurring 1 in 10,000 took 10 years to recognize.

DISADVANTAGES OF SUCCINYLCHOLINE CLASSIFIED BY MECHANISM OF ACTION

"If everything looks all right, you have overlooked something."

Indeed, the long and extensive list of complications of succinylcholine began to accumulate right after its clinical debut. Lee and Katz[6] in 1980 classified the numerous complications of succinylcholine by mechanism of action, a revised version of which appears in Table 4. Most, if not all, serious complications of succinylcholine result from its intended agonistic mechanism of action. The agonistic action manifests not only as depolarization of the skeletal muscle but also as direct activation of cardiac cholinergic receptors. The depolarizing mechanism of action of succinylcholine on the skeletal muscle, shared with decamethonium, is in itself new and unique. Few other drugs in popular clinical use are intended to act by a massive, simultaneous, and sustained agonistic mechanism of action. Paralysis by depolarizatin of the skeletal muscle is, so to speak, comparable to unconsciousness by depolarization of the neurons. Thus, succinylcholine produces relaxation somewhat like electricity produces coma.

PROLONGED NEUROMUSCULAR BLOCK

"Anything that can go wrong, will go wrong."

Following are brief descriptions of some of the major disadvantages of succinylcholine, presented for historical interest in roughly chronologic order of recognition. A recent review by Durant and Katz is recommended for further reading.[7]

In their first American clinical report on succinylcholine in 1952, Foldes et al already included an addendum that stated, "Since this paper was submitted for publication, several cases of prolonged repiratory depression after the use of succinylcholine have been reported." That same year, several reports related prolonged neuromuscular block to excessive doses of succinylcholine and to low plasma cholinesterase activity. Today, it is well known that prolonged neuromuscular block may result from normal subjects receiving excessive doses of succinylcholine, deficient plasma cholinesterases, inhibited cholinesterases, and atypical plasma cholinesterases. Resistance to succinylcholine due to increased activity of plasma cholinesterase is relatively rare. Table 5 lists conditions with abnormal plasma cholinesterase activity classified by cause.

Alles and Hawes were the first to show that plasma cholinesterase (pseudocholinesterase) and tissue cholinesterase (true cholinesterase, RBC cholinesterase) are different enzymes. Kalow and Lindsay in 1955 devised a method of assay of plasma cholinesterase using benzoylcholine as substrate, and Kalow and Genest in 1957 described "dibucaine number" as a method of differentiating atypical (E_1^a) from typical (E_1^u) usual plasma cholinesterases. Subsequently, other methods of detecting other atypical plasma cholinesterases have been described.

While typical plasma cholinesterase hydrolyzes succinylcholine readily, and also hydrolyzes benzoylcholine, its ability to hydrolyze benzoylcholine is inhibited by dibucaine. Atypical plasma cholinesterases hydrolyze succinylcholine poorly; E_1^a and E_1^f hydrolyze benzoylcholine, but their ability to hydrolyze benzoylcholine is resistant to inhibition by dibucaine (E_1^a) or fluoride (E_1^f); E_1^s, on the other hand, appears "silent," having little effect on succinylcholine or benzoylcholine. For a complete review on cholinesterase and succinylcholine, see monograph by Viby Mogensen.[8]

Table 4
Disadvantages of Succinylcholine (Classified by Mechanism of Action)*

Depolarization (endplate and muscle)
Fasciculation and increased abdominal pressure
Contracture
Denervated, extraocular, and jaw muscles
Potassium efflux and cardiac consequences
Muscle pain
Changing nature of block
Tachyphylaxis and slow recovery
Other agonistic actions
Tachycardia and hypertension, other dysrhythmias
Sinus bradycardia and arrest
Idiosyncratic responses
Failure to metabolize succinylcholine
Atypical plasma cholinesterase
Exaggerated multisystem reactions
Malignant hyperthermia
Muscular dystrophies
Active metabolites
Drug interactions and complicating medical conditions
Cardiac dysrhythmias
Hyperkalemia in burn, renal failure, etc
Other electrolyte imbalances
Cardiac glycosides
Contracture and cardiac dysrhythmias
Major neurologic lesions
Muscular dystrophies
Reduced metabolism of succinylcholine
Physiologic, eg, pregnancy, obesity, age extremes
Cholinesterase inhibition
Increased metabolism of succinylcholine
Increased neuromuscular sensitivity, eg, myasthenia gravis, Mg
Reduced neuromuscular sensitivity, eg, myasthenia gravis

*Data taken from Lee and Katz.[6]

PHASE II BLOCK

Historically, Jenden and colleagues[9] (1954) first described in vitro, using rabbit lumbrical muscle model exposed to a fixed concentration of decamethonium, two phases of neuromuscular block separated by an interposing period of spontaneous partial recovery. Many clinical and nonclinical observations, some controversial, have since been made on the mechanism, dose requirement, time requirement, neuromuscular response characteristics, reversibil-

Table 5
Abnormal Plasma Cholinesterase Activities Classified by Cause

I. Reduced activity on succinylcholine
   A. Diminished plasma cholinesterase
      1. Pregnancy, newborn, old age
      2. Liver disease, malignancy, burn, etc
      3. Glucocorticoids, estrogens, and contraceptive pills
   B. Inhibited plasma cholinesterase
      1. Irreversible inhibition
         Pesticides, cytotoxic compounds, echothiophate
      2. Reversible inhibition
         a. Edrophonium, neostigmine, pyridostigmine, hexafluorenium, tetrahydroaminoacrin
         b. Propanidid, pancuronium, trimethaphan, local anesthetics, aprotinine, MAO inhibitors, etc
   C. Atypical plasma cholinesterases
      1. E_1^a, ability to hydrolyze benzoylcholine resistant to inhibition by dibucaine
      2. E_1^f, resistant to inhibition by fluoride
      3. E_1^s, little hydrolysis on any substrates

II. Increased activity on succinylcholine
   A. Chronic dialysis, obesity, hyperlipemia, psychoses, etc
   B. Atypical (hyperactive) plasma cholinesterases

ity, and treatment of phase II block, as well as on its relationship to tachyphylaxis.[6,9–15] Terminology of the changing nature of succinylcholine-induced neuromuscular block is often a matter of personal choice. We feel that in the clinical setting, depolarizing, repolarizing, antidepolarizing, nondepolarizing, and desensitizing mechanisms of action of succinylcholine-induced neuromuscular block are too specific and difficult to prove. We, therefore, prefer to number the changing phases as phase I and phase II.

Given sufficient time, continuous neuromuscular depression with succinylcholine will result in phase II block. While normal subjects require a large dose of succinylcholine to develop a clear phase II block, "atypical" subjects will show signs of phase II block when they first emerge from the prolonged block following a single "usual" dose of succinylcholine. Obviously, duration rather than dose is the true determinant of development of phase II block.

Controversies in dose requirement and reversibility of phase II often arise from controversies in definitions and recognitions of phase II block. In the past, when tetanic fade and posttetanic facilitation were used as indicators of phase II block, investigators rarely concurred on how the tetanic responses were to be elicited, for how long, and how often. They also disagreed on how much fade constituted significant fade. The fact that tetanic and posttetanic responses are distorted by the stimulation itself further complicates the problem. When reversibility with cholinesterases was used as an indicator, investigators differed in their starting point of reversal, and so forth. From a historical point of view these difficulties in interpretation are quite understandable in view of the multitude of variables and factors involved in each parameter.

In 1975, Lee applied train-of-four stimulation to the study of phase II block. This method permits continuous repeated determination of fade without distorting the true picture of neuromuscular block. It also permits instantaneous correlation between magnitude of block and fade. Since fade changes not only with the nature of block but also with the magnitude of block, it is essential that train-of-four ratio always be referred to the magnitude of block at the time the ratio is determined. Recent studies have confirmed that train-of-four is suitable for diagnosis of phase II block and for prediction of its reversibility. It has replaced tetanus and posttetanic changes as the method of study of phase II block. Among all these controversies and complexities, it is interesting to note that the dose requirement for phase II block reported in the past two decades started out as greater than 10 mg/kg, diminished to the very first dose, and settled for 2 to 8 mg/kg recently.

How anesthesiologists feel about phase II block and tachyphylaxis plays an important role in determining what they use succinylcholine for and how they use it. In the past, some anesthesiologists intentionally used large doses of succinylcholine infused over long periods of time to produce prolonged relaxation to facilitate postoperative ventilatory control of their patients. In the future, clear-cut phase II block will become a curiosity, observable only when unintentionally created in patients with atypical plasma cholinesterases. Clinically, the main concern about phase II block is whether rapid spontaneous recovery will occur or, failing that, whether the residual block can rapidly be terminated. In the presence of uncertainty, anesthesiologists will simply limit their succinylcholine doses to stay clear of phase II block. Obviously, when succinylcholine begins to show tachyphylaxis, it is time to seek other methods of relaxation.

TACHYPHYLAXIS

Tachyphylaxis to succinylcholine was also once controversial regarding its dose requirement, magnitude, and position in the time course of continuous succinylcholine administration. Looking back, one realizes that if desensitization occurs, succinylcholine as an agonist loses potency by at least one definition. If repolarization occurs, or a nondepolarizing block develops in spite of continuous succinylcholine administration, one can say that succinylcholine probably loses its ability to depolarize. Furthermore, once a nondepolarizing block develops, the antidepolarizing effect is probably going to antagonize the depolarizer itself. Therefore, tachyphylaxis most likely occurs.

However, it is theoreticaly possible that during the period of observation, the developing nondepolarizing block may exactly compensate for the diminishing depolarizing block, resulting in a constant paralysis.

Generally speaking, tachyphylaxis, if observable, will probably be seen during the transition period between phase I and phase II. The reason is that the nondepolarizing block, being longer lasting, will show progressive cumulation later on and succinylcholine will appear to regain potency if administered by a constant infusion. In humans, "self-antagonism" of succinylcholine against its own nondepolarizing block was proposed as a unique mechanism of tachyphylaxis to succinylcholine.[10] Churchill-Davidson et al observed tachyphylaxis as one of the five stages of development of phase II block; depolarization, tachyphylaxis, Wedensky inhibition, "fade and potentiation," and nondepolarization.[16] The occurrence of tachyphylaxis in humans during exposure to constant infusion of succinylcholine corresponds to the original observation by Jenden et al made in vitro during continuous exposure of rabbit lumbrical muscle to a constant concentration of decamethonium.[6,8–10]

With hindsight, one can now partially explain the great variability and confusion in the magnitude of tachyphylaxis observed by various investigators in the past three decades. First of all, changing sensitivity is normally most observable with any relaxant when the magnitude of block changes around 50% block level. However, not many observations were made around this level of block. Secondly, when bolus injection of additional succinylcholine is made during phase II block, the effect of the bolus is in itself biphasic; an excitation often precedes a subsequent block. The size of the bolus dose itself might thereby alter the results observed. Thirdly, any study of tachyphylaxis must cover the changing block from the point of highest sensitivity to the point of lower sensitivity to determine the true magnitude of change. This is not always possible. Fourthly, varying the infusion rate of succinylcholine might not produce a true corresponding change in the level of block in phase II. While a sudden increase in infusion rate might not effectively increase the block, a sudden withdrawal of infusion might not result in rapid recovery either. All of these complicating factors may influence the observability, magnitude, and occurrence of tachyphylaxis. They make it difficult to attribute the results to the presumed biologic variables. Figure 1 represents a personal overview of train-of-four, tachyphylaxis, phase II block, and reversibility with edrophonium during a constant infusion of succinylcholine at a rate that initially produces an 80% to 90% block.[6,10,11]

MALIGNANT HYPERTHERMIA

Denborough and Lovell in 1960 and Denborough et al in 1962 first described a form of repeated anesthetic deaths in a family.[17] Malignant hy-

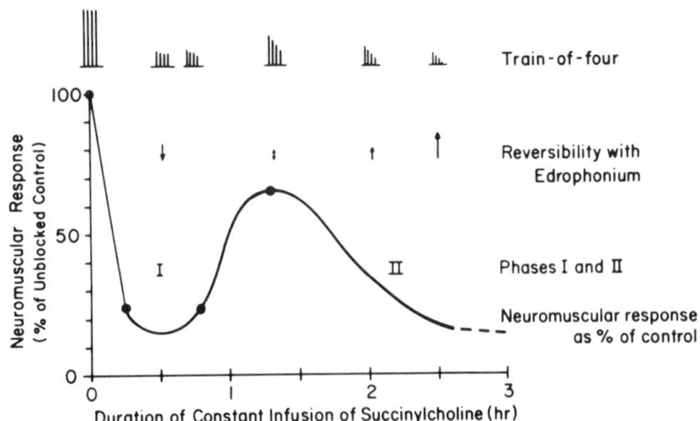

Figure 1. Semidiagrammatic overview of changing phases of neuromuscular block in humans observed during constant infusion of succinylcholine. In phase I, succinylcholine is potent, train-of-four fades little, and edrophonium increases the block. During transition, tachyphylaxis may occur. In phase II, the predominating slow-recovering residual block accumulates. It is characterized by train-of-four fade and increasing reversibility of the block with edrophonium.

perthermia has since been recognized as a highly fatal hypermetabolic syndrome. Variations of the syndrome include fulminant fatal hyperpyrexia on one extreme, and very mild nonmalignant normothermic chemical changes indicative of some abnormal muscle metabolism on the other. Succinylcholine is one of the most common precipitating factors of malignant hyperthermia and triggers some of the most characteristic attacks. Halothane and many other drugs also trigger malignant hyperthermia in genetically susceptible humans as well as in pigs, horses, and cats.

In 1937, Guedel wrote that he encountered six cases of fulminant and fatal hyperthermia under ether anesthesia in his own services in twenty years. Succinylcholine was not yet clinically available, and malignant hyperthermia was not recognized as such at that time. Coincidentally, the first malignant hyperthermia patient of Denborough and Lovell was very afraid of anesthesia because ten of his relatives had died of ether anesthesia since 1922, long before the era of halothane and succinylcholine. For a complete review, see Gronert.[18]

POTASSIUM EFFLUX

Lowenstein in 1966 and Tolmie et al in 1967 pointed out the danger of using succinylcholine in patients with burns.[19,20] Large potassium efflux with the resultant hyperkalemia was subsequently recognized as the cause of cardiac dysrhythmias and arrest in these patients. In patients with borderline hyperkalemia, even a small increase in serum concentration of potassium is significant. For a review on succinylcholine-induced hyperkalemia, see Gronert.[21]

SPASTIC RESPONSE FOLLOWING SUCCINYLCHOLINE

Eakins and Katz in 1966 described the action of succinylcholine on the tension of extraocular muscle.[22] Skeletal muscles of avians and evolutionally lower animals usually respond to depolarizing block by spasm, not flaccidity. Mammalian extraocular muscles respond similarly. The increased tension may increase the intraocular pressure; the increased pressure may in turn cause loss of eye content in the case of open injury to the eye. Samples of some porcine, feline, and equine species, and some human beings, develop malignant hyperthermia when exposed to appropriate triggering agents. When this happens, spasm is often observed following succinylcholine, especially in the jaw.

MISCELLANEOUS OBSERVATIONS

Sinus bradycardia and sinus arrest sometimes follow rapid intravenous injection of succinylcholine, especially in children when large bolus doses are repeated in three to five minutes. Resuscitation of the sinus arrest in otherwise healthy individuals is usually successful.

Patients with major central or peripheral nervous system lesions may respond to succinylcholine by spasm or by potassium efflux, or both.[23] Patients with some muscular dystrophies may respond to succinylcholine similarly. They may also suffer cardiac irregularities and arrest due to direct action of succinylcholine or indirect action of potassium efflux on the heart.

SUCCINYLCHOLINE TODAY

Succinylcholine appears to have a unique ability to weather a multitude of storms in the marketplace. It has caused not only some of the most frequent but also some of the most fatal complications encountered in modern anesthesia. As mentioned previously, many of these complications are unique to succinylcholine. However, succinylcholine has never been recalled or suspended from the market.

A simple survey revealed that in June 1983, nearly 80% of all patients undergoing general anesthesia at Harbor/UCLA Medical Center (Torrance, Calif) received succinylcholine. This figure is surprisingly high even to myself. Harbor/UCLA Medical Center has an unusually large proportion of emergent operations, including trauma and obstetric surgeries. Our usage of succinylcholine might be unusually high because of a larger number of patients undergoing ''crash'' rapid-sequence inductions. However, in spite of all the notoriety of its adverse effects and the objections of many anesthesiologists, succinylcholine no doubt continues to be widely used. Table 6 shows that approximately 2,000 kg of succinylcholine is being sold in the United States alone. Assuming a round figure of 100 mg per session, that is 20 million sessions of anesthesia per year involving succinylcholine. Admittedly, some of the drug sold may have been wasted, therefore the true figure may be lower.

Research activities with succinylcholine are also popular. A recent study revealed that succinylcholine increased the plasma levels of norepinephrine in humans.[24] Other studies confirmed the usefulness of train-of-four in the monitoring of tachyphylaxis and phase II block and in the management of continuous administration of succinylcholine in adults and in children.[13,14] Only self-antagonism of succinylcholine-induced phase II block by the phase I depolarizing effect of succinylcholine itself has not been followed-up by independent observers in humans.[10] Study on phase II block of succinylcholine in laboratory animals is difficult because of unusually large species and muscle variabilities (unpublished data of the author).

ADVANTAGES OF SUCCINYLCHOLINE

One then wonders what desirable features of succinylcholine so admirably keep it in popular demand for so many years. The only outstanding advantage of succinylcholine, in my opinion, is its short duration of action.

Table 6
Sales of Succinylcholine*

1978–79	1,763 kg
79–80	2,132 kg
80–81	2,233 kg
81–82	1,985 kg
82–83	1,909 kg

*All brands, United States.
Courtesy of IMS America, Ltd., U.S. Hospital Sales, Ambler, PA 19002.
Market data Copyright IMS America 1978–1983.

Table 7
Advantages of Succinylcholine

Short duration of action
Rapid onset
Low cost
Safety

Table 7 lists some other advantages. Foldes et al cited several other advantages.[5] However, except the short duration of action and the rapid onset, all of succinylcholine's advantages have been approximated, equaled, or surpassed by other neuromuscular relaxants in current use. Even its rapid onset of action is also partly dependent on its short duration of action. In other words, rapid onset of action of succinylcholine depends not only on its intrinsic character of rapid action but also on the practice of giving more than enough of it to quickly flood the receptor sites, so to speak. When intentionally overdosing in this manner, one counts on subsequent rapid recovery.

Will this single advantage of succinylcholine continue to keep it on the market in the future? Specifically, will atracurium and vecuronium replace succinylcholine? The answer is everybody's educated guess.

FUTURE INDICATIONS: A PERSONAL VIEW

It is often said that if succinylcholine were to be presented to the Food and Drug Administration for approval today, it would have no chance. Looking back, anything that can go wrong has gone wrong. However, hindsight is always sharper. Historically, except for the prolonged paralysis, all other major complications had taken many years to become recognized. For example, malignant hyperthermia was not recognized as a medical entity, and succinylcholine was not associated with malignant hyperthermia until nearly 10 years after its clinical use. Without succinylcholine, knowledge of malignant hyperthermia probably would accumulate more slowly. If succinylcholine were first introduced in the 1970s, a fulminant malignant hyperthermia might not have been encountered during the investigational stage, and less fulminant cases probably might have been attributed to halothane. Therefore, malignant hyperthermia might not have prevented the approval of succinylcholine even if introduced in the 1970s.

Now that succinylcholine is available and its advantages and disadvantages well known, what would be its future indications as speculated today? All neuromuscular relaxants serve the same purpose, to relax and to paralyze. They share the same concerns: safety, cost, and ease of use. All relaxants reaching the marketplace have met criteria of effectiveness and safety. They may differ in range and severity of acceptable side effects such as tachycardia

Table 8
Indications for Neuromuscular Relaxants

I. One-time relaxation	
A. Subparalyzing dose	Laryngospasm Electroconvulsive therapy Cardioversion test dose pre-treatment
B. Paralyzing dose	SEIZURE (episodic) Intubation (routine) INTUBATION (rapid) BRIEF TREATMENT, eg, setting fracture BRIEF EXAMINATION, eg, simple endoscopy
II. Sustained relaxation	
A. Short duration	EXTENDED IB SHORT surgical procedures, eg, triple endoscopy with biopsy, D & C with conization
B. 30–75 min	Various surgical operations, eg, laparoscopy
C. Long duration	Long surgical operations, status epilepticus, tetanus, intensive respiratory care

Note: Strong indications for succinylcholine are spelled out in capital letters. Competitive indications are initialed with capital letters. Weak indications are printed in lower case letters.

and hypotension, which may even be desirable under certain circumstances. Acceptance of these factors being prerequisite, the other factor, ie, ease of use, becomes the major determinant of popularity of a muscle relaxant. Easy to use means easy to produce, easy to maintain, and easy to terminate neuromuscular block. Matching the ease of use to the indications determines the distribution of use among relaxants, and thus the future of succinylcholine. Table 8 shows one method of classification of the indications of muscle relaxant in general.

The strong indications for succinylcholine probably will remain as such until a neuromuscular relaxant shorter acting and more rapidly onsetting and offsetting than atracurium and vecuronium comes into clinical use. These indications either require an onset more rapid than atracurium and vecuronium can deliver, or a duration shorter than atracurium and vecuronium can easily provide. They require profound relaxation of a short duration. EXTENDED IB (see Table 8) consists primarily of procedures that take longer than expected. For example, following a scheduled simple laryngoscopy, the surgeon decides to do a biopsy and has to wait a few minutes for the instrument. Under this circumstance, it is logical to continue with succinylcholine if it has been working well.

Competitive indications are where succinylcholine may compete with other relaxants. While other relaxants may serve the purpose adequately, they usually require more precise and therefore more difficult dose determination to provide a short but profound relaxation. Where precise control of duration and profound relaxation are not important, atracurium or vecuronium may be preferred. One example is laryngospasm during nonemergent induction for a two-hour surgery. Another example is a 75-minute surgery where relaxation is not important in the last 30 minutes, such as cesarean sections where succinylcholine is suitable for rapid intubation and either succinylcholine or atracurium is suitable for maintenance. After the baby is delivered and the uterus put back into the abdomen, relaxants may not be needed any longer.

Pretreatment for amelioration of fasciculation by small "self-taming" dose of succinylcholine and maintenance of relaxation after induction for long surgical procedures are examples of weak indications for succinylcholine. R.L. Katz has long criticized the conversion of an excellent short-acting relaxant into a poor provider of long relaxation (personal communication). The author feels that reversibility of phase II block may be at most a saving grace at times and that it definitely is not to be used casually as an excuse for prolonged use of succinylcholine.

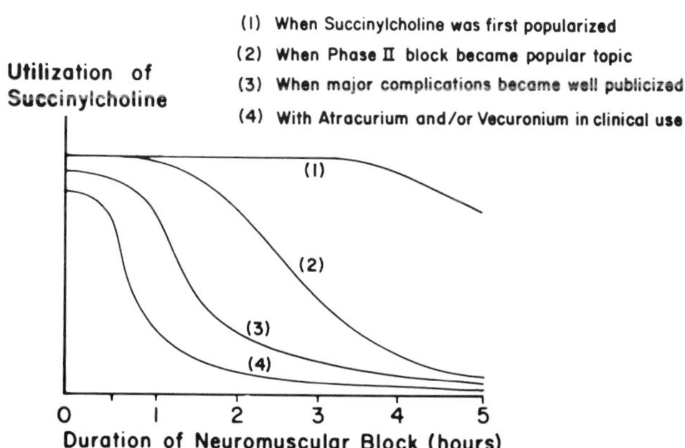

Figure 2. Diagrammatic illustration of the past, present, and projected future utilization of succinylcholine in roughly chronologic order. Curves 1, 2, 3, and 4 are shown on relative x-y scales, the present being between curves 3 and 4. Time zero means single-dose administration of succinylcholine. When the ideal short-acting and rapid-onsetting relaxant is available, curve 4 will shrink to zero in both dimensions (Lee, personal view).

CONCLUSION

So, is it time for "so long, Sux!"?

I would answer, "not yet." A drug capable of generating so many controversies, surviving so many crises, so uniquely short acting and rapid in onset, and inexpensive will not just die. Atracurium and vecuronium are not short-acting enough and rapid enough in onset to totally replace succinylcholine. They compete not only with succinylcholine but also with other relaxants. Succinylcholine may not even drastically fade away. With no new major crisis in sight, the worst with succinylcholine appears to be over. It will settle for less, but it will survive quite well until a clinically acceptable new nondepolarizing neuromuscular blocking drug of comparable duration of action and rapidity of onset takes over its role in clinical anesthesia practice (Fig 2). This "ideal" relaxant[25] will then replace succinylcholine, which in 1952 "approximated most closely the definition of the ideal muscle relaxant."[5] The once popular slogan, "So long, Sux!" has proven at least 5 years premature.

REFERENCES

1. Griffith HR, Johnson GE: The use of curare in general anesthesia. Anesthesiology 3:418–420, 1942
2. Bowman WC: Peripherally acting muscle relaxants, in Parnham MJ, Bruinvels J (eds): Discoveries in Pharmacology, vol 1: Psycho- and Neuro-pharmacology. Amsterdam, New York, Oxford, Elsevier Science Publishers BV, 1983, p 106
3. Hunt R, de M Taveau R: On the physiological action of certain cholin derivatives and new methods for detecting cholin. Br Med J 2:1788–1791, 1906
4. Beecher HK, Todd DP: A Study of the Deaths Associated With Anesthesia and Surgery. Springfield, Ill, Charles C Thomas, 1954
5. Foldes FF, McNall PG, Borrego-Hinojosa JM: Succinylcholine: A new approach to muscular relaxation in anesthesiology. N Engl J Med 247:596–600, 1952
6. Lee C, Katz R: Neuromuscular pharmacology, a clinical update and commentary. Br J Anaesth 52:173–188, 1980
7. Durant NN, Katz RL: Suxamethonium. Br J Anaesth 54:195–208, 1982
8. Viby Mogensen J: Cholinesterase and Succinylcholine. A monograph of 30 pages, Laegeforeningens forlag, 1982
9. Jenden DJ, Kamijo K, Taylor DB: The action of decamethonium on the isolated rabbit lumbrical muscle. J Pharmacol Exp Ther 103:229–240, 1954
10. Lee C: Self-antagonism: A possible mechanism of tachyphylaxis in suxamethonium-induced neuromuscular block in man. Br J Anaesth 48:1097–1102, 1976
11. Ramsey FM, Lebowitz PW, Savarese JJ, et al: Clinical characteristics of long-term succinylcholine neuromuscular blockade during balanced anesthesia. Anesth Analg 59:110–116, 1980
12. Lee C: Succinylcholine neuromuscular block reexamined (reply by Ramsey FM, Lebowitz PW, Savarese JJ, et al). Anesth Analg 59:663–634, 1980
13. Donati F, Bevan DR: Long-term succinylcholine infusion during isoflurane anesthesia. Anesthesiology 58:6–10, 1983

14. Goudsouzian NG, Liu LMP: The neuromuscular response of infants to a continuous infusion of succinylcholine. Anesthesiology 60:97–101, 1984
15. Cook DR, Fischer CG: Characteristics of succinylcholine neuromuscular blockade in neonates. Anesth Analg 57:63–66, 1978
16. Churchill-Davidson HC, Christie TH, Wise RP: Dual neuromuscular block in man. Anesthesiology 21:144–149, 1960
17. Denborough MA, Forster JFA, Maplestone PA, et al: Anesthetic deaths in a family. Br J Anaesth 34:395–396, 1962
18. Gronert GA: Malignant hyperthermia. Anesthesiology 53:395–425, 1980
19. Lowenstein E: Succinylcholine administration in the burned patient. Anesthesiology 27:494–496, 1966
20. Tolmie JD, Joyce TH, Mitchell GD: Succinylcholine danger in the burned patient. Anesthesiology 28:467–470, 1967
21. Gronert GA: Pathophysiology of hyperkalemia induced by succinylcholine. Anesthesiology 43:89–99, 1975
22. Eakins KE, Katz RL: The action of succinylcholine on the tension of extraocular muscle. Br J Pharmacol 26:205–211, 1966
23. Tobey RE: Paraplegia, succinylcholine and cardiac arrest. Anesthesiology 32:359–364, 1970
24. Nigrovic V, McCullough LS, Wajskol A, et al: Succinylcholine-induced increases in plasma catecholamine levels in humans. Anesth Analg 62:627–632, 1983
25. Savarese JJ, Kitz RJ: Does clinical anesthesia need new neuromuscular blocking agents? Anesthesiology 42:236–239, 1975

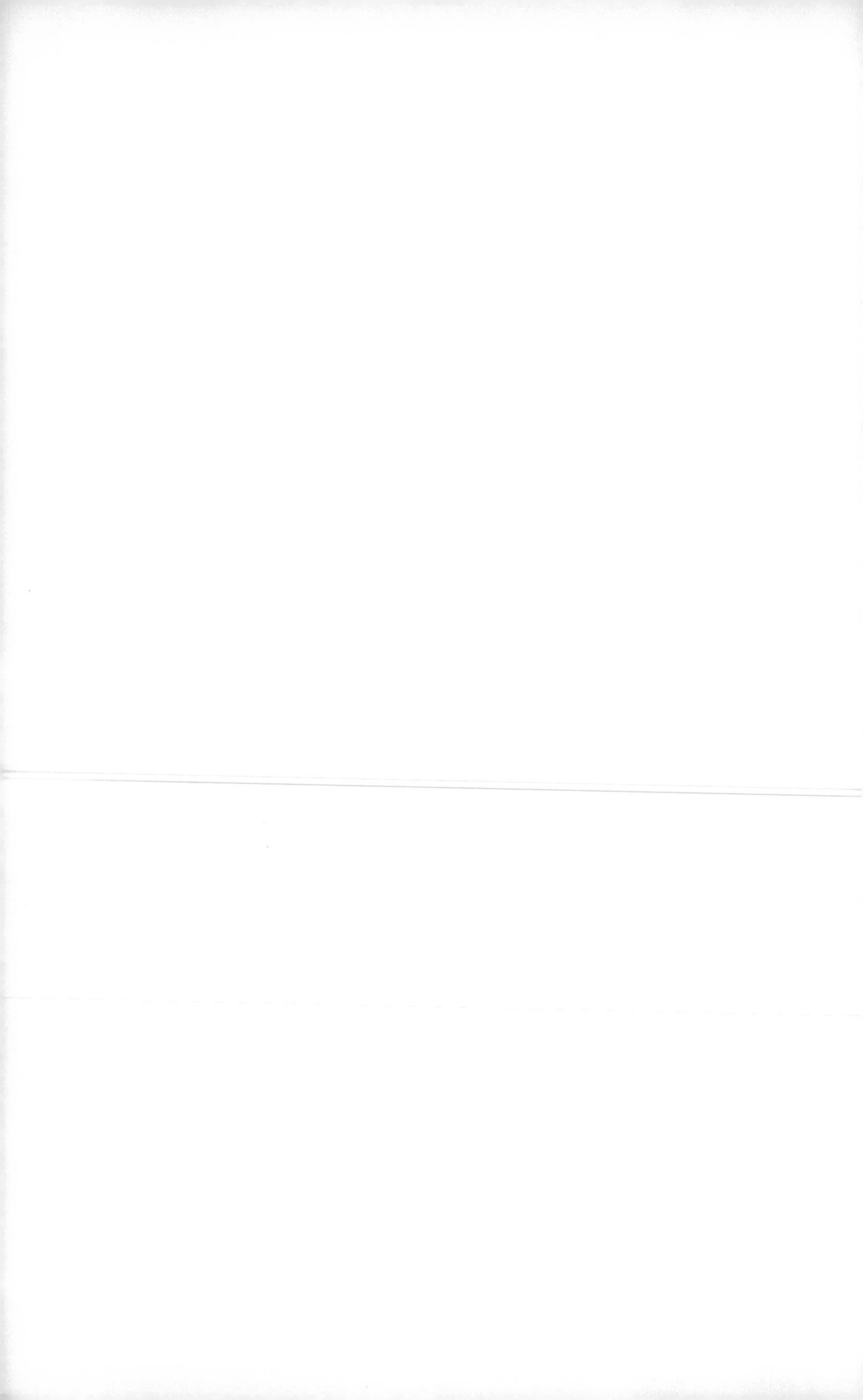

James P. Payne

6

Atracurium

Apart from the discovery of general anesthesia itself in 1846, the introduction of curare into clinical practice nearly 100 years later by Griffith and Johnson[1] in 1942 has probably had a greater impact on the development of surgery than any other single factor. Before 1846, major surgery was a ghastly and horrific business that almost certainly had a brutalizing effect on those who practiced it. In nearly every case it involved a degree of mutilation, and even for minor surgery the risks were not negligible. It is sometimes forgotten that the fundamental difference between the wound caused by the surgeon's scalpel and that inflicted by the mobster's knife is essentially one of motive. Without the protection of anesthesia, the end result could be the same, and certainly the anesthetist's ability to shield the patient from the effects of injury made surgery more acceptable to the population at large.

Initially that protection was limited to the elimination of pain and to keeping the patient unconscious and motionless. However, as surgeons became more venturesome and began to explore the various body cavities, the need developed for a better understanding of the physiologic responses involved; the matter was further complicated by the introduction of other drugs for specific purposes in the management of anesthesia. As a result the anesthetist has gradually became established as the clinical pharmacologist in the surgical team and as such his or her duties have been extended to encompass other responsibilities including the provision of easier operating conditions for the surgeon. The range and complexity of modern surgery is such that the anesthetist is expected not only to render the patient unconscious but also to paralyze muscles and if necessary to take control of respiration. In addition, the replacement of body fluids and the restoration of blood loss fall within the

MUSCLE RELAXANTS
ISBN 0-8089-1784-6

anesthetist's ambit, and he or she may also be asked to induce hypotension, lower the body temperature, and even arrest the heart in order to provide better operating conditions for the surgeon and safer operating conditions for the patient. There can be little doubt that this new era in surgery was made possible by the advent of curare, which provided the impetus to enable a new generation of anesthetists to develop a more scientific approach to their specialty.

Despite the advantages of curare, its properties are far from ideal, and its relatively nonspecific actions made its use hazardous in some circumstances. It is not surprising, therefore, that chemists, pharmacologists, and anesthetists soon began a search for a more specific substitute with all the advantages of curare and none of its drawbacks. With the reintroduction of the depolarizing drug suxamethonium in 1951 (it had first been described in 1906 but its neuromuscular blocking properties were missed because it was tested in curarized cats!) some measure of success was achieved. But the new drug brought its own problems because of its mode of action, and over the years a succession of compounds has been introduced but none completely satisfactorily. In particular, the competitive blocking agents all had an onset of block that was significantly slower than that seen with suxamethonium, and certain other deficiencies became apparent in clinical practice. Among other factors, they lacked the degree of specificity needed for an ideal blocking agent and their metabolism was unduly influenced by the presence of certain pathologic disturbances. Nevertheless, the experience gained with these compounds led to a greater understanding of their mode of action at the neuromuscular junction so that the possibility of designing and synthesizing a specific compound tailored to meet the needs of the clinician became more realistic. In 1983 Stenlake and colleagues[2] described their approach to this problem. In an unrelated study it had been shown that a plant derivative vaguely related to curare was able to undergo an unexpectedly facile degradation in mild alkali by a process well known to chemists, the Hofmann elimination pathway. This observation alerted Stenlake and associates to the possibility of designing a new class of short-acting neuromuscular blocking drugs that could be destroyed in vivo by a purely chemical pathway activated by the mild alkaline conditions that pertain at physiologic pH.

THE DEVELOPMENT OF ATRACURIUM

The chemical degradation of quaternary ammonium salts by the Hofmann elimination pathway usually takes place in the presence of strong alkali at the boiling point of water. The elimination is bimolecular and requires the removal of one of the β hydrogens and the rupture of the αC–N bond as shown in Fig 1. Such a reaction is promoted by electron withdrawal as a result of the

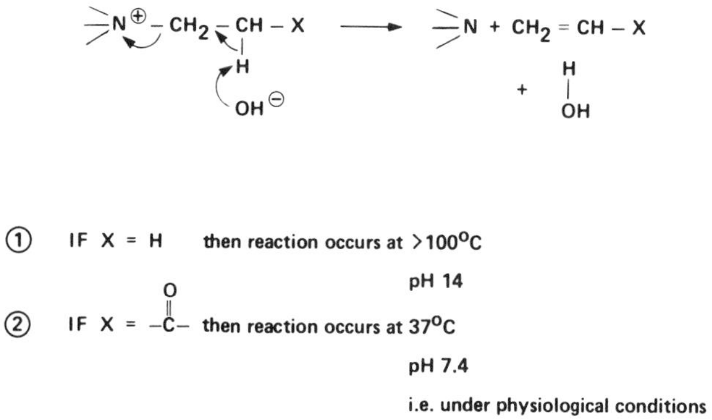

$$>\overset{\oplus}{N}-CH_2-\underset{\underset{OH^{\ominus}}{H}}{CH}-X \longrightarrow >N + CH_2=CH-X + H-OH$$

① IF X = H then reaction occurs at >100°C
pH 14

② IF X = $-\overset{O}{\overset{\|}{C}}-$ then reaction occurs at 37°C
pH 7.4
i.e. under physiological conditions

Figure 1. Conditions required for Hofmann elimination. (Reprinted with permission from Stenlake, Advances in Pharmacology and Therapeutics, 1979, Pergamon Press, Ltd.[7])

positive charge on the quaternary nitrogen. Its course and rate are dependent on steric and electron factors, and the occupation of the β carbon by electron-attracting substituents further weakens the βC–H bonds. Under these circumstances elimination occurs at a pH and temperature within the normal physiologic range.

Based on this concept, Stenlake and his colleagues had as their objective the synthesis of a bisquaternary compound with the necessary structural features to provide a competitive blocking drug with a highly specific action on the neuromuscular junction. Their task was not easy. What was needed was a compound incorporating appropriate electron-attracting β substituents to allow biodegradation to inactive compounds at normal pH and temperature in the body while at the same time providing sufficient stability at lower pH and temperature to favor manufacture and storage on a commercial basis.

Various series of compounds were made and tested. Ultimately, atracurium, which is destroyed in vivo by a unique combination of Hofmann elimination and ester hydrolysis, was selected (Fig 2) for further study, and its pharmacologic properties were investigated in detail in the laboratory. These investigations by Hughes and Chapple[3] established that atracurium was a potent competitive neuromuscular blocking agent in a wide range of experimental animals. It was significantly more potent in dogs than in cats and rhesus monkeys, although the time course of neuromuscular blockade was similar in all three species. Paralysis was easily reversed by anticholinesterase drugs and enhanced by inhalation agents such as halothane. Vagal blockade only occurred with doses substantially higher than those required for full neuromuscular paralysis, and sympathetic effects were minimal. Accordingly, the drug was selected for further study in humans and it was first used clinically in January 1979.

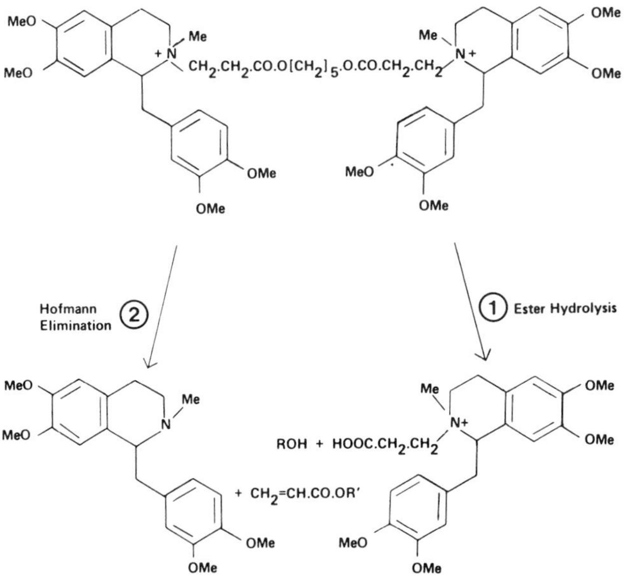

Figure 2. Chemical structure of atracurium. The arrows indicate the likely metabolic pathways. (Reproduced with permission from Hughes and Chapple.[3])

CLINICAL PHARMACOLOGY

The initial quantitative evaluation of the neuromuscular blocking properties of atracurium was carried out on 28 patients about to undergo elective urologic surgery and from whom informed consent had been obtained.[4,5] No premedication was given and anesthesia was induced with 5% thiopentone 400 to 600 mg given intravenously (IV) followed by 60% to 66% nitrous oxide in oxygen for maintenance, supplemented as required by thiopentone and fentanyl IV. Simultaneous recordings of the tetanic and single twitch contractions of the adductor pollicis muscles were obtained by supramaximal stimulation of each ulnar nerve at the wrist every 12 seconds, one with tetanic bursts of 50 Hz for 1 second and the other with single shocks. A polyethylene cannula was inserted percutaneously into the radial artery to allow the collection of serial blood samples and the continuous recording of BP. The ECG was recorded throughout and the heart rate was derived from the recording at regular intervals. In some patients the central venous pressure was recorded from a catheter inserted through the left brachial vein until its tip lay in the region of the right atrium.

In the first ten patients the IV injection of atracurium was limited to 0.2 mg kg^{-1}. At that dose the tetanic response was depressed to a level barely perceptible; the twitch response, however, was more resistant and the twitch height remained at approximately 25% of control. When the dose was raised to 0.3 mg kg^{-1}, the tetanic response was obliterated and the twitch was only just present. With doses in excess of 0.3 mg kg^{-1}, blockade of both the tetanic and single twitch responses was complete and the earlier differences in sensitivity ceased to be important. However, whereas the onset of maximum block of both responses was shortened as the dose of atracurium was increased through the range from 0.2 to 0.6 mg kg^{-1}, the onset of maximum block of the tetanic response was always faster than that of the single twitch and continued to be so over the total dose range. Once the dose was increased above 0.6 mg kg^{-1} there was no further shortening of either response. On the question of duration of maximum block of these responses, both tetanic block and twitch block were directly related to the dose of drug used, but particularly in the lower dose range, block of the single twitch was significantly shorter than that of the tetanus. This difference became less apparent as the dose was increased. During recovery the two components of the tetanic response, the peak height of the contraction and the sustained contraction, were restored at different rates. Initially the tetanic response was essentially that of a single twitch, but shortly thereafter the fade began to disappear and latterly the peak height contraction was overtaken by the sustained response into which the peak height became fused. With a dose of 0.2 mg kg^{-1} the block was of medium duration, but it was rapidly antagonized with neostigmine 2.5 mg given IV, repeated if necessary.

At these dose levels of atracurium the cardiovascular variables remained unchanged, and when the dose was increased to 0.6 mg kg^{-1} in eight additional patients the resulting transient fall in BP and the equally transient increase in heart rate remained insignificant. No changes were seen either in the ECG or in central venous pressure.

In the next six patients who received an initial dose of 0.3 mg kg^{-1}, three were subsequently given three to six incremental doses of 0.05 mg kg^{-1} when recovery of the single twitch had reached 50% of the control response. In the remaining three patients the incremental doses were raised to 0.1 mg kg^{-1} and they were given when recovery of the peak tetanic contraction had reached 50% of the control contraction. In all instances a consistent pattern emerged in terms of the degree of block achieved and the time taken to reach 50% recovery. In each patient the magnitude of the block and the rate of recovery were consistent and dose related. Such a uniform recovery pattern implies a lack of cumulative effects certainly within the dose range studied.

When the recovery of the peak tetanic contraction after a dose of atracurium just sufficient to produce complete paralysis was compared with the recovery after similar doses of more established neuromuscular blocking agents, it was clear that the recovery after atracurium was significantly faster (Fig 3). The relationships were expressed quantitatively by calculating the rate

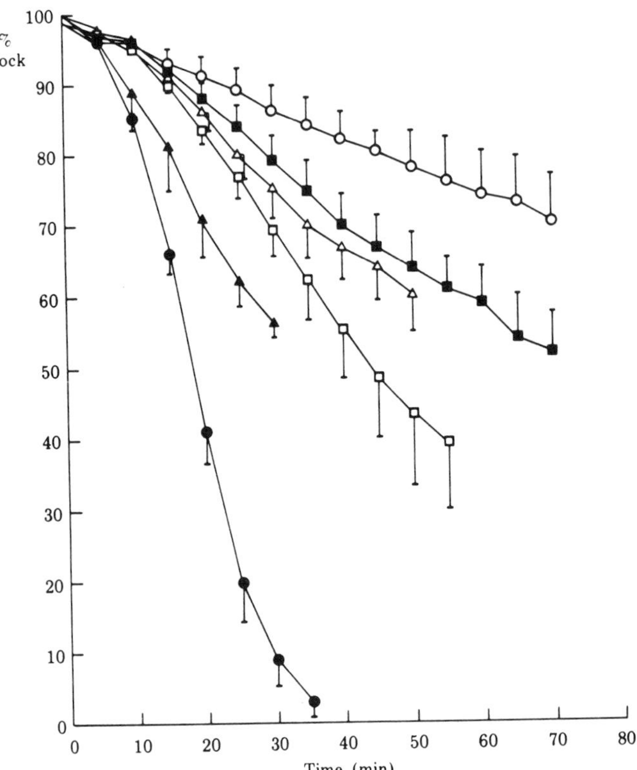

Figure 3. Recovery of the peak tetanic contraction of the adductor pollicis muscle after neuromuscular paralysis by IV doses of the following: (○) dimethyl tubocurarine 0.1 to 0.3 mg kg^{-1} (n = 6); (■) tubocurarine 0.2 to 0.5 mg kg^{-1} (n = 6); (△) panucronium 0.05 to 0.06 mg kg^{-1} (n = 5); (□) fazadinium 0.4 to 0.8 mg kg^{-1} (n = 6); (▲) gallamine 1.0 to 1.5 mg kg^{-1} (n = 3); (●) atracurium 0.2 mg kg^{-1} (n = 5). Each point represents the mean value in a number of patients (n) and vertical lines indicate SEM. (Reproduced with permission from Payne and Hughes.[5])

constants for recovery of the sustained tetanus after each drug (Fig 4), and again it was clear that the recovery process after atracurium was faster than after the other drugs in terms of this response. In this context it is known that competitive blocking drugs, in addition to their action at the motor endplate, also act presynaptically to depress the output of acetylcholine. It is suggested that the failure to sustain a tetanus during block reflects this reduced output, and the fact that different neuromuscular blocking drugs have different recovery profiles implies that such effects are not uniform.

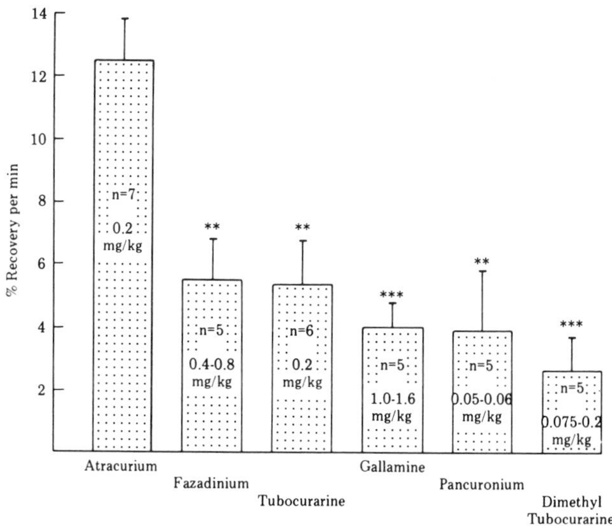

Figure 4. Rate constants for recovery of the sustained tetanus of the adductor pollicis muscle from neuromuscular blockade by atracurium. (Reproduced with permission from Payne and Hughes.[5])

A further observation was that the effect on the tetanic but not on the twitch response of a given dose of atracurium was enhanced in the presence of halothane, and presumably other volatile anesthetics behave likewise. Although this aspect has not been fully explored, from existing evidence it can be inferred that when the tetanic block is enhanced its recovery time is correspondingly slowed. However, it is also true that once the recovery process has begun, the recovery rate after atracurium proved to be independent of the dose given. It remains to be determined whether this is a unique feature of atracurium block and if it can be modified by volatile anesthetics.

The absence of any observed effect on the single twitch reflects the relative insensitivity of this response and merely reinforces the argument that when neuromuscular blocking drugs are under investigation examination of the pattern of the tetanic response is more informative than the scanning of twitch effects.

Evidence of histamine release has occasionally been reported in anesthetised patients, and it has been argued that the drug should be avoided in patients with a history of allergic diathesis. However, scrutiny of available records suggests that the risk is slight, if not negligible, and most anesthetists probably do not regard the possibility of histamine release as a problem.

Reference has already been made to atracurium's unique form of breakdown in the body and, particularly, to the formation of laudanosine. Some clinicians have expressed concern that this tertiary amine might penetrate the brain and give rise to certain undesirable effects. That possibility is extremely remote. There is good chemical evidence that very little laudanosine is formed in vivo and what is formed has no detectable clinical effect, presumably because of the very rapid excretion of metabolites of atracurium in the bile. Moreover, no pathologic evidence of damage to the CNS has ever been detected at autopsy in experimental animals, even after many days of repeated overdosage with atracurium.

PHARMACOKINETICS AND PHARMACODYNAMICS

Clinicians are notoriously reluctant to become involved with attempts to determine the pharmacokinetic and pharmacodynamic patterns of the drugs they use. This is unfortunate because the information is essential for a proper understanding of drug effects, and the anesthetist is better placed than most to make such studies. Most clinicians merely prescribe drugs and may not see the patient again for days and even weeks thereafter. The anesthetist prescribes drugs, some of which are extremely potent and potentially lethal, administers them personally, and remains with the patient until their effects have worn off. But the brainwashing has been effective insofar as our colleagues have tended to accept that such complex phenomena are subjects only for specialist consideration. If it were remembered that pharmacokinetics merely describes what the body does to drugs and that pharmacodynamics depicts what the drugs do to the body, the matter might be seen in better perspective.

On the basis of these definitions, the relationship between the kinetic behavior of atracurium and its dynamic responses has been investigated in a series of relatively simple studies in patients. Preliminary experiments in cats established a consistent pattern in the dose-response relationships as assessed by the depression of the single twitch response when plotted against the plasma concentration of the drug. Accordingly, the study was extended to humans. Three different methods of dosage were employed in order to assess accurately the degree of block obtained. This involved the use of single bolus injections, continuous infusions, and a divided dose technique similar to that commonly used in animal studies. The studies were carried out as previously described on patients about to undergo elective surgery and from whom informed consent had been obtained. A standard pattern of anesthesia was adopted, and once intubation had been achieved, simultaneous recordings of the tetanic and single twitch contractions of the adductor pollicis muscles were obtained.

In the case of the bolus injections, which were varied over a threefold range from 0.3 to 0.9 mg kg^{-1}, blood samples were taken at regular intervals during the activity of the drug and plasma concentrations were determined by a high-precision liquid chromatography (HPLC) method. The corresponding heights of the tetanic and single twitch responses were measured and the results were plotted against the plasma concentrations. In order to display the results compactly, it proved convenient to normalize the plasma concentrations to the equivalent of a dose of 1 mg kg^{-1}. In the case of the IV infusions a similar pattern was followed, and again the data were normalized to give plasma concentrations equivalent to those obtained from an infusion of 0.01 mg kg^{-1} min^{-1}.[6] The infusions themselves were given for either 30- or 60-minute periods (Fig 5)[8]. The divided dose technique was employed to establish a dose-response relationship in individual patients. For this purpose a relatively small dose of atracurium 0.05 mg kg^{-1} was given at three-minute intervals until approximately a 95% block of the single twitch response had been obtained.

What immediately became apparent in these studies was that a bolus dose of 0.1 mg kg^{-1} equivalent to a plasma level of 1 μg mL^{-1} was sufficient to produce a 95% block of the tetanic response. The twitch response was more resistant; with that dose the block was rarely greater than 50% and in some patients did not exceed 25%.

The quantitative results obtained from the patients given atracurium by infusion and preceded by a bolus injection demonstrated that the total dose required to obtain paralysis over 30 minutes was of the order of 0.004 mg kg^{-1} min^{-1}, which corresponds to a plasma level of approximately 0.6 μg mL.$^{-1}$ When the infusion was extended to one hour, the dose required to maintain tetanic block was increased to 0.006 mg kg^{-1} min^{-1}. At the end of 60 minutes the corresponding plasma level was about 0.9 μg mL^{-1}. When the plasma concentrations of atracurium were examined, it became obvious that when infusions were used, approximately 40 minutes were needed to reach a plateau (Fig 6) and that the effect obtained was directly related to the rate and

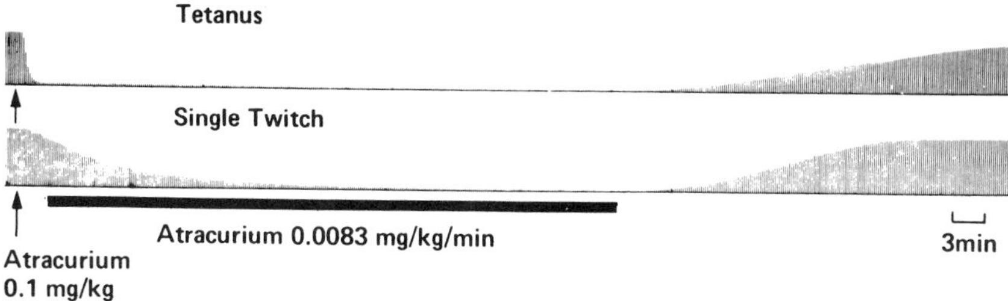

Figure 5. Recording of the tetanic and single twitch responses of the adductor pollicis muscles from a patient who received an initial bolus dose of atracurium 0.1 mg kg^{-1} followed by an infusion at a rate of 0.0083 mg kg^{-1} min^{-1} for 60 minutes. (Reproduced with permission from Hughes and Payne.[8])

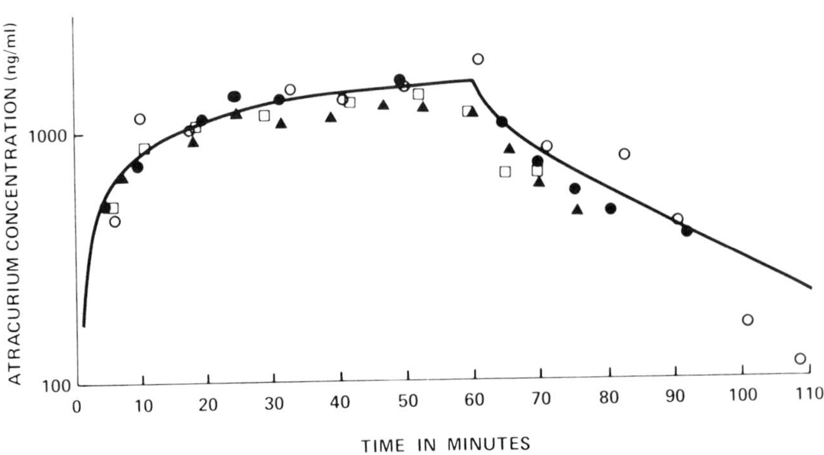

Figure 6. Logarithmic plot of atracurium plasma concentrations against time for four patients receiving infusions for one hour. Dose rates and symbols are 0.001 (□), 0.002 (▲), 0.004 (●), and 0.008 (○) mg kg^{-1} min^{-1}, but concentrations have been scaled equivalent to a dose rate of 0.01 mg kg^{-1} min^{-1}. (Reproduced with permission from Weatherley et al[6])

concentration of the infusion (Fig 7). At the highest concentration (0.01 mg kg^{-1} min^{-1}), equivalent to a plasma concentration of about 1.5 μg mL^{-1}, tetanic block was complete whereas an infusion of 0.002 mg kg^{-1} had a plasma equivalent of 0.3 μg mL^{-1} and no discernible effect on the tetanus.

In summary, it has been shown that after bolus injections of atracurium the concentration of the drug in plasma is directly related to the dose given and that, furthermore, the effect produced is directly related to the plasma concentration. During continuous infusions of the drug it has been established that there is close relationship between the plasma concentration and the extent of the block and that the plasma concentration only slowly reaches a plateau. This presumably reflects the half-life of the drug and its mode of elimination. What is also important is that recovery from neuromuscular block after an atracurium infusion follows the same pattern as that seen after bolus injections and is just as rapid. The implication of this seems to be that atracurium may have special advantages for use as an infusion in long surgical procedures.

On the basis of the pharmacokinetic and pharmacodynamic data just described, it was possible to construct and test a model (Fig 8) that in principle could be used to predict the profile with time of either the tetanic or single twitch response for any regimen of atracurium.[6] The ability to use such a model to predict the pattern of drug responses had a direct value in research, but it also has a more general application in that it provides a useful tool to teach basic pharmacologic principles in the clinical environment.

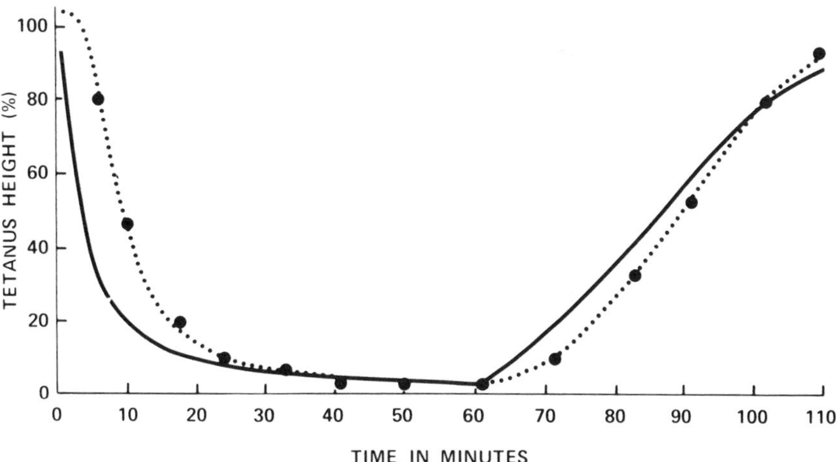

Figure 7. Results of adjusting tetanus parameters to give best fits to plasma concentrations (solid line) or to effect compartment concentrations (dotted line) using the first 0.008 mg kg^{-1} min^{-1} infusion tetanus measurements (●). (Reproduced with permission from Weatherley, et al.[6])

CLINICAL USE

In the dosage quoted, atracurium has proved to be an effective neuromuscular blocking agent of medium duration and without absolute contraindications for use in a wide range of surgical conditions. The drug is prepared as the besylate in a strength of 10 mg mL^{-1} of solution. Each ampule contains 5 mL and it is normally stored at a temperature of 2 to 8 °C. Under these conditions it has a shelf life of about 2 years.

Although most clinicians in the United Kingdom initially used the dose range of 0.3 to 0.6 mg kg^{-1}, it seems likely that a dose of 0.5 mg kg^{-1} will come to be accepted partly because the calculation of total dosage is simple and partly because in practice there is no significant difference between the dose of 0.5 mg kg^{-1} and that of 0.6 mg kg^{-1}.

Since atracurium became available for general use in the United Kingdom in December 1982, the drug has been given to more than 250,000 patients. Thus, there is now a sufficient range of experience to produce a reasonable assessment of its suitability as a skeletal muscle relaxant with special reference to the ease of tracheal intubation, the extent and duration of relaxation, the convenience of reversal, and the absence of unwanted effects.

Undoubtedly, the first requirement of a neuromuscular blocking drug in clinical practice is its suitability for intubation. The problem with this criterion is the number of other factors involved. The anatomy of the larynx, the speed

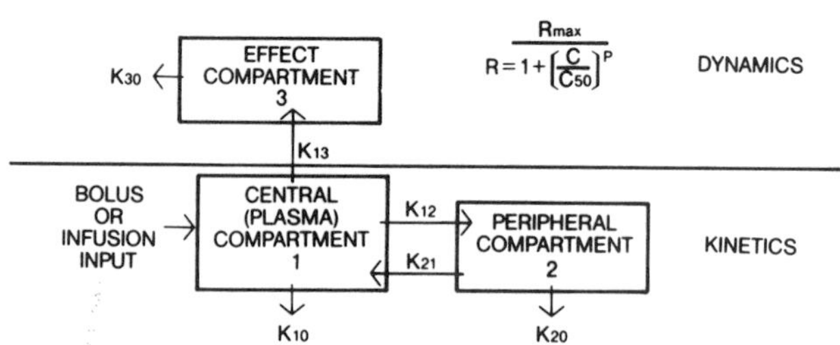

Figure 8. The pharmacokinetic and pharmacodynamic model for atracurium IV. Kinetic effects are represented below the horizontal line by the conventional two-compartment open model with the additional elimination rate constant, k_{20}, from the peripheral compartment. Dynamic effects are represented by the effect compartment 3 and the linking equation shown. The k_{13} input to the effect compartment is arbitarily small, but k_{30}, total elimination from the effect compartment, R_{max}, the maximal response (approximately 100%), C_{50}, and s in the Hill equation are optimally fitted by computer program. (Reproduced with permission from Weatherley et al.[6])

of circulation, and the individual patient response are just as important as the drug used, and the technical skill and experience of the anesthetist further influence the rapidity and smoothness of intubation. Despite these variables there appears to be general agreement that with a dose of 0.5 mg kg^{-1} it should be possible to carry out a smooth and atraumatic intubation in nearly every patient in two minutes or less from the time of injection. In some patients this will be accomplished within one minute.

The same dose provides full abdominal muscle relaxation and paralyzes completely the muscles of respiration. The duration of relaxation depends on the physical state of the patient, the site of operation, and the particular anesthetic technique in use. Normally, adequate relaxation can be expected over a period from 20 to 40 minutes. Spontaneous breathing recovers early and rapidly within a few minutes of signs that the single twitch of the train-of-four is reappearing. This rapid recovery has been regarded as a disadvantage by some anesthetists who have complained that unless a careful watch is kept on the patient the rapid return of muscle activity could embarrass the surgeons and themselves. However since the main purpose of their employment is to care for the patient, it is difficult to accept such comments as valid criticism; they could equally be regarded as criticism of the professional standards of the individuals concerned.

A particular advantage of atracurium is the consistent pattern of response seen with incremental doses. The predictable response in terms of the extent of the block and the speed of recovery implies a lack of cumulative effects within the dose regimen described (Fig 8) and offers an alternative approach to the use of volatile anesthetic agents to extend the depth and duration of relaxation. However, many anesthetists prefer the latter approach since the volatile agents offer a degree of flexibility not available with IV drugs.

Because recovery from block with atracurium is fairly rapid, induced reversal with anticholinesterases is not always necessary and many anesthetists choose to avoid the use of such drugs. Nevertheless, paralysis is rapidly antagonized by neostigmine with a dose of 2.5 mg, and even if block is complete, recovery is prompt if the dose is increased to 5 mg. Other anticholinesterases such as edrophonium and pyridostigmine have also been used, but their efficacy remains to be established in comparison with neostigmine even if theoretically they would appear to have advantages.

Adverse reactions after atracurium have not been a problem in anesthetic practice in the United Kingdom, although a variety have been reported including cutaneous reactions such as urticaria, rashes, localized erythema, and flushing as well as hypotension, bradycardia, and bronchospasm, not all of which could be definitely attributed to the drug. The incidence of reported adverse reactions in the United Kingdom is 0.11%, none of which were life-threatening and some of which were essentially frivolous. Nonetheless, when a new drug has been introduced into clinical practice it is incumbent on all who use it to report unwanted effects, even if later analysis does not incriminate the drug.

In addition to its obvious value in the general field, atracurium offers specific advantages in certain specialized practice such as (1) obstetric and pediatric anesthesia, (2) surgery of the elderly and the critically ill, particularly those patients in renal or hepatic failure, and (3) in cardiac surgery including cardiopulmonary bypass procedures.

In patients undergoing caesarian section, suxamethonium is still the drug of choice for intubation, but atracurium is now more widely used for the maintenance of surgical relaxation. In the mother, abdominal relaxation is excellent and most patients recover full respiratory function spontaneously, but in those who need it reversal with neostigmine 2.5 mg given IV is rapid and effective. Placental transfer of atracurium is insignificant, and no adverse effects attributable to the drug have been reported on Apgar scores nor has there been any deterioration in the time to sustained respiration.

The general rule in pediatric anesthesia that when dosage is determined on a weight basis infants and small children need greater amounts of competitive neuromuscular blocking drugs to achieve the same degree of muscle relaxation when similar anesthetic techniques are in use seems to hold true for atracurium. Despite that proviso, in practice the infant or child dose does not differ materially from the adult requirement. In the range of 0.4 to 0.6 mg kg^{-1}, conditions for intubation are satisfactory and muscle relaxation is adequate during the ensuing 30 minutes; an incremental dose of 0.1 mg kg^{-1} will extend this period for about 15 minutes, and there is no evidence of cumulative effects if further increments are needed.

Age carries its own risks when surgery under general anesthesia is contemplated, and these risks are compounded when the patient is seriously ill. Because of disturbances in metabolism and in fluid balance commonly found in the elderly, such patients are less capable of handling the various drugs to which they are exposed; thus it is important to ensure that drug dosage is kept to a minimum and, in particular, that cumulation is avoided. Patients in renal and hepatic failure are specially vulnerable and it is therefore a singular advantage that the breakdown of atracurium proceeds independently of renal and hepatic activity. In the case of patients in kidney failure, it has been shown that the pattern of atracurium elimination does not differ significantly from that in normal patients even after repeated dosage spread over several hours. In patients with liver failure the pattern is similar; the elimination half-life of the drug remains unchanged when compared with normal patients and provides further evidence that the elimination of atracurium is not conditional on the physiologic status of the patient.

The use of atracurium by IV infusion in cardiopulmonary bypass surgery combined with induced hypothermia offers another example of how the properties of the drug can be exploited in the management of anesthesia. When atracurium is used by IV infusion, a steady level of neuromuscular block can be maintained for the duration of the infusion with less drug than is needed with bolus injections, and the rate of recovery is not substantially different. Moreover, during the phase of induced hypothermia, significantly slower infusion rates provide satisfactory operating conditions in keeping with the fact that the metabolism of atracurium is reduced when the temperature is lowered.

In essence, atracurium meets the need for a neuromuscular blocking drug of medium duration. It has enough flexibility to allow it to have a wide range of applications, although the relatively slow onset of action characteristic of competitive blocking agents restricts its use, for example, for emergency intubation. In this respect only suxamethonium has the speed of onset for this purpose, and despite its other disadvantages it seems unlikely that it will be displaced by any of the new drugs thus far described.

EDITOR'S NOTE

There are at present two schools of thought concerning the use of succinylcholine versus atracurium or vecuronium for emergency intubation. One view, just expressed, is that succinylcholine is the drug of choice. Another view is that the patient with the "full stomach" can safely be given atracurium or vecuronium for rapid-sequence intubation if a small dose of either drug is given and followed two to three minutes later by a larger dose. In the case of atracurium, a dose of 0.1 mg/kg followed in two to three minutes by 0.4

mg/kg will usually permit endotracheal intubation within one minute after the larger dose. In the case of vecuronium, the initial dose of 0.02 mg/kg followed in two to three minutes by 0.08 mg/kg will usually permit endotracheal intubation within one minute after the larger dose. Numerous variations on the theme with different doses and time intervals have been proposed and will be studied. The question of whether succinylcholine or one of the atracurium or vecuronium recipes is better will only be answered with time, and even then each of the possibilities may have its adherents.

REFERENCES

1. Griffith HR, Johnson GE: The use of curare in general anesthesia. Anesthesiology 3:418–420, 1942
2. Stenlake JB, Waigh RD, Urwin J, et al: Atracurium: Conception and inception. Br J Anaesth 55:3–10S, 1983
3. Hughes R, Chapple DJ: The pharmacology of atracurium: A new competitive neuromuscular blocking agent. Br J Anaesth 53:31–44, 1981
4. Hunt TM, Hughes R, Payne JP: Preliminary studies with atracurium in anesthetized man. Br J Anaesth 52:238P, 1980
5. Payne JP, Hughes R: Evaluation of atracurium in anaesthetized man. Br J Anaesth 53:45–54, 1981
6. Weatherley BC, Williams SG, Neill EAM: Pharmacokinetics, pharmacodynamics and dose-response relationships of atracurium administered i.v. Br J Anaesth 55:39–45S, 1983
7. Stenlake JB: Advances in Pharmacology and Therapeutics. Oxford, New York, Pergamon Press, 1979, p 303
8. Hughes R, Payne JP: Clinical assessment of atracurium using the single twitch and tetanic responses of the adductor pollicis muscles. Br J Anaesth 55:47–52s, 1983

FURTHER READING

1. Ali HH, Savarese JJ, Basta SJ, et al: Clinical pharmacology of atracurium: A new intermediate acting nondepolarizing relaxant. Semin Anesth 1:57–62, 1982
2. Atracurium editorial: Lancet 1:394–395, 1983
3. British Journal of Anaesthesia: Symposium on atracurium. Br J Anaesth 55(suppl):1–139s, 1983
4. Katz RL, Stirt J, Murray AL, et al: Neuromuscular effects of atracurium in man. Anesth Analg 61:730–734, 1982
5. Miller RD: Is atracurium an ideal neuromuscular blocking drug? Anesth Analg 61:721–722, 1982

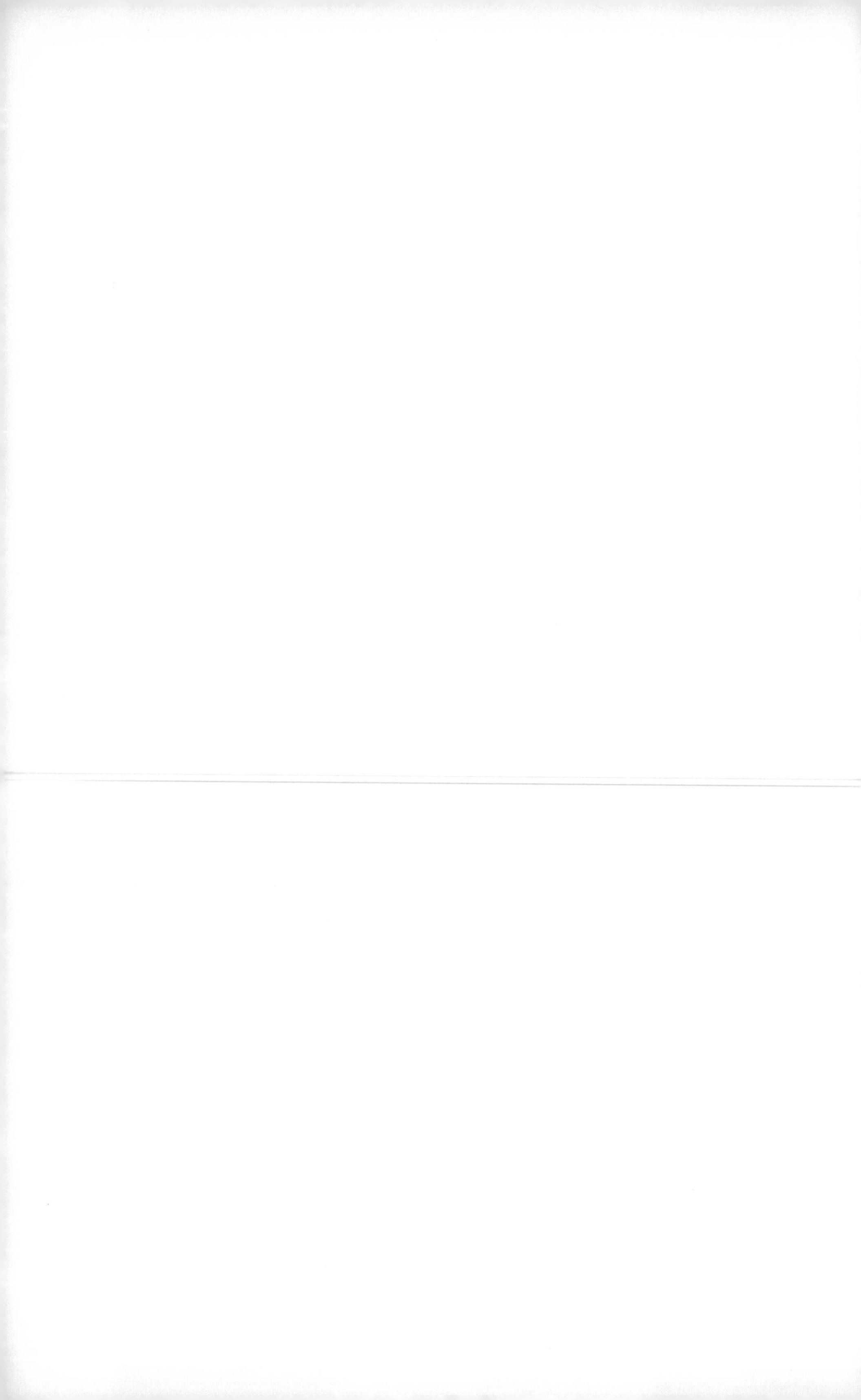

Ronald D. Miller

7

Vecuronium

Vecuronium (ORG NC45, Norcuron, Organon, Inc, West Orange, NJ) is one of two nondepolarizing neuromuscular blocking drugs that have durations of action between those of succinylcholine and pancuronium; atracurium is the other new blocking drug and is discussed by Payne in this issue. Our group has extensively reviewed the clinical pharmacology of vecuronium.[1,2] This report will represent a summary of those studies.

DEVELOPMENTAL CHEMISTRY

Savage et al[3] manipulated the steroid nucleus that led to the development of the bisquaternary pancuronium (Fig 1). Vecuronium is a monoquaternary neuromuscular blocking drug. Two nitrogen atoms are required for both neuromuscular blockers to retain potency. Also, the acetylcholine fragments in the ring D of both pancuronium and vecuronium make them among the most potent of all the steroid muscle relaxants studied.[3] This rigid-trapped fragment probably interacts with the nicotinic cholinergic receptor and must have a low affinity for muscarinic receptors. Although both vecuronium and pancuronium are hydrophilic, vecuronium is slightly more lipophilic because it is a monoquaternary rather than bisquaternary compound. However, this increased lipophilicity cannot alone account for the markedly different pharmacologic profile of vecuronium as compared with pancuronium.

MUSCLE RELAXANTS
ISBN 0-8089-1784-6

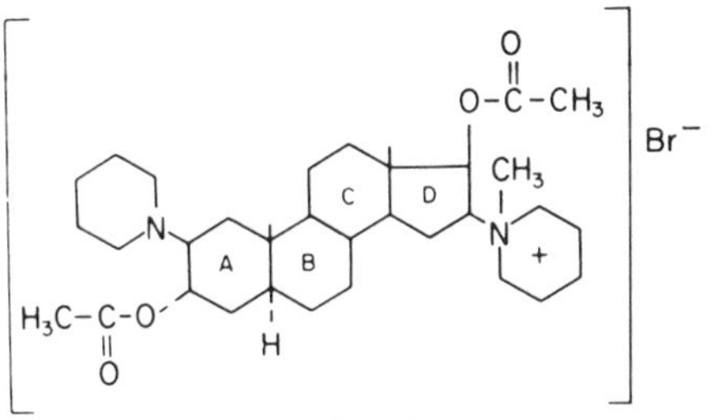

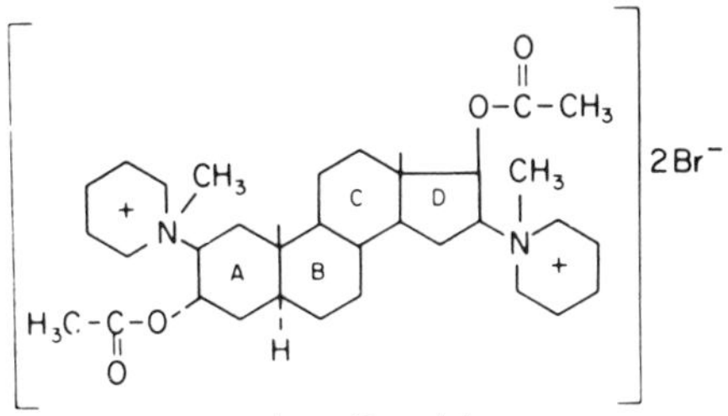

Vecuronium Bromide

Pancuronium Bromide

Figure 1. Comparative chemical formulas for pancuronium and vecuronium. (Reprinted with permission from Miller et al.[1])

POTENCY

The potency of vecuronium is equal to or slightly greater than that of pancuronium; the ratio of their potencies ranges from 1.0 to 1.74.[4–11] Because of several factors including different anesthetics and methods of nerve stimulation, the ED_{90} or ED_{95} (ie, the dose of neuromuscular blocking drug that depress twitch tension 90% or 95%) varies considerably ranging from 0.023 to 0.044 mg · kg^{-1}.[4,12] If the clinician remembers that vecuronium's potency is similar to that of pancuronium, an appropriate dose can be chosen.

ONSET TIME AND DURATION OF ACTION

The doses of vecuronium that depress twitch tension less than 100% have onset times (time from administration of muscle relaxant to its peak effect) ranging from four to eight minutes[4–9,11,13–19] (Table 1). Because larger doses depress twitch tension 100%, onset time appears to be shorter. For example, four times the ED_{95} of vecuronium has an onset time of 1.3 minutes.[15] Despite markedly increasing the dose, vecuronium never has an onset time as short as that of succinylcholine. The onset time of vecuronium can be shortened by

Table 1
Time Course of Action of Vecuronium*

Dose (mg/kg)	Onset Time (min)	Percent Depression of Twitch Tension	Duration (min)
0.01	6.7	25	14
0.014	6.3	36	16
0.02	6.0	36	27
0.07	3.8	100	34
0.14	2.8	100	104

*Data taken from Fahey et al.[4] Reprinted with permission.[55]

giving a small nonparalyzing dose prior to the intubating dose (Katz RL, Foldes F: personal communication). For example, if vecuronium, 0.1 mg/kg intravenously (IV), is preceded three minutes earlier by the IV administration of 0.01 mg/kg of vecuronium, the onset time from the larger dose (and intubating time) will be less than 1.5 minutes.

Vecuronium has a duration of action (time from vecuronium administration to 90% or 95% recovery of control twitch tension) that is about 50% to 67% shorter than that of pancuronium.[4,6,8,9,11] For doses depressing twitch tension less than 100%, duration of action is about 15 to 30 minutes.[4,5,8,9,11,17] When three times the ED_{95} of vecuronium was given, duration of action was 53[17] and 60[5] minutes. Comparable doses of pancuronium produce a neuromuscular blockade of approximately two to three hours.

CUMULATIVE EFFECTS

Vecuronium is said to have little or no cumulative effect, which means that the duration of action of a given dose of vecuronium does not increase with repetitive doses. Specifically, Fahey et al[4] administered a given dose of vecuronium to patients and observed its effect. When twitch tension had recovered to 25% of control, the same dose was given with the same resulting duration of action. The same duration of action from repetitive doses implies a lack of cumulative effect. Similar results were found by Buzello and Nöldge.[20]

The claim that a muscle relaxant has no cumulative effect requires further clarification. Recovery of neuromuscular function parallels the decrease in plasma concentration (this does not apply to atracurium). Following a single dose of vecuronium or pancuronium, plasma concentration falls rapidly because of redistribution from the central to the peripheral compartment. With subsequent doses, muscle relaxant in the peripheral compartment limits this distribution phase and the decrease in plasma concentration results from elimination or metabolism. Thus, both pancuronium, and to a lesser extent vecuronium, can be demonstrated to have cumulative effects.

PHARMACOKINETICS

Unlike pancuronium, metocurine, d-tubocurarine, or gallamine, vecuronium does not depend heavily on the kidney for its elimination. Only 10% to 25% of an injected dose of vecuronium is excreted in the urine,[21–23] the predominant route of elimination probably being the bile.[21] Because only small amounts of vecuronium's metabolites have been detected by methods such as thin-layer chromatography,[22] most of the drug excreted in the urine and bile is unchanged.[21] In humans, vecuronium has a more rapid clearance (5.2 ± 0.7 ml · kg^{-1} · min^{-1}; mean ± SD) and a shorter elimination half-life (71 ± 20 minutes) than pancuronium (1.8 ± 0.4 ml · kg^{-1} · min^{-1}; 140 ± 25 minutes)[24] (Table 2). Thus, these two characteristics probably account for the shorter duration of action of vecuronium.

FACTORS THAT INFLUENCE THE PHARMACOKINETICS OR PHARMACODYNAMICS OF VECURONIUM

Anesthesia

Vecuronium is influenced less by the choice and concentration of anesthetic than are d-tubocurarine and pancuronium. Enflurane and isoflurane augment a d-tubocurarine and pancuronium neuromuscular blockade about twice as much as does an equipotent concentration of halothane.[25–27] For example, the ED_{50}s of d-tubocurarine and pancuronium are 1.70 and 0.27 mg/m^2, respectively, during isoflurane anesthesia, and 5.60 and 0.49 mg/m^2, respectively, during halothane anesthesia.[26,27] In contrast, a vecuronium-induced neuromuscular blockade is augmented by enflurane and isoflurane only 20% to 30% greater than that produced by halothane or nitrous oxide-narcotic anesthesia.[16,18,28]

Changes in the end-tidal concentration of inhaled anesthetics also have a lesser influence on neuromuscular blockades produced by vecuronium than those produced by other nondepolarizing neuromuscular blockers. Increasing the anesthetic concentration from 1.2 MAC to 2.2 MAC decreases the ED_{50} of vecuronium 51%, 33% and 18% during enflurane, isoflurane and halothane anesthesia, respectively.[18] Yet, the ED_{50}s of d-tubocurarine and pancuronium decreased 62% and 57%, respectively, for similar increases in the halothane concentration, and 30% and 70%, respectively, for similar increases in the isoflurane concentration.[29]

Age

Infants and Children

The potency of vecuronium is similar in pediatric and adult patients. During halothane and nitrous oxide anesthesia, the ED_{50} of vecuronium was 16.5 μg/kg in infants (< 1 year), 19.0 μg/kg for children (1 to 8 years), and 15.0 μg/kg for adults.[30] Goudsouzian et al[31] found ED_{50} values of 33 μg/kg and 23 μg/kg for children (2 to 9 years) and adolescents (10 to 17 years), respectively. The higher ED_{50} values in the latter study may be partly explained by the use of the cumulative method rather than the single bolus method for producing dose-response curves.

The duration of a neuromuscular blockade induced by vecuronium (70 μg/kg) appears to be longer in infants (73 ± 27 minutes) than in children (35 ± 6 minutes) or adults (53 ± 7 minutes).[30] Goudsouzian et al[31] did not study infants but found similar durations of action in children and adolescents. The longer duration of action in infants may be related to the larger volume of distribution in infants resulting in more vecuronium in the peripheral compartment, which is inaccessible to the organs of clearance. Also, age-related changes in biliary clearance may account for vecuronium's longer duration of action in infants.

The Elderly

d'Hollander et al found that less vecuronium was required to sustain a steady state of paralysis, and recovery from neuromuscular blockade was longer in elderly patients (> 60 years) than in younger patients.[32] Yet, Rupp et al[33] found that in elderly patients (> 70 years), the plasma concentration of vecuronium required to depress twitch height 50% was the same when compared with their younger counterparts. Conversely, plasma clearance and the volume of distribution decreased in the elderly, probably because of decreased extracellular fluid and muscle mass. However, elimination half-life did not change in the elderly, suggesting that neuromuscular blockade should not be prolonged in the elderly. The differences between the Rupp et al[33] and d'Hollander et al[32] studies indicate that more research is required to better define the influence of age on the neuromuscular blockade produced by vecuronium.

Succinylcholine

Prior administration of succinylcholine probably enhances the neuromuscular blockade from vecuronium.[9,34] However, there is lack of agreement among various investigators. d'Hollander et al[35] found that succinylcholine augmented both the magnitude and duration of a vecuronium-induced neuromuscular blockade. This augmentation would occur if vecuronium had been given within 30 minutes of succinylcholine administration. Krieg et al[34] found that vecuronium given after succinylcholine caused a 19% greater depression of twitch tension than did vecuronium given without a prior dose of succinylcholine. Yet, Fisher and Miller[36] found that prior administration of succinylcholine did not alter a vecuronium-induced neuromuscular blockade. Clearly, the response to vecuronium varies when given after succinylcholine.

Acid-Base Balance

In cats, Funk et al[37] found that acidosis augmented and alkalosis lessened a vecuronium-induced neuromuscular blockade. In humans, Gencarelli et al[38] found that the timing of changes in end-tidal P_{CO_2} was important in relation to its influence on vecuronium. During an end-tidal P_{CO_2} of 25, 41, or 56 mm Hg, neither the magnitude nor the recovery time from a vecuronium-induced neuromuscular blockade changed. However, when vecuronium was infused at a constant rate and then the end-tidal P_{CO_2} was changed, respiratory acidosis augmented and respiratory alkalosis lessened twitch tension (Fig 2). Thus, if

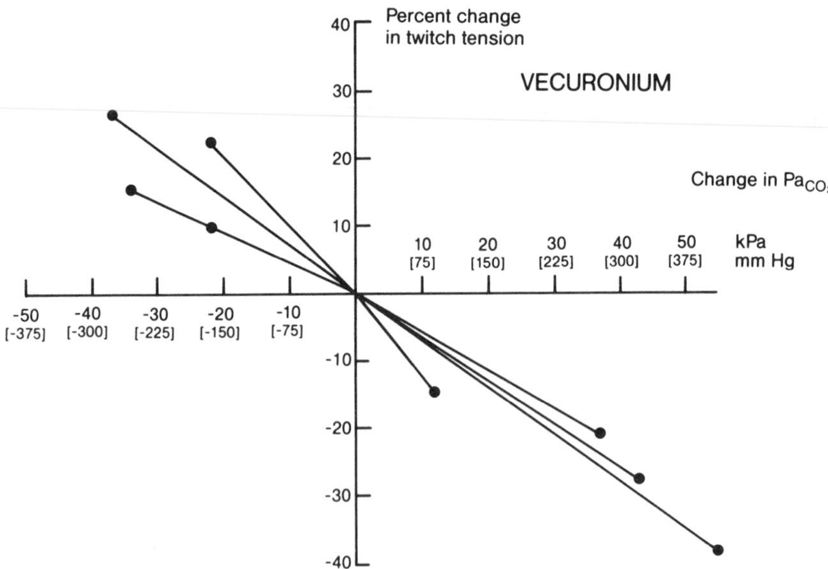

Figure 2. The relationship between acute changes in Pa_{CO_2} and subsequent changes in twitch tension in patients receiving vecuronium. Each point represents the data for one patient. (Reprinted with permission from Gencarelli et al.[38])

respiratory acidosis occurs during a vecuronium-induced neuromuscular blockade, an augmented and prolonged blockade may result.

CARDIOVASCULAR EFFECTS

The two major cardiovascular effects from older nondepolarizing blockers are tachycardia (eg, pancuronium and gallamine) and hypotension from histamine release (eg, d-tubocurarine and metocurine). In contrast, vecuronium has little or no cardiovascular effects. For example, Booij et al[39] gave three times the ED_{90} of vecuronium IV to dogs and found no change in heart rate, BP, or cardiac output. Marshall et al[40] found that doses of vecuronium up to 20 times greater than those required for neuromuscular blockade produced no cardiovascular changes in cats and dogs. Lastly, vecuronium does not release histamine.[41]

Gregoretti et al[42] administered vecuronium, 0.1 mg/kg IV, to patients anesthetized with enflurane or halothane. The only cardiovascular change was a slight decrease in heart rate (from 76 to 63 beats per minute) during halothane anesthesia. However, the control heart rate was obtained before both vecuronium and halothane were administered. The authors concluded that when vecuronium is used, its lack of vagolytic activity may allow drug- or reflex-induced bradycardia to occur more easily during surgery and anesthesia. Yet, Engbaek et al[43] found no change in heart rate, arterial BPs, or systolic time intervals from vecuronium, 57 μg/kg IV, given to patients also anesthetized with halothane. To severely test vecuronium's apparent lack of cardiovascular effects, Morris et al[44] gave 0.28 mg/kg (12 times the ED_{90}) of vecuronium IV to patients anesthetized with halothane who were about to undergo coronary artery bypass grafting. Heart rate and arterial BP did not change. Cardiac output decreased 9% and systemic vascular resistance decreased 12%.[44] Also, Gencarelli et al[45] gave vecuronium, 0.10 to 0.14 mg/kg as an IV bolus, to three patients undergoing removal of a pheochromocytoma with small increases in plasma catecholamine concentrations in blood but no change in any measured cardiovascular variables.

ANTAGONISM

There have been no reports of difficulty in antagonizing a vecuronium-induced neuromuscular blockade with anticholinesterase drugs. Fahey et al[4] found that less neostigmine was required to antagonize a neuromuscular blockade induced by vecuronium than one induced by pancuronium. However, this conclusion was based on data obtained from administration of intermittent boluses of neostigmine. Possibly because a neuromuscular blockade by vecuronium would terminate spontaneously more rapidly than one by pancuronium, less neostigmine would be required with vecuronium. To compensate for the possibility that this pharmacokinetic characteristic would lessen the neostigmine requirement, Gencarelli and Miller[46] continuously infused either pancuronium or vecuronium and found no difference in the neostigmine dose required for antagonism. They concluded that vecuronium and pancuronium are effectively and equally (independent of their pharmacokinetics) antagonized by neostigmine. Baird et al[47] found that edrophonium, 0.5 to 1.0 mg/kg IV, rapidly (ie, one to two minutes) restored a vecuronium depressed twitch to within 80% of the control height but that an additional six to eight minutes was required for complete restoration of neuromuscular function, as judged by the train-of-four.

SPECIAL CLINICAL SITUATIONS

Cardiac Surgery and Cardiopulmonary Bypass

Because it has little or no cardiovascular effect, vecuronium may be an ideal neuromuscular blocking drug for cardiac surgery.[44] Still, is it appropriate to rely on drugs that have a relatively short duration for a situation that requires several hours of paralysis? In other words, why not administer the longer acting metocurine or pancuronium instead of the shorter acting vecuronium? The duration of action of vecuronium could be extended by giving very large doses. For example, Morris et al[44] gave vecuronium, 0.28 mg/kg, to patients undergoing cardiopulmonary bypass. This high dose has a duration of neuromuscular blockade of about 174 minutes.[4] Also, very large doses of vecuronium can be given with no cardiovascular effects.

The lack of cardiovascular effects associated with large doses of vecuronium can be a disadvantage when the high-dose fentanyl approach to anesthesia is used. Pancuronium is commonly satisfactorily used because its vagolytic effect counteracts the tendency of fentanyl to produce bradycardia. Thus, when vecuronium is given with high-dose fentanyl anesthesia (especially cardiac anesthesia), heart rate often decreases.[48]

Hypothermia and cardiopulmonary bypass also can alter the amount of vecuronium required for neuromuscular blockade. Buzello et al[49] found that before cardiopulmonary bypass, pancuronium acted about two times longer than vecuronium. However, during hypothermic bypass, the durations of action of pancuronium and vecuronium increased 1.8-fold and fivefold, respectively. Thus, during hypothermic bypass, pancuronium and vecuronium had similar durations of action. Consequently, we conclude that hypothermic cardiopulmonary bypass is associated with a marked increase in the duration of neuromuscular blockade from vecuronium.

Obstetrics

Vecuronium has been successfully used in patients undergoing cesarean section. Baraka et al[50] gave vecuronium, 0.05 mg/kg, to patients undergoing cesarean section after recovery from an initial dose of succinylcholine had occurred. The mean duration of neuromuscular blockade was 19 minutes. Furthermore, Apgar scores did not differ for infants delivered before vecuronium administration (N = 9) and those delivered after vecuronium administration (N = 19). Dailey et al[51] confirmed that vecuronium has difficulty crossing the placental barrier. Specifically, when a 0.04 mg/kg dose of vecuronium or pancuronium was given to the mother, 8.5 to 26.4 ng/mL and 12.2 to 34.2 ng/mL, respectively, of drug was found in umbilical cord venous blood. The ratio of the drug concentration in umbilical cord venous blood to that in maternal venous blood was 0.11 for vecuronium and 0.19 for pancuronium. In a similar study, Demetriou et al[52] found a ratio of 0.11 for vecuronium. Lastly, plasma clearance of vecuronium is more rapid in pregnant patients, probably because of cardiovascular and fluid shifts during pregnancy.[51] Although the increased clearance rate during pregnancy would presumably result in a shorter neuromuscular blockade, this assumption has not been verified.

Renal Disease

Because vecuronium does not depend heavily on the kidney for its elimination, duration of neuromuscular blockade should not be prolonged in patients with renal failure. This conclusion has indeed been confirmed with large doses (0.28 mg/kg) of vecuronium[23] (Tables 2 and 3).

Table 2
Comparative Pharmacokinetics of Vecuronium and Pancuronium in Anesthetized Humans*

Drug	Renal Function	Distribution t½ (min)	Elimination t½ (min)	$V_{D_{ss}}$ (mL/kg)	Clearance (mL/kg/min)
Vecuronium	Normal	8.5	80	194	3.0
Vecuronium	Absent	10.5	97	239	2.5
Pancuronium	Normal	20.0	140	260	1.8
Pancuronium	Absent	12.0	257	296	0.8

$V_{D_{ss}}$ = volume of distribution at steady state.
*Data taken from Fahey et al[23] and Cronnelly et al.[24] Reprinted with permission.[55]

Table 3
Pharmacodynamics of Vecuronium (0.14 mg/kg) in Patients With and Without Renal Function*

Renal Function	Onset Time (min)	Duration (min)	Recovery Time (min)
Normal	2.1	103	21
Absent	1.8	104	29

*Data taken from Fahey et al.[23] Reprinted with permission.[55]

Liver Disease

Because vecuronium is significantly eliminated in the bile, one might predict that liver disease would prolong a vecuronium-induced neuromuscular blockade. After vecuronium, 0.2 mg/kg IV, was given to patients with cirrhosis, elimination half-life increased from 58 to 84 minutes, and plasma clearance decreased 50%.[53] Also, the duration of neuromuscular blockade increased from 62 to 130 minutes.[53] However, protein binding of vecuronium was not altered by the presence of cirrhosis.[54] Thus, the duration of neuromuscular blockade produced by vecuronium will be increased in patients with impaired hepatic function.

SUMMARY

Vecuronium provides additional flexibility to the clinician using neuromuscular blocking drugs. The shorter duration of action, the lack of significant cardiovascular effects, and the lack of dependence on the kidney for elimination provide clinical advantages over, or alternatives to, currently available nondepolarizing neuromuscular blocking drugs.

REFERENCES

1. Miller RD, Rupp SM, Fisher DM, et al: Clinical pharmacology of vecuronium and atracurium. Anesthesiology (in press)
2. Miller RD: Clinical pharmacology of vecuronium. Pharmacotherapy (in press)
3. Savage DS, Sleigh T, Carlyle I: The emergence of Org NC 45, 1-[(2β,3α,5α,16β,17β)-3, 17-bis(acetyloxy)-2-(1-piperidinyl)-androstan-16-yl]-1-methylpiperidinium bromide, from the pancuronium series. Br J Anaesth 52(suppl):3S–9S, 1980
4. Fahey MR, Morris RB, Miller RD, et al: Clinical pharmacology of ORG NC45 (Norcuron™): A new nondepolarizing muscle relaxant. Anesthesiology 55:6–11, 1981

5. Agoston S, Salt P, Newton D, et al: The neuromuscular blocking action of Org NC 45, a new pancuronium derivative, in anaesthetized patients. A pilot study. Br J Anaesth 52(suppl): 53S–59S, 1980
6. Crul JF, Booij LHDJ: First clinical experiences with Org NC 45. Br J Anaesth 52(suppl):49S–52S, 1980
7. Baird WLM, Herd D: A new neuromuscular blocking drug, Org NC 45. A pilot study in man. Br J Anaesth 52(suppl):61S–62S, 1980
8. Buzello W, Bischoff G, Kuhls E, et al: The new non-depolarizing muscle relaxant Org NC 45 in clinical anaesthesia: Preliminary results. Br J Anaesth 52(suppl):62S–64S, 1980
9. Krieg N, Crul JF, Booij LHDJ: Relative potency of Org NC 45, pancuronium, alcuronium and tubocurarine in anaesthetized man. Br J Anaesth 52:783–788, 1980
10. Walts LF, Stirt JA, Katz RL: A comparison of neuromuscular blocking effects of norcuron and pancuronium. Anesthesiology 55:A210, 1981
11. Gramstad L, Lilleaasen P, Minsaas B: Comparative study of atracurium, vecuronium (Org NC 45) and pancuronium. Br J Anaesth 55(suppl):95S–96S, 1983
12. Nagashima H, Yun H, Radnay PA, et al: Influence of anesthesia on human dose-response of Org-NC45. Anesthesiology 55:A202, 1980
13. Ørding H, Viby Mogensen J: Dose-response curves for OR NC 45 [sic] and pancuronium. Acta Anaesthesiol Scand 25(suppl):73, 1981
14. Swen J: Org NC 45: Initial experiences. Br J Anaesth 52(suppl):66S–67S, 1980
15. Viby-Mogensen J, Jørgensen BC, Engbaek J et al: On Org NC 45 and halothane anaesthesia. Preliminary results. Br J Anaesth 52(suppl):67S–69S, 1980
16. Duncalf D, Nagashima H, Hollinger I, et al: Relaxation with Org-NC45 during enflurane anesthesia. Anesthesiology 55:A203, 1981
17. Fragen RJ, Robertson EN, Booij LHDJ, et al: A comparison of vecuronium and atracurium in man. Anesthesiology 57:A253, 1981
18. Rupp SM, Miller RD, Gencarelli PJ: Vecuronium-induced neuromuscular blockade during enflurane, halothane and isoflurane in humans. Anesthesiology 60:102–105, 1984
19. Foldes FF, Nagashima H, Boros M, et al: Muscular relaxation with atracurium, vecuronium and Duador under balanced anaesthesia. Br J Anaesth 55(suppl):97S–103S, 1983
20. Buzello W, Nöldge G: Repetitive administration of pancuronium and vecuronium (Org NC 45, Norcuron) in patients undergoing long lasting operations. Br J Anaesth 54:1151–1157, 1982
21. Upton RA, Nguyen T-L, Miller RD, et al: Renal and biliary elimination of vecuronium (ORG NC 45) and pancuronium in rats. Anesth Analg 61:313–316, 1982
22. Sohn YJ, Bencini A, Scaf AHJ, et al: Pharmacokinetics of vecuronium in man. Anesthesiology 57:A256, 1982
23. Fahey MR, Morris RB, Miller RD, et al: Pharmacokinetics of Org NC45 (Norcuron) in patients with and without renal failure. Br J Anaesth 53:1049–1053, 1981
24. Cronnelly R, Fisher DM, Miller RD, et al: Pharmacokinetics and pharmacodynamics of vecuronium (ORG NC45) and pancuronium in anesthetized humans. Anesthesiology 58:405–408, 1983
25. Fogdall RP, Miller RD: Neuromuscular effects of enflurane, alone and combined with d-tubocurarine, pancuronium, and succinylcholine, in man. Anesthesiology 42:173–178, 1975
26. Miller RD, Eger EI II, Way WL, et al: Comparative neuromuscular effects of Forane and halothane alone and in combination with d-tubocurarine in man. Anesthesiology 35: 38–42, 1971
27. Miller RD, Way WL, Dolan WM, et al: Comparative neuromuscular effects of pancuronium, gallamine, and succinylcholine during Forane and halothane anesthesia in man. Anesthesiology 35:509–514, 1971
28. Foldes FF, Bencini A, Newton D: Influence of halothane and enflurane on the neuromuscular effects of Org NC 45 in man. Br J Anaesth 52(suppl):64S–65S, 1980

29. Miller RD, Way WL, Dolan WM, et al: The dependence of pancuronium- and d-tubocurarine-induced neuromuscular blockades on alveolar concentrations of halothane and Forane. Anesthesiology 37:573–581, 1972
30. Fisher DM, Miller RD: Neuromuscular effects of vecuronium (ORG NC45) in infants and children during N_2O, halothane anesthesia. Anesthesiology 58:519–523, 1983
31. Goudsouzian NG, Martyn JJA, Liu LMP, et al: Safety and efficacy of vecuronium in adolescents and children. Anesth Analg 62:1083–1088, 1983
32. d'Hollander A, Massaux F, Nevelsteen M, et al: Age-dependent dose-response relationship of Org NC 45 in anaesthetized patients. Br J Anaesth 54:653–657, 1982
33. Rupp SM, Fisher DM, Miller RD, et al: Pharmacokinetics and pharmacodynamics of vecuronium in the elderly. Anesthesiology 59:A270, 1983
34. Krieg N, Hendricks HHL, Crul JF: Influence of suxamethonium on the potency of Org NC 45 in anaesthetized patients. Br J Anaesth 53:259–262, 1981
35. d'Hollander AA, Agoston S, De Ville A, et al: Clinical and pharmacological actions of a bolus injection of suxamethonium: Two phenomena of distinct duration. Br J Anaesth 55:131–134, 1983
36. Fisher DM, Miller RD: Interaction of succinylcholine and vecuronium during N_2O-halothane anesthesia. Anesthesiology 59:A278, 1983
37. Funk DI, Crul JF, van der Pol FM: Effects of changes in acid-base balance on neuromuscular blockade produced by ORG-NC 45. Acta Anaesthesiol Scand 24:119–124, 1980
38. Gencarelli PJ, Swen J, Koot HWJ, et al: The effects of hypercarbia and hypocarbia on pancuronium and vecuronium neuromuscular blockades in anesthetized humans. Anesthesiology 59:376–380, 1983
39. Booij LHDJ, Edwards RP, Sohn YJ, et al: Cardiovascular and neuromuscular effects of Org NC 45, pancuronium, metocurine, and d-tubocurarine in dogs. Anesth Analg 59:26–30, 1980
40. Marshall RJ, McGrath JC, Miller RD, et al: Comparison of the cardiovascular actions of Org NC 45 with those produced by other non-depolarizing neuromuscular blocking agents in experimental animals. Br J Anaesth 52(suppl):21S–32S, 1980
41. Basta SJ, Savarese JJ, Ali HH, et al: Vecuronium does not alter serum histamine within the clinical dose range. Anesthesiology 59:A273, 1983
42. Gregoretti SM, Sohn YJ, Sia RL: Heart rate and blood pressure changes after ORG NC45 (vecuronium) and pancuronium during halothane and enflurane anesthesia. Anesthesiology 56:392–395, 1982
43. Engbaek J, Ørding H, Sørensen B, et al: Cardiac effects of vecuronium and pancuronium during halothane anaesthesia. Br J Anaesth 55:501–505, 1983
44. Morris RB, Cahalan MK, Miller RD, et al: The cardiovascular effects of vecuronium (ORG NC45) and pancuronium in patients undergoing coronary artery bypass grafting. Anesthesiology 58:438–440, 1983
45. Gencarelli PJ, Roizen MF, Miller RD, et al: ORG NC45 (Nocuron™) and pheochromocytoma: A report of three cases. Anesthesiology 55:690–693, 1981
46. Gencarelli PJ, Miller RD: Antagonism of Org NC45 (vecuronium) and pancuronium neuromuscular blockade by neostigmine. Br J Anaesth 54:53–56, 1982
47. Baird WLM, Bowman WC, Kerr WJ: Some actions of Org NC 45 and of edrophonium in the anaesthetized cat and in man. Br J Anaesth 54:375–385, 1982
48. Salmenperä M, Peltola K, Takkunen O, et al: Cardiovascular effects of pancuronium and vecuronium during high-dose fentanyl anesthesia. Anesth Analg 62:1059–1064, 1983
49. Buzello W, Schluermann D, Schindler M, et al: Hypothermic cardiopulmonary bypass and neuromuscular blockade by pancuronium and vecuronium. Anesthesiology (in press)
50. Baraka A, Noueihed R, Sinno H, et al: Succinylcholine-vecuronium (Org NC 45) sequence for cesarean section. Anesth Analg 62:909–913, 1983

51. Dailey PA, Fisher DM, Shnider SM, et al: Pharmacokinetics, placental transfer, and neonatal effects of vecuronium and pancuronium administered during cesarean section. Anesthesiology (in press)
52. Demetriou M, Depoix J-P, Diakite B, et al: Placental transfer of Org NC 45 in women undergoing caesarean section. Br J Anaesth 54:643–645, 1982
53. Lebrault C, Berger JL, d'Hollander AA, et al: Pharmacokinetics and pharmacodynamics of vecuronium (ORG NC45) in patients with cirrhosis. Anesthesiology (submitted for publication)
54. Duvaldestin P, Henzel D: Binding of tubocurarine, fazadinium, pancuronium and Org NC 45 to serum proteins in normal man and in patients with cirrhosis. Br J Anaesth 54:513–516, 1982
55. Miller RD: Vecuronium: A new nondepolarizing neuromuscular blocking agent. Clinical pharmacology, pharmacokinetics, cardiovascular effects and use in special clinical situations. Pharmacotherapy 4:238–247, 1984

Ralph P.F. Scott
John J. Savarese

8

The Cardiovascular and Autonomic Effects of Neuromuscular Blocking Agents

A variety of studies over the years have highlighted the deficiencies common to most neuromuscular blocking agents. In particular, they lack the degree of specificity that the ideal blocking agent should show for the neuromuscular junction. This is especially true with respect to cardiovascular side effects. These cardiovascular effects are generally due either to stimulation or inhibition of peripheral autonomic sites, to release of histamine and possibly other vasoactive substances from vascular mast cells, or to increases in serum potassium levels secondary to motor endplate depolarization.

Several agents have been introduced over the last three decades with varying degrees of specificity. As the mode of action of these drugs has become better understood, the possibility of designing compounds that more clearly meet the demands of the clinician has become increasingly realistic. The accumulated knowledge in the field of neuromuscular blockade is now such that medicinal chemists are able to produce effective neuromuscular blocking drugs more predictably with less reliance on chance than is the case with any other class of drugs. Consequently, most unwanted activity can be avoided altogether by appropriate molecular design, and any new compounds that do produce unwanted effects can often be discarded at an early stage in preclinical testing.

A careful examination of the advantages and disadvantages of the present neuromuscular blockers will lead to the conclusion that a nondepolarizing succinylcholine or a pancuronium without cardiovascular side effects would

MUSCLE RELAXANTS
ISBN 0-8089-1784-6

provide significant improvements. The introduction of atracurium and vecuronium marked an exciting stage in the development of agents with cardiovascular stability. However, these two drugs both fall into the intermediate-duration class, and work is continuing to find agents with similar cardiovascular stability but with shorter and longer durations of action.

PHARMACOLOGY OF THE AUTONOMIC NERVOUS SYSTEM

Acetylcholine acts on both muscarinic and nicotinic receptors (Table 1). Muscarinic receptors are present in various smooth muscles, cardiac muscles, and exocrine glands; nicotinic receptors are located in autonomic ganglia and at the skeletal neuromuscular junction. Cholinoceptors are also found on the esteratic receptors of acetylcholinesterase and plasma cholinesterase.

In order for neuromuscular blocking agents to interact with the recognition sites of the cholinoceptors at the neuromuscular junction, the drugs must bear some chemical relationship to acetylcholine (Fig 1). Consequently, there is a possibility that they might compete with or mimick acetylcholine at other cholinoceptive sites.

Table 1
Cholinoceptive Sites

Site	Activator or Substrates	Inhibitor
Nicotinic receptors	Nicotine, tetramethylammonium	d-tubocurarine
Neuromuscular junction	Succinylcholine, decamethonium	All nondepolarizing neuromuscular blocking agents
Autonomic ganglia	Dimethylphenylpiperazinium	Hexamethonium, d-tubocurarine
Muscarinic receptors (bowel, bladder bronchi, sinus node of the heart, pupillary sphincter)	Muscarine	Atropine, gallamine, pancuronium
Esteratic receptors		
Active site of acetyl-cholinesterase	Acetylcholine, methacholine	Neostigmine, pyridostigmine, benzoquinonium
Active site of plasma-cholinesterase	Benzoylcholine, butyrylcholine, succinylcholine	Hexaflurenium, tetrahydrodaminocrine, pancuronium

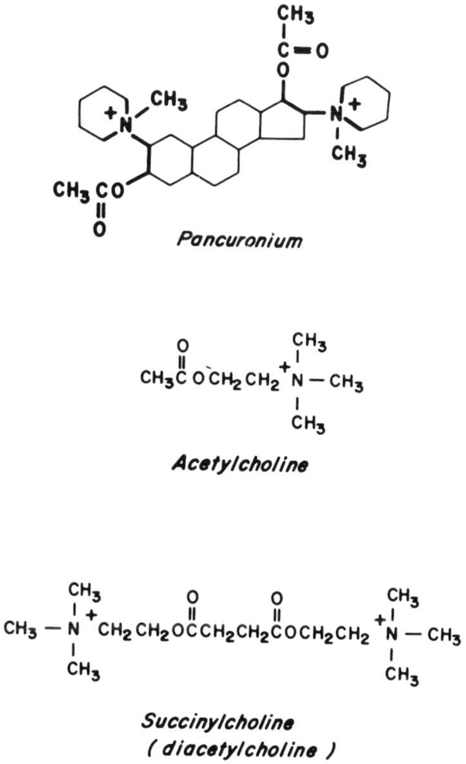

Pancuronium

Acetylcholine

Succinylcholine
(diacetylcholine)

Figure 1. Structural relationship of acetylcholine to two neuromuscular blocking agents. Succinylcholine (diacetylcholine) is simply two molecules of acetylcholine linked through the acetate methyl groups. Pancuronium may be viewed as two acetylcholine-like fragments (outlined in dark print) properly orientated conformationally on a bulky rigid inflexible steroid nucleus.

INTERACTION OF NEUROMUSCULAR BLOCKING AGENTS AT DIFFERENT CHOLINOCEPTIVE SITES

Autonomic Ganglia

Tubocurarine (Fig 2) blocks ganglionic nicotinic receptors and produces some ganglionic blockade in a dose range similar to that required to produce neuromuscular blockade. It may have a slightly greater action on parasympathetic than on sympathetic ganglia.[1] Autonomic reflexes arising in the course of surgical operations may be impaired by this ganglion blocking action,[2] and this action may contribute to hypotension.[3] Recent evidence, however, suggests that the role of ganglionic blockade in the hypotensive action of tubocurarine is less important in its ability to release histamine.[4]

Fazadinium (not available in the United States, but used in Europe) also

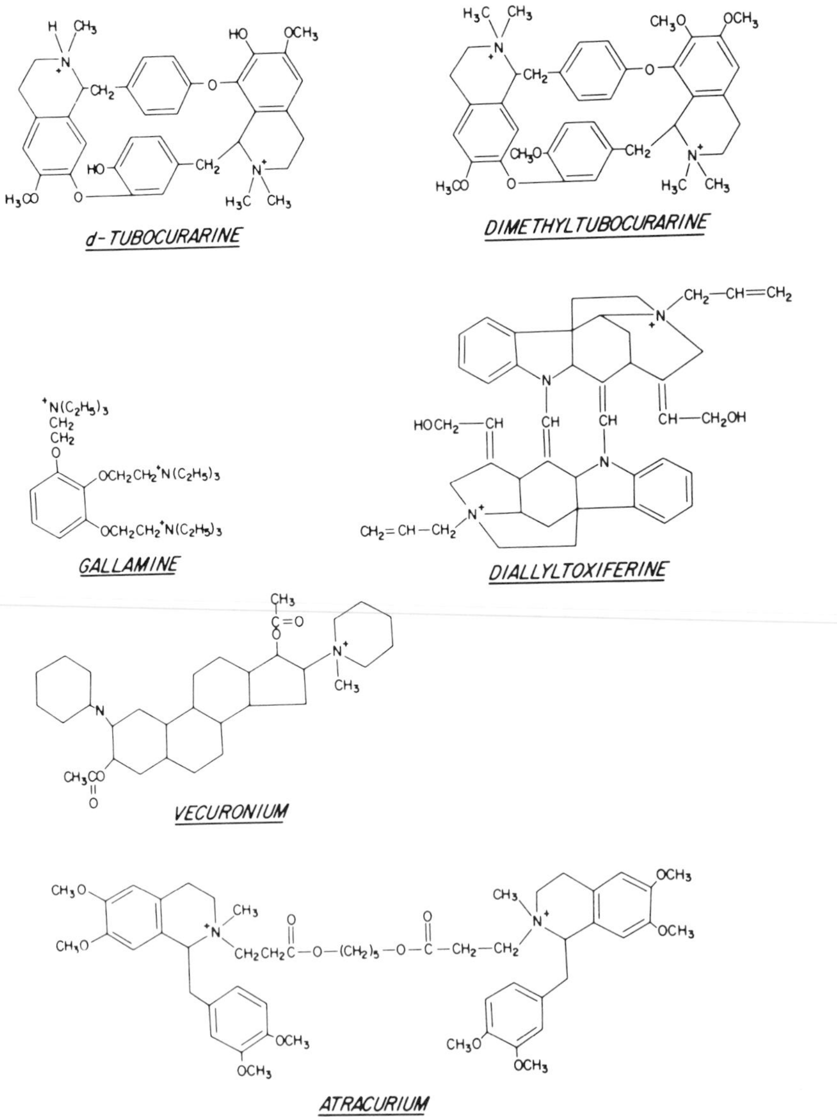

d-TUBOCURARINE

DIMETHYLTUBOCURARINE

GALLAMINE

DIALLYLTOXIFERINE

VECURONIUM

ATRACURIUM

Figure 2. The chemical structure of some common nondepolarizing neuromuscular blocking agents.

has some ganglion-blocking activity in animals,[5] and large doses may cause a decrease in arterial pressure in humans.[6]

Metocurine and alcuronium (not available in the United States) are weaker ganglion blockers, and other neuromuscular blocking drugs (gallamine, pancuronium, atracurium, vecuronium) have no ganglion blocking activity in the doses used clinically.

Succinylcholine has a weak ganglion stimulant action[7] that appears to be of little practical importance.

Muscarinic Receptors

Evidence has accumulated in recent years that muscarinic receptors are probably not a homogenous group. By definition they are all stimulated by muscarine and blocked by atropine, but they may differ in their interactions with other agonists and antagonists. Figure 3 is a diagrammatic representation of the main components of the autonomic nervous system with respect to the heart. For the purpose of the diagram, these muscarinic cholinoceptors have been labeled M_1, M_2, and M_3, but this is not a strict classification and is probably an oversimplification.[8]

An early indication that muscarinic receptors may not all be identical in character came from the work of Riker and Wescoe[9] who showed that galla-

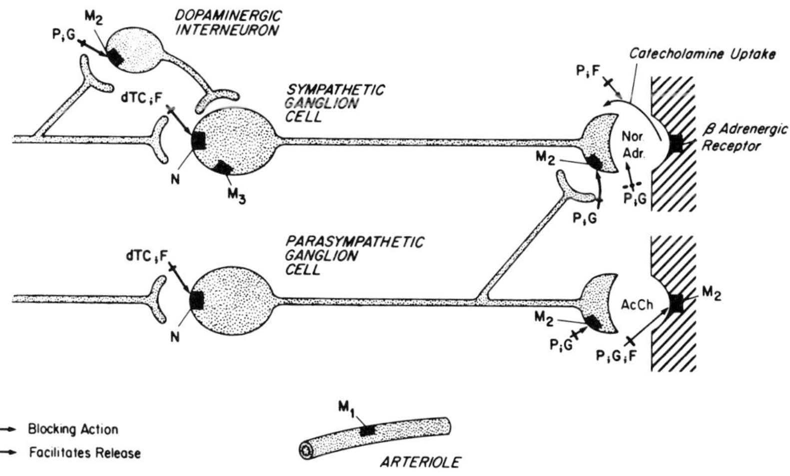

Figure 3. Diagrammatic representation of the autonomic nervous system with respect to the heart, and sites of action of some neuromuscular blocking drugs on this system. The muscarinic receptors have been divided into three subclasses (M_1, M_2, M_3). Abbreviations: N = nicotinic receptor; P = pancuronium; G = gallamine; F = fazadinium; dTc = d-tubocurarine.

mine, although generally free from atropine-like activity in smooth muscle, nevertheless blocked muscarinic receptors in the cat heart and consequently inhibited the cardiac vagus. In Fig 3, the cardiac muscarinic receptors are included in the M_2 group to distinguish them from the more usual type labeled M_1. Other workers have since shown that pancuronium,[10] fazadinum,[5] alcuronium,[11] and stercuronium[12] also block the cardiac muscarinic receptors in doses approximating those required to produce muscle relaxation.

Arterioles also have muscarinic receptors but these receptors are not innervated. They resemble most of the noncardiac muscarinic receptors in their agonist and antagonist selectivity and are labeled M_1 in Fig 3. The vasodepressor response to methacholine, although blocked by atropine, is not affected by pancuronium, showing that the muscarinic receptors involved in the arterioles are not the same type as in the sinoatrial node.

Pancuronium and gallamine also have effects within the sympathetic nervous system. It is believed that vagal nerve terminals impinge not only upon the nodal and atrial cells of the heart but also upon the sympathetic nerve endings where they act to inhibit the release of noradrenaline.[13] The cholinoceptors on the sympathetic nerve endings are of the muscarinic type (M_2), and there is indirect evidence that they are blocked by gallamine and pancuronium.[14]

The small dopaminergic interneurons on sympathetic ganglia (Fig 3) are activated through muscarinic receptors (M_2) stimulated by acetylcholine that is released from collaterals of the preganglionic cholinergic fibers. Dopamine release from these cells onto the postganglionic neurons hyperpolarizes them and therefore suppresses ganglionic transmission.[15] These cholinoceptors may also be blocked by pancuronium and gallamine and may therefore facilitate transmission through the ganglia by inactivating the inhibitory modulating influence of the dopaminergic cell loop.[16]

Transmission through sympathetic ganglia is mediated by acetylcholine acting on nicotinic receptors. There are, however, muscarinic cholinoceptors present on sympathetic ganglia whose physiologic function is as yet unknown. They are labeled M_3 as they differ from M_1 and M_2 receptors in their sensitivity to different agonists and antagonists.[17] They are not blocked by gallamine or pancuronium.

It should be noted that pancuronium and gallamine may cause noradrenaline release by a mechanism that is quite independent of muscarinic blockade.[18] Also, pancuronium and fazadinium have been shown to block noradrenaline reuptake into sympathetic nerve endings both in cardiac muscle and in smooth muscle in guinea pigs and rats.[19–21]

While the main mechanism by which pancuronium and gallamine depress cardiovagal activity in the cat is by blocking postjunctional muscarinic receptors, other workers have concluded that the main site of action of these two drugs in blocking the guinea pig cardiac vagus is on the postganglionic nerve terminals.[22]

It can be concluded from the foregoing discussion that the combination of any of the aforementioned actions of gallamine, pancuronium, and fazadinium may account for the cardiovascular effects of these drugs. There is considerable species difference with regard to the relative importance of these effects. It is not known which effect is predominant in humans, but it is likely that the relative importance varies from patient to patient according to such factors as the pre-existing autonomic balance, the type of premedication given, the anesthetic used, and any concurrent drug therapy.

STRUCTURE ACTIVITY RELATIONSHIPS

The chemical relationship of acetylcholine to two neuromuscular blockers is shown in Fig 1. Succinylcholine is essentially two molecules of acetylcholine linked through the acetate methyl groups.

Depolarizing agents such as succinylcholine generally stimulate nicotinic and muscarinic receptors in imitation of the role of acetylcholine. Removal of the carboxyl groups of succinylcholine results in decamethonium, which has markedly weaker autonomic stimulating properties than succinylcholine.[23]

Bulky molecules such as pancuronium with a rigid ring system cannot activate or stimulate the receptors themselves but instead block the acetylcholine and receptor reaction and so produce a nondepolarizing block by competitive receptor inhibition. Pancuronium is the nondepolarizing relaxant most closely related structurally to acetylcholine (Fig 1). The acetylcholine-like fragments of pancuronium confer upon the steroidal molecule its high neuromuscular blocking activity, its vagolytic property, and its plasma cholinesterase inhibiting action.

d-tubocurarine (Fig 2), originally believed to be a bisquaternary, has now been shown to be a monoquaternary compound with a tertiary amine group in equilibrium with a proton at physiologic pH.[24] In general, bisquaternary compounds do not possess strong ganglionic blocking or histamine releasing properties. Methylation of d-tubocurarine to produce metocurine or dimethyltubocurarine (a bisquaternary compound) reduces the histamine releasing and ganglion blocking activities associated with d-tubocurarine and results in a muscle relaxant that is three times less potent than d-tubocurarine in blocking sympathetic and parasympathetic ganglia.[11, 25]

Gallamine (a triquaternary compound) has marked vagolytic properties probably due to the presence of three positively charged nitrogen atoms.[9, 11]

Vecuronium is simply pancuronium without the quaternary methyl group in the 2, piperidino substitution (Figs 1 and 2). This seemingly minor chemical difference is responsible for all the considerable pharmacologic differences between vecuronium and pancuronium. The absence of this methyl group reduces the acetylcholine-like characteristics of the molecule in the area of ring A of the steroidal nucleus, thereby lessening its vagolytic property without loss of neuromuscular blocking activity. The ring D substituents are retained intact from pancuronium and are responsible for high neuromuscular blocking potency but not for the vagolytic effect.

DEMONSTRATION OF AUTONOMIC EFFECTS OF NEUROMUSCULAR BLOCKING AGENTS IN WHOLE ANIMALS

There are no appropriate means for testing the autonomic effects of relaxants in humans, and most of our knowledge of these actions is derived from experiments performed in isolated organ systems or in whole animals such as the cat. In the cat, measurement of neuromuscular and autonomic function may be accomplished simultaneously. Neuromuscular function is assessed by recording the twitch response of the tibialis anterior (or other appropriate muscle) evoked indirectly via stimulation of the sciatic or perineal nerve. Vagal function is measured by quantitation of the bradycardia and hypotension elicited by stimulation of the vagus nerve. Sympathetic ganglionic responses are assessed by preganglionic stimulation of a sympathetic trunk central to the superior cervical ganglion and recording the evoked contraction of the nicitating membrane (Fig 4).

MARGIN OF SAFETY

The separation of neuromuscular blocking action from autonomic effects can be described for each drug as its autonomic margin of safety. This indicates the number of multiples of a dose of relaxant producing 95% neuromuscular blockade that must be administered in order to produce side effects. The higher the autonomic margin of safety the lower the probability of occurrence of a side effect. The following quotients are used:

$$\frac{\text{ED}_{50}\text{ (ganglion block)}}{\text{ED}_{95}\text{ (neuromuscular block)}}$$

$$\frac{\text{ED}_{50}\text{ (cardiac vagal block)}}{\text{ED}_{95}\text{ (neuromuscular block)}}$$

$$\frac{\text{ED}_{50}\text{ (histamine release)}}{\text{ED}_{95}\text{ (neuromuscular block)}}$$

Calculation of autonomic margins of safety for neuromuscular blocking drugs in humans is not possible because suitable means for quantitating autonomic responses in humans are not available. There is considerable indication, however, that if a neuromuscular blocking agent produces an autonomic effect in the cat within or near its neuromuscular dose range, the neuromuscular blockade in humans will be accompanied by cardiovascular changes corresponding to those autonomic actions (Table 2).

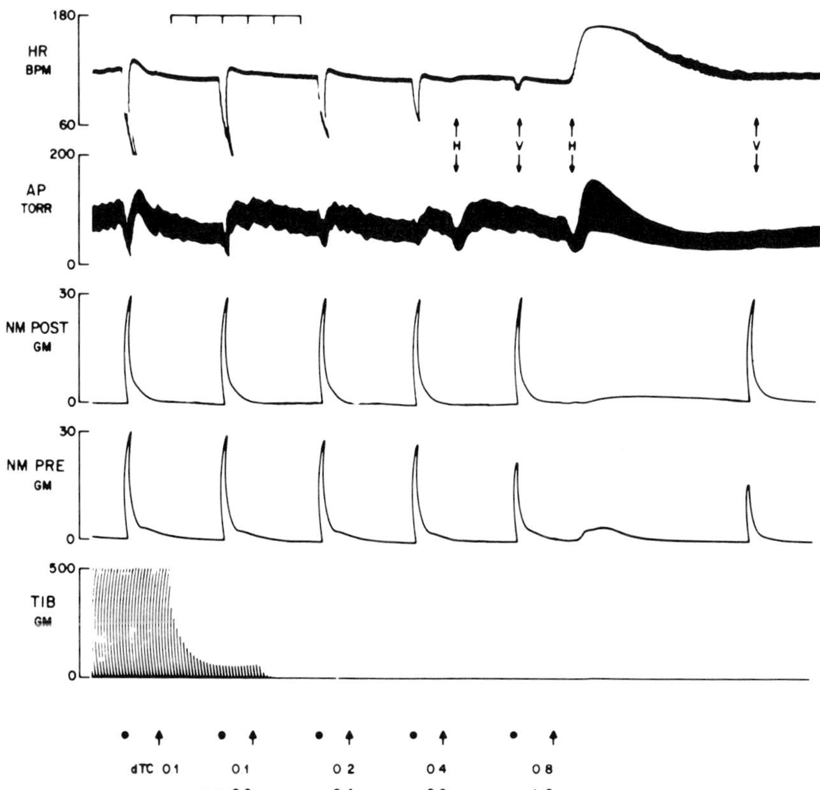

Figure 4. Simultaneous recording of autonomic and neuromuscular function in a cat anesthetized with chloralose. Recordings are (top to bottom) of heart rate, femoral arterial pressure, contractions of the left and right nictitating membranes elicited preganglionically and postganglionically, and tibialis anterior muscle twitch. At times indicated by dots below the graphs, stimulation of the right vagus nerve and both sympathetic trunks (left postganglionically and right preganglionically) was applied at 20 Hz for 10 seconds. At times indicated by arrows below graphs, d-tubocurarine in doses indicated (mg/kg) was given IV. Lower figures indicate cumulative dosage. Note that vagal response (bradycardia and hypotension), ganglionic response (preganglionically stimulated nictitating membrane), and neuromuscular response are all inhibited at a cumulative dose of 0.8 to 1.6 mg/kg. Marker H between the upper two graphs indicates cardiovascular changes suggestive of histamine release. Marker V indicates points of vagal stimulation with little or no response.

Table 2
Autonomic Margin of Safety of Nondepolarizing Relaxants in Humans

Drug	Neuromuscular Block*	Autonomic Margin of Safety†		Margin of Safety for Histamine Release‡
		Ganglion Block	Vagal Block	
d-tubocurarine	0.51	2.94	0.59	1
Metocurine	0.28	18.6	2.86	2
Pancuronium	0.07	328.6	2.86	High
Alcuronium	0.25	18.0	1.84	High
Vecuronium	0.056	89.2	40.6	High
Atracurium	0.28	35.7	8.7	3

*ED_{95} in humans (mg/kg).

†Autonomic margin of safety $= \frac{ED_{50}\text{ for autonomic inhibition in the cat}}{ED_{95}\text{ for neuromuscular block in humans}}$

‡Margin of safety for histamine release $= \frac{ED_{50}\text{ for histamine release in humans}}{ED_{95}\text{ for neuromuscular block in humans}}$

The ED_{95} for neuromuscular block for some of the nondepolarizing relaxants in humans under nitrous oxide has been determined. These values together with the ED_{50}s for ganglion and vagal block derived in the cat (since these cannot be determined in humans) were used to calculate the values in the table. The ED_{50} for histamine release, however, can be calculated in humans using an isotope radioenzymatic assay.

HISTAMINE RELEASE

All basic compounds may disrupt mast cells and cause histamine release if the dose is large enough.[26] Effects among neuromuscular blocking drugs appear to be most pronounced with tubocurarine, possibly because of its free hydroxyl groups, which are thought to enhance histamine releasing potency.[27]

The lack of a sensitive, reliable assay for plasma histamine previously made it difficult to document its role in drug-induced cardiovascular changes. However, the development of a radioenzymatic technique has greatly enhanced the ability to detect histamine in clinically important situations.[28–31]

The histamine releasing ability of tubocurarine occurs within the clinical dose range, and this is almost certainly the most important cause of the transient hypotension observed following administration of this drug. The margin of safety for ganglionic blockade is considerably higher, the duration of which tends to parallel neuromuscular blockade.

A study in humans[32] demonstrated a good correlation between the dose of tubocurarine administered and the amount of histamine released. There is also a correlation between the level of plasma histamine and the extent of hypotension. When plasma levels are elevated to about 200% of control values, there appears to be a significant change in heart rate and arterial BP. More recently it has been shown that atracurium will also release histamine at the extreme upper end of the clinical dose range[33] (0.6 mg/kg), and this is associated with cardiovascular changes. The ability of atracurium to release histamine relative to its neuromuscular blocking potency is approximately one half that of dimethyltubocurarine and less than one third of tubocurarine.

A number of clinical strategies have been applied to attenuate the adverse reaction to histamine release produced by tubocurarine and other muscle relaxants including atracurium. It appears that small differences in plasma levels of a histamine releasing drug can produce large changes in the amount of histamine liberated. It has been shown that slowing the rate of administration of muscle relaxants can prevent this rise in histamine levels and the subsequent hemodynamic changes.[34,35]

Furthermore, there are data suggesting that the prophylactic use of H_1 and H_2 antagonists can also attentuate the cardiovascular response to histamine caused by these drugs.[36–38]

Gallamine, pancuronium and vecuronium have minimal potential for releasing histamine in clinical doses.

AUTONOMIC ACTIONS OF INDIVIDUAL MUSCLE RELAXANTS AND THEIR CIRCULATORY EFFECTS UNDER GENERAL ANESTHESIA (TABLE 3)

d-Tubocurarine

d-Tubocurarine inhibits both sympathetic and parasympathetic functions at a dose range close to amounts necessary to block neuromuscular transmission (Fig 5). This is the classical nicotinic ganglion blocking effect of d-tubocurarine easily demonstrable in the cat (Fig 4) (or dog).[11,39]

Vagal blockade by d-tubocurarine occurs at parasympathetic ganglia. The bradycardic response to direct muscarinic receptor activators such as methacholine is not inhibited, but the bradycardia produced by stimulation of the vagus nerve is prevented.[11,39] In the absence of histamine release, d-tubocurarine does not generally produce clinically important changes in heart rate, although it probably favors a slight bradycardia during maintenance of anesthesia. The histamine releasing, and to a lesser extent the ganglion blocking, action of d-tubocurarine produce a fall in peripheral resistance.[40] If no

Table 3
Effects of 100% Blocking Dose of Nondepolarizing Muscle Relaxants in Humans Under Halothane Anesthesia

				Under Anesthesia			
Drug	Ganglion Block	(Muscarinic) Vagal Block	Histamine Release	SVR	CO	BP	HR
Tubocurarine	**	—	***	↓	↓	↓	—
Metocurine	*	—	**	↓	—	↓	—
Pancuronium	—	**	—	—	↑	↑	↑
Gallamine	—	***	—	—	↑	↑	↑
Alcuronium	*	*	—	↓	↑	↓	↑
Fazadinium	**	**	—	↓	↑	↓	↑
Vecuronium	—	—	—	—	—	—	—
Atracurium	—	—	—	—	—	—	—

Abbreviations: SVR = systemic vascular resistance; CO = cardiac output; BP = blood pressure (mean arterial pressure); HR = heart rate.

One asterisk (*) = mild; two asterisks (**) = moderate; three asterisks (***) = major.

important change in heart rate occurs, the cardiac output may fall, particularly in the presence of an anesthetic technique that includes a mild cardiac depressant anesthetic vapor.

In the absence of significant myocardial depression, ie, under nitrous oxide-narcotic anesthesia, stroke volume may increase due to improved ventricular emptying, and there may be little or no fall in cardiac output despite the occurrence of moderate hypotension.[41]

A negative inotropic action of d-tubocurarine originally attributed to the preservative[42] has been disproved.[43]

Metocurine

Metocurine may also block sympathetic and parasympathetic ganglia in the same manner as its parent compound, d-tubocurarine.[39] It is, however, approximately three times less potent than d-tubocurarine in this respect.[39] It is also a more potent neuromuscular blocking agent than d-tubocurarine, so that its neuromuscular blocking action is separated by a wide dose range from its autonomic effects.[11] In the dog, only at eight times the ED_{95}, did metocurine produce hemodynamic changes similar to those observed with d-tubocurarine at ED_{95}. The safety margin in the dog is eight times greater.[45]

Brief (5 to 15 minutes) increases in heart rate may result when large bolus doses of metocurine (0.4 mg/kg or more) are given rapidly. Heart rate increases in this situation are probably manifestations of systemic histamine release by this drug.

In the absence of histamine release, metocurine does not produce clinically important changes in heart rate, although a slight bradycardia may occur during maintenance of anesthesia.

Metocurine may also produce clinical hypotension, but the incidence and severity of this side effect are probably much less than in the case of d-tubocurarine.[46] In healthy patients under nitrous oxide-narcotic anesthesia,

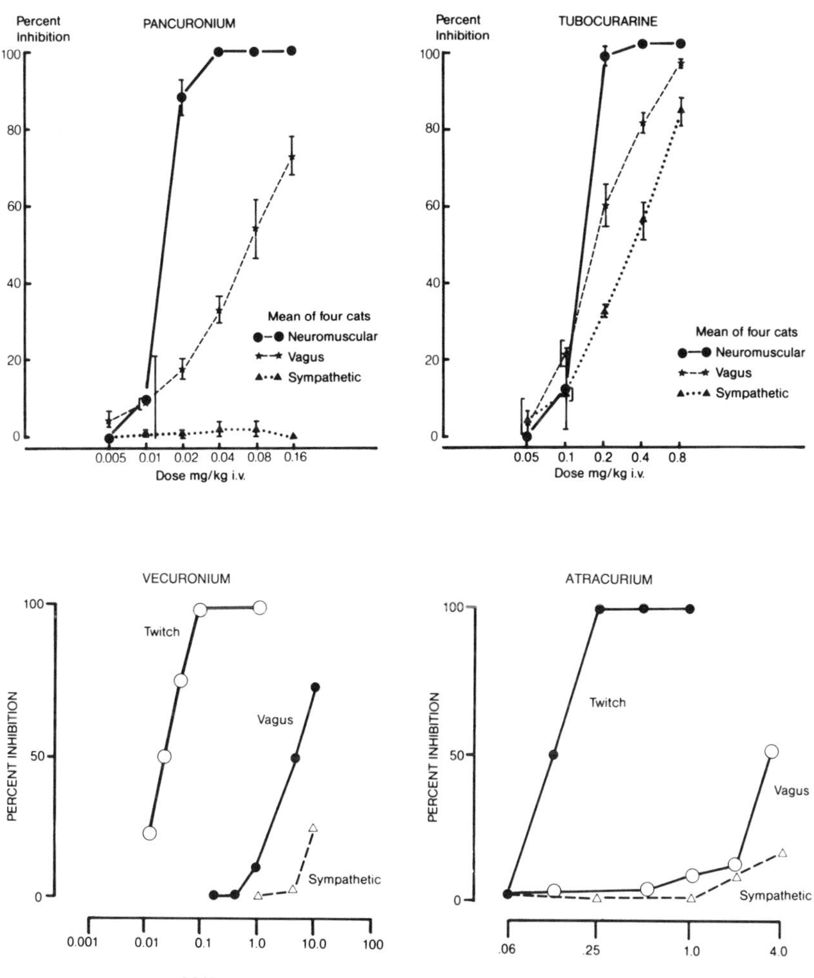

Figure 5. Dose-response curves for neuromuscular and autonomic function inhibition in cats following pancuronium, tubocurarine, and vecuronium, and in monkeys following atracurium. Note that vecuronium and atracurium cause insignificant autonomic inhibition at doses considerably in excess of that required to produce 100% depression of the single twitch. (Data modified from Durant et al[103] and from Hughes et al.[11,25,80])

metocurine 0.4 mg/kg given as a rapid bolus produced an average 7% fall in mean arterial pressure.[46] This hypotensive effect was considered to be due to histamine release in 33% of those who received this high dose (an amount more than adequate for tracheal intubation).[46] When administered more slowly[47] and to sicker patients[48] in other studies, significant cardiovascular changes have not been noted.

There is little change in cardiac output in normal humans under halothane anesthesia[102] when doses of 0.2 mg/kg are administered.

Pancuronium

The possible cardiac actions of pancuronium have already been outlined. Pancuronium has an atropine-like effect that is limited to cardiac muscarinic receptors.[10,11] Experimentally, bradycardia due to vagal stimulation or secondary to acetylcholine or methacholine are blocked (Fig 5).

Increased serum catecholamine levels in humans have been measured after administration of pancuronium.[49] Repetitive doses of pancuronium bromide 0.2 mg/kg in the dog produce a vasopressor effect that undergoes rapid tachyphylaxis and is restored by noradrenaline infusion. The restorative effect by noradrenaline was prevented by treatment with an adrenergic neurone pump inhibitor. Furthermore, treatment with catecholamine-depleting agents guanethidine and reserpine eliminated the vasopressor response. These data suggest a tyramine-like release of catecholamines at adrenergic nerve endings by pancuronium, ie, an indirect sympathomimetic effect.

Workers have also noted an inhibition of neuronal uptake of noradrenaline by pancuronium in the rat.[21]

In humans, pancuronium increases heart rate principally by blocking vagal muscarinic receptors in the sinus node.[50,11] Its indirect sympathomimetic effect is probably less important. In support of this theory, atropine prophylaxis has been found to reduce pancuronium-induced tachycardia.[51]

Pancuronium generally produces less dramatic increases in heart rate[51,52] than gallamine and the tachycardia has not been shown to be dose dependent in humans but inversely related to the control heart rate.[51] The vagolytic effect of pancuronium is probably weak within the dose range required for clinical neuromuscular blockade and usually results in heart rates of 70 to 90 beats per minute in the average patient. Marked tachycardia may occur in a small percentage of patients. This unexpected response may be due to its indirect sympathomimetic action.

A rise in arterial pressure of 10 to 20 mm Hg following the administration of pancuronium is common,[40] particularly under nitrous oxide in the absence of potent anesthetic vapors. The increased heart rate resulting in an increased cardiac output in the absence of any fall in peripheral resistance is the probable mechanism involved. Some workers have suggested that pancuronium has a weak inotropic effect on cardiac muscle.[53] However, other studies using dog models showed no direct influence on cardiac contractility, the increases in left ventricular dp/dt max and the cardiac output following pancuronium being dependent on heart rate.[54]

As a consequence of a 25% average increase in heart rate, Kelman and Kennedy noted a mean 8.6% increase in cardiac output in patients under nitrous oxide-phenoperidine anesthesia.[52] The control heart rate in a series of ten patients averaged 57 beats per minute. A similar change in hemodynamics with less percentage increases in heart rate was recorded by Stoelting in patients under halothane.[40]

Gallamine

Gallamine's atropine-like effect is limited to the cardiac muscarinic receptors.[9] Experimentally, both vagal-induced bradycardia and bradycardia secondary to acetylcholine or methacholine are blocked.[11] Its indirect sympathomimetic effects are probably less important than its vagolytic effect.

The tachycardia caused by gallamine has been shown to be dose dependent, reaching a maximum at approximately 1 mg/kg.[55,56] Nearly 100% increases in heart rate may occur if the patient's baseline heart rate is slow to begin with (in the range of 50 to 60 beats per minute). Gallamine probably does not produce complete vagal blockade at this dose or at higher doses since atropine, given after maximum gallamine-induced tachycardia has been obtained, will produce a further small increase in heart rate.[55] Gallamine-induced tachycardia generally persists beyond the neuromuscular blocking action such that decreased heart rate when gallamine is being used for operative relaxation has been used as a reliable indicator of diminishing neuromuscular blockade.[57]

As a result of the increased heart rate, a rise in arterial pressure of 10 to 20 mm Hg is common, particularly under nitrous oxide anesthesia in the absence of potent anesthetic vapors.[56]

Tachycardia without any important change in peripheral resistance leads to increased cardiac output when the drug is given to normal humans. Cardiac output increases are in the range of 25% to 50% after 0.5 to 2 mg/kg and tend to be greater under nitrous oxide-narcotic anesthesia than under halothane.[56] The release of catecholamines in the heart by this drug may contribute slightly to its effect on cardiac output.[18]

Alcuronium

Alcuronium has a weak ganglion blocking action and a relatively weak vagolytic effect that occurs at muscarinic receptors.[11,58] This weak vagolytic effect may produce slight increases in heart rate most notably when the baseline heart rate is slow.[11,59] Kennedy and Kelman,[60] for example, found a 9% increase in heart rate after 0.15 mg/kg of alcuronium was given to patients under nitrous oxide-phenoperidine anesthesia. Alcuronium has been implicated as a cause of hypotension when large doses are given to humans,[61–63] most notably in relatively ill patients.[62] This hypotensive effect may be due to the ganglion blocking action since histamine release by alcuronium has been reported only once. Other studies have found that alcuronium has little effect on arterial pressure.[60,65]

Fazadinium

Fazadinium has strong muscarinic, vagolytic, and ganglion blocking properties that occur closer to the neuromuscular blocking dose range than those of alcuronium[5,11,66] These properties combine to produce a fall in peripheral resistance and an increase in cardiac output. A modest dose less than necessary for intubation, 0.5 mg/kg, produced a 41% increase in cardiac output and a 28% fall in peripheral resistance in a group of patients under phenoperidine-nitrous oxide anesthesia.[67]

Succinylcholine

Succinylcholine stimulates both autonomic ganglia and muscarinic receptors,[7] mimicking the action of acetylcholine at these sites.

The most common change in heart rate after the administration of succinylcholine is an increase most notably in adults given small doses of atropine as premedication.[68–70] The mechanism in this case is stimulation of autonomic ganglia manifested as tachycardia because the vagal result of ganglionic stimulation, bradycardia, is prevented by atropine.

Sinus bradycardia occurs most commonly in nonatropinized relatively sympathotonic individuals[71] (eg, children) and is due to stimulation of cardiac muscarinic receptors in the sinus node. Sinus bradycardia has also been noted in adults and appears more commonly after a second dose when the drug is given approximately five minutes after the first.[72,73] It has been suggested that the higher incidence of bradycardia after a second dose of succinylcholine[74] may be due to the hydrolysis products of succinylcholine (succinylmonocholine and choline) sensitizing the heart. Thiopental, atropine, ganglion blocking drugs, and nondepolarizing relaxants have all been used to prevent the bradycardia.

Many authors have reported increased arterial pressure secondary to succinylcholine administration particularly during prolonged infusion from maintenance and relaxation.[7] This may represent a clinical manifestation of its ganglion stimulating action.

Vecuronium

Since the early studies on the pancuronium series, the importance of cardiovascular side effects among neuromuscular blocking agents has been apparent. Vecuronium was selected for study from a series of analogs on the grounds that it was the compound most likely to be capable of producing neuromuscular blockade without concomitant side effects.

Results obtained in anesthetized cats and dogs (Fig 5) have demonstrated that vecuronium even in doses 20 times greater than those required for neuromuscular blockade has no effect on heart rate, arterial pressure, autonomic ganglia, α- or β-adrenal receptor or baroreceptor reflex activity.[75,76] Studies in pithed rats and guinea pig atria have further shown that vecuronium has little effect on cardiac muscarinic receptors or on noradrenaline reuptake mechanisms.[75]

In both experimental animals and in humans, it has shown minimal potential for histamine release.[77,78]

Eighteen adult patients under nitrous oxide-narcotic anesthesia demonstrated no significant change in heart rate or arterial pressure with doses of vecuronium up to 150 μg/kg, which is three times the 95% blocking dose.[78]

Equipotent doses of pancuronium and vecuronium were compared in 20 patients receiving halothane anesthesia. Pancuronium 0.08 mg/kg caused a significant increase in heart rate, an insignificant change in arterial pressure, and significant changes in systolic time intervals. The equipotent dose of vecuronium 0.057 mg/kg caused no significant changes in heart rate, arterial pressure, or systolic time interval.[79]

Atracurium

Dose-response curves for atracurium obtained from results in anesthetized cats, dogs, and rhesus monkeys (Fig 5) demonstrate that there is a wide separation between the doses required for neuromuscular paralysis and those that inhibit autonomic mechanisms.[76,80]

In cats, significant hypotension and slight bradycardia were evident after 4 mg/kg intravenously (IV), but this dose was 16 times that required for full neuromuscular paralysis. Similar results were found in rhesus monkeys. In dogs, atracurium 2 mg/kg reduced mean arterial pressure to 53% of the control value, but this dose was eight times that required for full neuromuscular paralysis. Atracurium at high concentrations had no inotropic or chronotropic effects on spontaneously beating guinea pig atria.

In humans anesthetized with nitrous oxide and enflurane, there was no significant change in heart rate, mean aterial pressure, right atrial pressure, or cardiac output following administration of 0.2 or 0.4 mg/kg of atracurium.[44]

In one study, a patient with coronary artery disease produced a typical histamine response at 0.3 mg/kg with marked cardiovascular changes.[81]

In humans under nitrous oxide-narcotic anesthesia, mean arterial pressure and heart rate showed no significant changes from control values until a dose of 0.6 mg/kg, double the full paralyzing dose.[82] Maximum heart rate and arterial pressure changes occurred one to two minutes after drug injection and returned to normal within approximately five minutes. These changes have been shown to be due to a dose-dependent release of histamine, and the increase in plasma histamine levels correlate with the heart rate and arterial pressure changes. These changes can be abolished by either slowing the rate of injection of atracurium to 75 seconds or by IV pretreatment with H_1 and H_2 blockers (chloropheniramine and cimetidine).[83]

Pipecuronium

Pipecuronium is a pancuronium analog[84] that is about 20% more potent than the parent compound.[85] Pipecuronium does not cause a tachycardia as does pancuronium, and in patients undergoing abdominal surgery, there was no significant change in BP, central venous pressure, pulmonary artery pressure, pulmonary artery wedge pressure, or cardiac index.[86]

RGH 4201

RGH 4201 (duador) has about half the duration of pancuronium. In animal experiments, there was a significant vagolytic effect. It also causes a significant increase in heart rate in humans.[87]

BWA 444U

BWA 444U is a benzylisoquinolium ester compound like atracurium but is metabolized by plasma cholinesterase. Its margin of safety for histamine release was less than that of atracurium so it has been withdrawn from further studies.[88]

BW 785U

BW 785U[34] is another drug in a series of ester compounds metabolized by plasma cholinesterase. It is a nondepolarizing agent with a rapid onset and short duration of action. Like d-tubocurarine, it produces a dose-related increase in plasma histamine. The associated increase in heart rate and reduction in BP occur within the neuromuscular blocking dose range.

BW 938U

BW 938U is a highly potent noncumulative, nondepolarizing ester with a wide cardiovascular/autonomic safety margin and an intermediate to long duration of action.

EFFECTS ON CARDIAC RHYTHM

Nondepolarizing Agents

The nondepolarizing agents generally do not in themselves produce cardiac dysrhythmias. In fact, there is evidence that d-tubocurarine increases the dose threshold for the production of epinephrine-induced arrhythmias in dogs under halothane[89] and nitrous oxide.[90]

Arrhythmias after administration of pancuronium or gallamine may occur as a result of (1) a sudden shift of autonomic balance toward the adrenergic side due to the vagal blocking effect of these drugs; (2) a possible indirect sympathomimetic effect, and (3) a relatively greater inhibition of the atrioventricular node than the sinus node.

These mechanisms may manifest themselves clinically as unifocal or multifocal premature ventricular contractions, ventricular tachycardia, or nodal (junctional) tachycardia. In the case of gallamine, junctional tachycardia may arise in patients with sinus node disease, the vagolytic effect causing a relatively greater increase in the spontaneous rate of activity of the atrioventricular node than the sinus node.

Succininylcholine

Succinylcholine is probably the only neuromuscular blocking agent that may itself precipitate cardiac dysrhythmias in humans under anesthesia. Succinylcholine stimulates all cholinergic autonomic receptors, nicotinic receptors in both sympathetic and parasympathetic ganglia, and muscarinic receptors in the sinus node of the heart. The development of cardiac dysrhythmias is a clinical manifestation of this generalized autonomic stimulation. Sinus bradycardia, junctional rhythms, and ventricular dysrhythmias ranging from unifocal premature ventricular contractions to ventricular fibrillation in special circumstances have all been well documented. However, many authors of clinical studies have noted these dysrhythmias in the presence of the intense autonomic stimulus of tracheal intubation, and it is not always entirely clear whether the cardiac irregularities are due to the action of succinylcholine alone or to the added presence of extraneous autonomic stimulation.

Nodal rhythms commonly occur as bradycardias and are probably due to the relatively greater stimulation of the sinus node than the atrioventricular node, the result being suppression of the sinus mechanism and emergence of atrioventricular node as the pacemaker. The incidence of junctional rhythm is higher[72,91] after a second dose of succinylcholine but can be prevented by prior administration of d-tubocurarine.[92]

Succinylcholine lowers the threshold of the ventricle to catecholamine-induced arrhythmias in the monkey[93] and the dog[89] under stable anesthetic conditions. Other autonomic stimuli such as endotracheal intubation, hypoxia, hypercarbia, and surgery are probably additive to the effect of succinylcholine and may provoke ectopic activity.

Ventricular escape beats may also occur after severe sinus and atrioventricular nodal slowing secondary to succinylcholine administration.

The depolarizing nature of the drug causes ventricular dysrhythmias by releasing potassium from skeletal muscle.[93] The rise in potassium in normal people following 1-mg/kg doses of the drug is about 0.5 mEq. However, greater increases may occur within one to two minutes of succinylcholine administration in the following groups: (1) burned patients[91]; (2) patients with extensive denervation of skeletal muscle due to injury or disease of the CNS[73]; (3) massively traumatized patients[94]; and (4) patients with severe intra-abdominal infection.[95] The period of danger usually begins within a few days in the burned and denervated patient and within a few hours in the traumatized patient. Studies in babboons[96] have shown that hyperkalemia following surgical denervation begins as early as four days after the establishment of the lesion and reaches a peak within 14 days. Patients at least 6 months past complete healing of burns are probably not at risk, nor are uremic patients.[97] Studies in dogs have suggested that patients with immobilization atrophy may not exhibit the hyperkalemic response.[98]

The use of succinylcholine is probably contraindicated in these various groups.

A modest dose of nondepolarizing relaxant (6 mg of d-tubocurarine, 40 mg of gallamine, 3 mg of metocurine, or 1 mg of pancuronium) administered three minutes before succinylcholine may attenuate but will not guarantee the absence of the hyperkalemic response, and thus choosing another relaxant is preferred.

DRUG INTERACTIONS WITH CARDIOVASCULAR EFFECTS

Succinylcholine lowers the threshold of the ventricle to catecholamine-induced arrhythmias. To this must be added the possible influence of drugs such as digitalis, tricyclic antidepressants, monoamineoxidase inhibitors, catecholamines, and anesthetic drugs such as halothane and cyclopropane, all of which may lower the ventricular threshold for ectopic activity or increase the arrhythmogenic effect of the catecholamines.

The nondepolarizing agents may also produce cardiovascular effects upon interaction with other drugs. A study in dogs[99] has shown that administration of pancuronium and imipramine may cause a tachycardia in an additive manner. The 80-μg/kg dose of pancuronium produced premature ventricular contractions and ventricular tachycardia that rapidly progressed to ventricular fibrillation in two of the ten dogs given imipramine 8 mg/kg/d and in four of the ten dogs given 16 mg/kg/d. The authors concluded that severe ventricular arrhthymias may occur as a result of administration of pancuronium in dogs anesthetized with halothane and receiving imipramine chronically.

In another study,[100] neither pancuronium nor d-tubocurarine affected the arrhythmogenic dose of adrenaline during halothane anesthesia in dogs. These findings indicate that the usual guidelines for the administration of adrenaline during halothane anesthesia are not affected by concomitant administration of these two nondepolarizing muscle relaxants. Gallamine and d-tubocurarine may decrease the incidence of epinephrine-induced arrhthymias as compared with succinylcholine, which may enhance adrenaline effects.

Occasionally, drug interactions may be advantageous. Combinations of pancuronium and metocurine not only potentiate neuromuscular blockade[101] but also minimize the heart rate change associated with pancuronium alone. At twice the ED_{95}, the heart rate increased significantly more in the pancuronium group than in the metocurine-pancuronium combination group.

REFERENCES

1. Guyton AC, Reeder RC: Quantitative studies on autonomic actions of curare. J Pharmacol Exp Ther 98:188, 1950
2. Burstein CL, Jackson A, Bishop HF, et al: Curare in the management of autonomic reflexes. Anesthesiology 11:409, 1950
3. McDowell SA, Clarke RSJ: A clinical comparison of pancuronium with d-tubocurarine. Anaesthesia 24:581, 1969
4. Moss J, Philbin DM, Rosow CE, et al: Histamine release by neuromuscular blocking agents in man. Klin Wochenschr 60:891–95, 1982
5. Marshall IG: The ganglion blocking and vagolytic actions of three short-acting neuromuscular blocking drugs in the cat. J Pharm Pharmacol 25:530, 1973
6. Blogg CE, Savege TM, Simpson JC, et al: A new muscle relaxant—AH 8165. Proc R Soc Med 66:1023, 1973
7. Paton WDM: The effects of muscle relaxants other than muscle relaxation. Anesthesiology 20:453, 1959
8. Birdsall NJM, Hulme EC: Biochemical studies on the muscarinic acetylcholine receptor. J Neurochem 27:7, 1976
9. Riker WF, Wescoe WC: The pharmacology of flaxedil with observations on certain analogs. Ann NY Acad Sci 54:573, 1951
10. Saxena PR, Benta IL: Mechanism of selective cardiac vagolytic action of pancuronium bromide. Specific blockade of cardiac muscarinic receptors. Eur J Pharmacol 11:332, 1970
11. Hughes R, Chapple DJ: Effects of non-depolarizing neuromuscular blocking agents on peripheral autonomic mechanisms in cats. Br J Anaesth 48:59, 1976

12. Li CK, Mitchelson F: The effects of stercuronium on cardiac muscarinic receptors. Eur J Pharmacol 51:251, 1978
13. Loffelholz K, Muscholl E: Inhibition of parasympathetic nerve stimulation of the release of adrenergic transmitter. Naunyn Schmiedebergs Arch Pharmacol 267:181, 1970
14. Vercruysse P, Bossuyt P, Hanegreefs G, et al: Gallamine and pancuronium inhibit pre-junctional and post-junctional muscarinic receptors in canine saphenous veins. J Pharmacol Exp Ther 209:225, 1979
15. Greengard P, Kebabian JW: Role of cyclic AMP in synaptic transmission in the mammalian peripheral nervous system. Fed Proc 33:1059, 1974
16. Gardier RW, Tsevdos EJ, Jackson DB, et al: Distinct muscarinic mediation of suspected dopaminergic activity in sympathetic ganglia. Fed Proc 37:2422, 1978
17. Marshall RJ: A new muscarinic agent: 1, 4, 5, 6-tetrahydro-5-phenoxy pyrimidine (AH 6405). Br J Pharmacol 39:191P, 1970
18. Brown BR, Crout JR: The sympathomimetic effect of gallamine on the heart. J Pharmacol Exp Ther 172:266, 1970
19. Marshall RJ, Ojewole JAO: Comparison of autonomic effects of some currently used neuromuscular blocking agents. Br J Pharmacol 66:77P, 1979
20. Quintana A: Effect of pancuronium bromide on the adrenergic reactivity of the isolated rat vas deferens. Eur J Pharmacol 46:275, 1977
21. Salt PJ, Barnes PK, Conway CM: Inhibition of neuronal uptake of noradrenalin in the isolated perfused rat heart by pancuronium and its homologues ORG 6368, ORG 7268 and ORG NC45. Br J Anaesth 52:313, 1980
22. Lee Son S, Waud BE: Effects of nondepolarizing neuromuscular blocking agents on the cardiac vagus nerve in the guinea pig. Br J Anaesth 52:981, 1980
23. Paton WDM, Zaimis EJ: Methonium compounds. Pharmacol Rev 4:219, 1952
24. Everett AJ, Cowe LA, Wilkonson S: Revision of the structures of (+) tubocurarine chloride and (+) chondrocurine. Chem Commun 1020–1021, 1970
25. Hughes R, Chapple DJ: Cardiovascular and neuromuscular effects of dimethyltubocurarine in anaesthetized cats and rhesus monkeys. Br J Anaesth 48:847, 1976
26. Paton WDM: Histamine release by compounds of single chemical structure. Pharmacol Rev 9:269, 1957
27. Buckett WR, Frisk-Holmberg: The use of neuromuscular blocking agents to investigate receptor structure requirements for histamine release. Br J Pharmacol 40:165, 1970
28. Beavan MA, Horakova Z: in Silva MR (ed): Handbook of Experimental Pharmacology, vol 18. Berlin, Springer-Verlag, 1978, pp 151
29. Snyder SH, Baldasserarini R, Axelrod J: A sensitive and specific isotope assay for tissue histamine. J Pharmacol Exp Ther 153:544, 1966
30. Iverson U, Iverson SD, Snyder SH: Handbook of Psychopharmacology. New York, Plenum, 1979, p 253
31. Beavan MA, Jacobsen S, Horakova Z: Modification of the enzymatic isotope assay of histamine and its application to measurement of histamine in tissues, serum and urine. Clin Chem Acta 37:91, 1972
32. Moss J, Philbin DM, Rosow CE, et al: Histamine release by neuromuscular blocking agents in man. Klin Wochenschr 60:891, 1982
33. Basta SJ, Savarese JJ, Ali HH, et al: Histamine releasing potencies of atracurium, di-methyltubocurarine, and tubocurarine. Br J Anaesth 55:105S, 1983
34. Rosow CE, Basta SJ, Savarese JJ, et al: BW 785U: Correlation of cardiovascular effects with increases in plasma histamine. Anesthesiology 53:S270, 1980
35. Basta SJ, Moss J, Savarese JJ, et al: Cardiovascular effects of BW A444U: Correlation with plasma histamine levels. Anesthesiology 50:A198, 1981
36. Lorenz W, Doenicke A: Histamine release in clinical conditions. Mt Sinai J Med 45:357, 1978

37. Lorenz W, Doenicke A, Schoning B, et al: Histamine release: H1 and H2 receptor antagonists for pre-medication in anaesthesia and surgery: A critical view based on randomised clinical trials with haemaccel and various anti-allergic drugs. Agents Actions 10:114, 1980
38. Philbin DM, Moss J, Rosow CE, et al: The use of H1 and H2 blockers with morphine: A double blind study. Anesthesiology 53:S67, 1980
39. Savarese JJ: The autonomic margin of safety of metocurine and d-tubocurarine. Abstracts of scientific papers, ASA Annual Meeting, San Francisco, 1976, pp 393–394
40. Stoelting RK: The hemodynamic effects of pancuronium and d-tubocurarine in anaesthetized patients. Anesthesiology 39:645, 1973
41. Antonio RP: Unpublished data, 1977
42. Dowdy EG, Holland WC, Yamanaka I: Cardioactive properties of d-tubocurarine with and without preservatives. Anesthesiology 34:256, 1971
43. Stoelting RK: Blood pressure responses to d-tubocurarine and its preservatives in anesthetized patients. Anesthesiology 35:315, 1971
44. Hilgenberg JC, Stoelting RK, Harris WA: Hemodynamic effects of atracurium during enflurane-nitrous oxide anesthesia. Br J Anaesth 55:82S, 1983
45. Antonio RP, Philbin DM, Savarese JJ: Comparative hemodynamic effects of d-tubocurarine and metocurine in the dog. Anesthesiology 51:S281, 1979
46. Savarese JJ, Ali HH, Antonio RP: The clinical pharmacology of metocurine: Dimethyltubocurarine revisited. Anesthesiology 47:277, 1977
47. Hughes R, Ingram G, Payne JP: Studies on di-methyltubocurarine in anesthetized man. Br J Anaesth 48:969, 1976
48. Zaidan J, Philbin DM, Antonio RP: Haemodynamic effects of metocurine in patients with coronary artery disease receiving propranolol. Anesth Analg 56:255, 1977
49. Nana A, Cardan E, Domokos M: Blood catecholamine changes after pancuronium. Acta Anaesthesiol Scand 17:83, 1973
50. Walts LF, McFarland W: Effect of vagolytic agents on ventricular rhythm during cyclopropane anesthesia. Anesth Analg 44:429, 1965
51. Miller RD, Eger EI II, Stevens WC: Pancuronium-induced tachycardia in relation to alveolar halothane, dose of pancuronium and prior atropine. Anesthesiology 42:352, 1975
52. Kelman GR, Kennedy BR: Cardiovascular effects of pancuronium in man. Br J Anaesth 43:335, 1968
53. Demenech SJ, Garcia CR, Sasian RJM: Pancuronium bromide: An indirect sympathomimetic agent. Br J Anaesth 48:1143, 1976
54. Fitzal S, Gilly H, Ilias W: Comparative investigation on the cardiovascular effects of ORG NC45 and pancuronium in dogs. Br J Anaesth 55:641–646, 1983
55. Eisele JH, Marta JA, Davis HS: Quantitative aspects of the chronotropy and neuromuscular effects of gallamine in anesthetized man. Anesthesiology 35:630, 1971
56. Stoelting RK: Hemodynamic effects of gallamine during halothane-nitrous oxide anesthesia. Anesthesiology 39:645, 1973
57. Longnecker DE, Stoelting RK, Morrow AG: Cardiac and peripheral vascular effects of gallamine in man. Anesth Analg 52:931, 1973
58. Waser PG, Harbeck P: Pharmacologie und klinishe anwendung des kurzduernden muscelrelaxans diallyl-nor-toxiferin. Anaesthesist 11:33, 1962
59. Savarese JJ: The autonomic margin of safety of alcuronium and pancuronium. Anesthesiology (in press)
60. Kennedy Br, Kelman GR: Cardiovascular effects of alcuronium in man. Br J Anaesth 42:625, 1970
61. Baraka A: A comparative study between diallyl nortoxiferine and tubocurarine. Br J Anaesth 39:624, 1967

62. Harrison GA: The cardiovascular effects and some relaxant properties of four relaxants in patients about to undergo cardiac surgery. Br J Anaesth 44:485, 1972
63. Hunter AR: Diallyl toxiferine. Br J Anaesth 36:466, 1964
64. Chan CS, Yeung ML: Anaphylactic reaction to alcuronium. Br J Anaesth 44:103, 1972
65. Foldes FF, Brown IM, Lunn JN: The neuromuscular effects of diallyl-nortoxiferine in anesthetized subjects. Anesth Analg 42:177, 1963
66. Brittian RT, Tyers MB: The pharmacology of AH 8165, a rapid acting, short lasting, competitive neuromuscular blocking drug. Br J Anaesth 45:837, 1973
67. Savege TM, Blogg CE, Ross L: The cardiovascular effects of AH 8165. Anaesthesia 28:253, 1973
68. Barreto RS: Effect of intravenously administered succinylcholine upon cardiac rate and rhythm. Anesthesiology 21:401, 1960
69. Lupprian KG, Churchill-Davidson HC: Effect of suxamethonium on cardiac rhythm. Br Med J 2:1174, 1960
70. Perez HR: Cardiac arrhythmias after succinylcholine. Anesth Analg 49:33, 1970
71. Leigh MD, McCoy DD, Belton KM: Bradycardia following intravenous administration of succinylcholine chloride to infants and children. Anesthesiology 18:698, 1957
72. List WFM: Succinylcholine-induced cardiac arrhythmia. Anesth Analg 50:361, 1971
73. Cooperman LH: Succinylcholine-induced hyperkalemia in neuromuscular disease. JAMA 213:1867, 1970
74. Schoenstadt DA, Whitcher CE: Observation on the mechanism of succinylcholine-induced cardiac arrhythmia. Anesthesiology 24:358, 1963
75. Marshall RJ, McGrath TC, Miller RD, et al: Comparison of the cardiovascular actions ORG NC45 with those produced by other nondepolarizing neuromuscular blocking agents in experimental animals. Br J Anaesth 52:21S, 1980
76. Sutherland GA, Squire IB, Gibb AJ, et al: Neuromuscular blocking and autonomic effects of vecuronium and atracurium in the anaesthetized cat. Br J Anaesth 55:1119–1126, 1983
77. Marshall IG, Agoston S, Booij LHDJ, et al: Pharmacology of ORG NC45 compared with other non-depolarizing neuromuscular blocking drugs. Br J Anaesth 52:11S, 1980
78. Crul JF, Booij LHDJ: First clinical experiences with ORG NC45. Br J Anaesth 52:49S, 1980
79. Engbaek J, Ording H, Sorensen B, et al: Cardiac effects of vecuronium and pancuronium during halothane anaesthesia. Br J Anaesth 55:501–505, 1983
80. Hughes R, Chapple DJ: The pharmacology of atracurium, a new competitive neuromuscular blocking agent. Br J Anaesth 53:31, 1981
81. Philbin DM, Machaj VR, Tomichek RC, et al: Hemodynamic effects of bolus injection of atracurium in patients with coronary artery disease. Br J Anaesth 55:131S, 1983
82. Basta SJ, Savarese JJ, Ali HH, et al: Histamine-releasing potency of atracurium, di-methyltubocurarine and tubocurarine. Br J Anaesth 55:105S, 1983
83. Scott RPF, Savarese JJ: Atracurium: Clinical strategies for preventing histamine release and attenuating the hemodynamic response. Anesthesiology 61:A287, 1984
Orleans, 1984 (in press)
84. Newton DEF, Richardson FJ, Rashkovsky DM, et al: Clinical neuromuscular blocking and cardiovascular effects of pipecuronium bromide. Volume of summaries, Sixth European Congress of Anesthesiologists, paper 538
85. Vimlati L, Tassonyi E: Circulatory effects of pipecuronium bromide, a new steroid muscle relaxant agent in humans. Volume of summaries, Sixth European Congress of Anesthesiologists, London, 1983, paper 339
86. Szenohradszky J, Marosi G, Kertesz A, et al: Clinical experience with pipecuronium bromide. Volume of summaries, Sixth European Congress of Anesthesiologists, London, 1983, paper 67
87. Boros M, Szenohradszky J, Marosi G, et al: Volume of summaries, Sixth European Congress of Anesthesiologists, London, 1983, paper 68

88. Savarese JJ, Ali HH, Basta SJ, et al: The clinical pharmacology of BWA 444U. Anesthesiology 58:333–341, 1983
89. Tucker WA, Munson ES: Effects of succinylcholine and d-tubocurarine on epinephrine-induced arrhythmias during halothane anesthesia in dogs. Anesthesiology 42:41, 1975
90. Wong KC, Wyte SR, Martin WE: Anti-arrhythmic effects of skeletal muscle relaxants. Anesthesiology 34:458, 1971
91. Bush GH, Graham HAP, Littlewood ANM: Danger of suxamethonium and endotracheal intubation in anaesthesia for burns. Br Med J 2:1081, 1962
92. Mathias JA, Evans-Prosser CDG, Churchill-Davidson HC: The role of nondepolarizing drugs in the prevention of suxamethonium bradycardia. Br J Anaesth 42:609, 1970
93. Bali IM, Dundee JW, Daggart JR: The source of increased plasma potassium following succinylcholine. Anesth Analg 54:680, 1975
94. Mazze RI, Escue HM, Houston JB: Hyperkalemia and cardiovascular collapse following succinylcholine injection in the traumatized patient. Anesthesiology 33:328, 1970
95. Kohlschutter B, Baur H, Roth F: Suxamethonium induced hyperkalemia in patients with severe intra-abdominal infection. Br J Anaesth 48:557, 1976
96. John DA, Tobey RE, Homer LD: Onset of succinylcholine-induced hyperkalemia following denervation. Anesthesiology 45:294, 1976
97. Koide M, Waud BE: Serum potassium concentrations after succinylcholine in patients with renal failure. Anesthesiology 36:142, 1972
98. Gronert GA, Theye RA: Effect of succinylcholine on skeletal muscle with immobilization atrophy. Anesthesiology 40:268, 1974
99. Edwards RP, Miller RD, Roizen MF: Cardiac responses to imipramine and pancuronium during anesthesia with halothane or enflurane. Anesthesiology 50:421–425, 1979
100. Schick LM, Chapin JC, Muson ES: Pancuronium, d-tubocurarine and epinephrine induced arrhythmias during halothane anesthesia in dogs. Anesthesiology 52:207–209, 1980
101. Lebowitz PW, Ramsey FM, Savarese JJ, et al: Potentiation of neuromuscular blockade in man produced by combination of pancuronium and metocurine or pancuronium and d-tubocurarine. Anesth Analg 59:604, 1980
102. Stoelting RK: Hemodynamic effects of di-methyl-tubocurarine during nitrous oxide-halothane anesthesia. Anesth Analg 53:513, 1974
103. Durant NN, Marshall IG, Savage DS, et al: The neuromuscular and autonomic blocking activities of pancuronium, ORG NC45, and other pancuronium analogues in the cat. J Pharm Pharmacol 31:831–836, 1979

Robert K. Stoelting

9

Choice of Muscle Relaxants in Patients With Heart Disease

Choice of a muscle relaxant (neuromuscular blocker) for patients with heart disease is determined by the likely circulatory effects that will be evoked by these drugs. Knowledge of these circulatory effects permits the anesthesiologist to logically select the muscle relaxant in an attempt to produce desirable drug interactions between the muscle relaxant and the known pathophysiology of the underlying heart disease. In many instances, administration of a muscle relaxant with minimal circulatory effects is considered ideal. Conversely, in some patients, the circulatory effects of muscle relaxants can be used in an attempt to improve stroke volume via drug-induced changes in heart rate and/or systemic vascular resistance.

CIRCULATORY EFFECTS OF MUSCLE RELAXANTS

Circulatory effects of muscle relaxants may reflect (1) stimulation or inhibition of peripheral autonomic nervous system activity; (2) release of histamine from mast cells; and/or (3) changes in the serum potassium concentration secondary to prolonged depolarization of the neuromuscular junction (Fig 1).[1–3] Circulatory changes that may occur as a result of these mechanisms acting alone or in combination include alteration of (1) systemic vascular resistance, (2) venous capacitance, (3) myocardial contractility, (4) heart rate, and (5) cardiac rhythm.

MUSCLE RELAXANTS
ISBN 0-8089-1784-6

Peripheral Autonomic Nervous System

Many of the circulatory effects of muscle relaxants can be explained on the basis of stimulation or inhibition of nicotinic and/or muscarinic cholinergic receptors in the peripheral autonomic nervous system. An important concept is that depolarizing muscle relaxants like succinylcholine mimic the

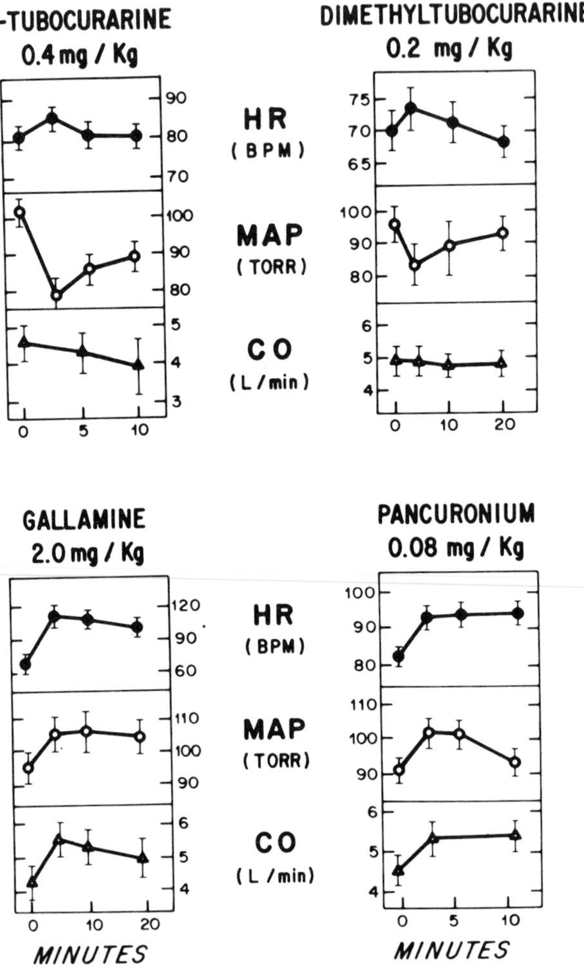

Figure 1. Summary of circulatory changes (mean ± SD) in the first ten minutes following administration of equipotent doses of nondepolarizing muscle relaxants to adult patients anesthetized with nitrous oxide and halothane. Abbreviations: HR = heart rate; MAP = mean arterial pressure; CO = cardiac output. (Data adapted from Stoelting.[1–3])

action of the neurotransmitter acetylcholine at cholinergic receptors while nondepolarizing muscle relaxants tend to block the effects of acetylcholine at these sites.

Structural similarity of muscle relaxants and acetylcholine may explain some circulatory effects. For example, the stimulatory effect of succinylcholine at cholinergic receptors is due structurally to trimethyl-substituted quaternary ammonium functions, the carboxyl groups, and the linearity and flexibility of the molecule. Succinylcholine is two molecules of acetylcholine linked through the acetate methyl groups. Pancuronium is the nondepolarizing muscle relaxant most closely related structurally to acetylcholine. The acetylcholine-like fragments of pancuronium confer upon this steroidal molecule its high neuromuscular blocking activity, its vagolytic property, and plasma cholinesterase-inhibitory action.[4]

The D-tubocurarine molecule contains only one permanent quaternary function, the other nitrogen being a tertiary amine in equilibrium with a proton at physiologic pH. Both the autonomic ganglion, and histamine-releasing properties of D-tubocurarine are probably due to the presence of the tertiary amine function. When D-tubocurarine is methylated at the tertiary amine and at the hydroxyl groups, the result is metocurine. Metocurine has much weaker autonomic ganglion-blocking and histamine-releasing properties than D-tubocurarine. None of the bisquaternary muscle relaxants possess potent autonomic ganglion-blocking or histamine-releasing properties.

Gallamine, a trisquaternary substance, is a potent vagolytic drug. This vagolytic property is due to the presence of three positively charged nitrogens.

The autonomic margin of safety depicts the difference between the dose of muscle relaxant producing desirable degrees of skeletal muscle relaxation and the dose that produces effects on the peripheral autonomic nervous system.[5] A narrow autonomic margin of safety is present when the doses of muscle relaxant that produce skeletal muscle relaxation and autonomic nervous system effects are similar (Fig 2). Conversely, a wide autonomic margin of safety means skeletal muscle relaxation can be produced by doses that have little or no impact on activity of the peripheral autonomic nervous system (Fig 2). Obviously, circulatory effects are likely to accompany the administration of a muscle relaxant with a narrow autonomic margin of safety.

D-Tubocurarine is the only nondepolarizing muscle relaxant that blocks both vagal and sympathetic nervous system pathways within the clinical dose range (eg, narrow autonomic margin of safety).[1] Ganglionic blockade is the manifestation of this effect on the autonomic nervous system. The histamine-releasing property of D-tubocurarine also occurs within the clinical dose range. In contrast to D-tubocurarine, metocurine has a wide autonomic margin of safety such that the dose necessary for skeletal muscle relaxation is well below that which produces autonomic ganglion blockade or evokes the release of histamine.[3]

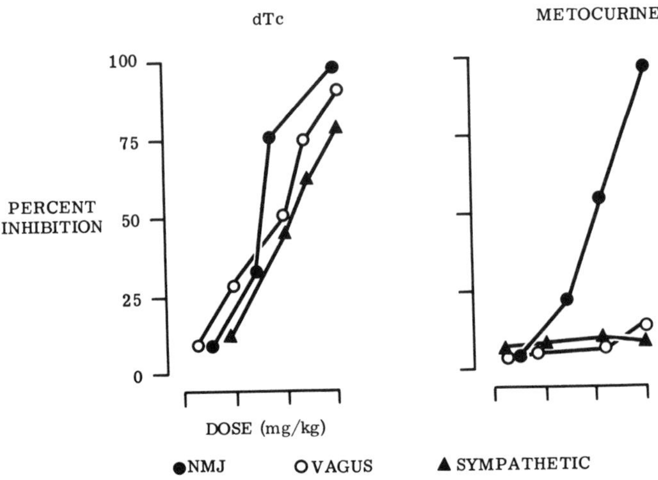

Figure 2. Schematic diagrams of the autonomic margin of safety (eg, difference between dose of muscle relaxant producing neuromuscular blockade and that producing circulatory effects due to autonomic nervous system effects) for long-acting nondepolarizing muscle relaxants. When the autonomic margin of safety is narrow, as with D-tubocurarine (DTc), it is predictable that circulatory changes will accompany clinical doses of the drug. Conversely, metocurine has a wide autonomic margin of safety and is less likely to produce circulatory changes.

Pancuronium and gallamine both block vagal muscarinic receptors.[4] The vagolytic property of gallamine overlaps the neuromuscular blocking action, whereas the only overlap of these two properties in the case of pancuronium occurs at the upper end of the neuromuscular dose-response curve. Neither drug possesses significant autonomic ganglion-blocking or histamine-releasing effects. Both drugs also produce a stimulation of sympathetic transmission that is mediated through blockade of muscarinic receptors in the sympathetic nervous system. Pancuronium and gallamine also facilitate transmissions of impulses through the sympathetic nervous system.[6] Blockade of muscarinic receptors, which are an important part of an inhibitory pathway through sympathetic ganglia, may remove the influence of this braking system and actually facilitate ganglionic transmission. In addition, inhibition of muscarinic receptors of sympathetic postganglionic nerve endings may facilitate release of the neurotransmitter. Pancuronium has been shown to both cause release of catecholamines and to inhibit their uptake by sympathetic nerves.[7] Gallamine has also been shown to evoke catecholamine release within the myocardium.

Atracurium and vecuronium do not alter the activity of the peripheral autonomic nervous system even at high doses (Fig 3).[8]

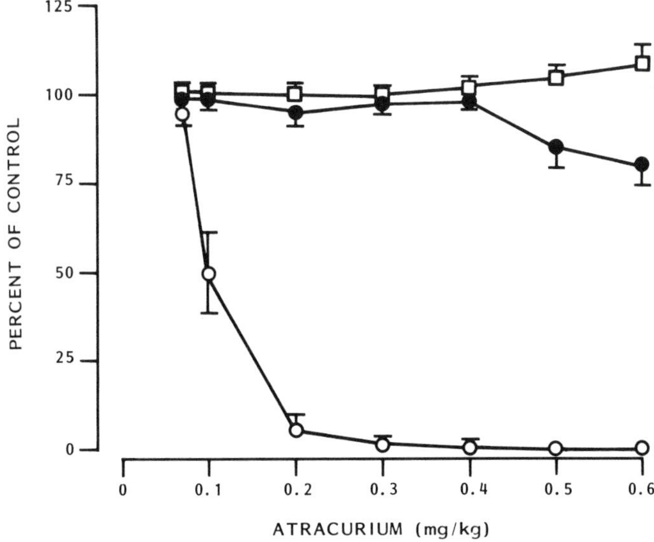

Figure 3. Doses of atracurium equivalent to two times the ED_{95} dose (0.4 mg/kg) did not produce significant alterations in HR and mean arterial pressure MAP when administered to adult patients anesthetized with nitrous oxide, thiopental, and fentanyl. Doses equivalent to two and a half (0.5 mg/kg) and three times (0.6 mg/kg) the ED_{95} produced statistically significant ($P < 0.05$) but transient and clinically insignificant circulatory changes. Data are mean ± SE. (Data adapted from Basta et al.[8])

Histamine Release

Histamine release manifests as (1) decreased BP due to a reduction in systemic vascular resistance at the arterioles and venules; (2) erythema of the skin most evident over the face and upper trunk; (3) H_2-mediated positive inotropic and chronotropic effects at the heart; (4) increased coronary blood flow; and (5) increased airway resistance particularly in susceptible individuals. Drug-induced histamine release does not involve immunologic mechanisms, but rather a nonspecific displacement of histamine from mast cells. Large doses of a histamine-releasing drug given as a bolus are particularly likely to evoke the release of histamine.[9] Conversely, the same dose administered over three minutes is less likely to evoke significant histamine release (Fig 4).[10]

Administration of D-tubocurarine 0.5 to 0.6 mg/kg as a 30-second bolus produces a fourfold to sixfold increase in the serum histamine concentration, which parallels the reduction in BP.[9] The hypotensive property of D-tubocurarine in humans is, therefore, almost entirely due to release of histamine. The autonomic ganglion-blocking effect in the clinical dose range is probably

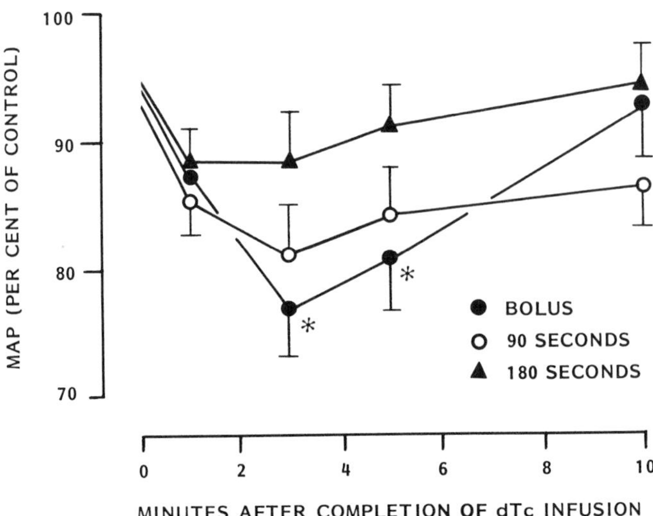

Figure 4. Reductions in MAP following administration of DTc 0.4 mg/kg to patients anesthetized with nitrous oxide and halothane were dependent on the rate of injection of the drug. All patients were anesthetized with nitrous oxide and halothane. Asterisk indicates $P < 0.05$ compared with control. (Reproduced with permission from Stoelting et al.[10])

negligible. Metocurine is three times less potent as a histamine releaser than D-tubocurarine.[3] Atracurium is about one third as potent as metocurine as a histamine-releasing drug.[8] Pancuronium and vecuronium do not evoke the release of histamine even at high doses.[11]

Tachycardia

Tachycardia caused by gallamine and pancuronium is dose related and cumulative. Gallamine probably produces complete vagal blockade within the neuromuscular blocking dose-range (Figs 1 and 2).[2] The vagolytic property of pancuronium within this range is less than that of gallamine, so that pancuronium is probably only partially vagolytic within the clinical range. Less increase in heart rate, therefore, results during its use than during use of gallamine (Figs 1 and 2).[1,2] The indirect sympathomimetic effects of both drugs probably contributes to the heart rate increase, particularly when cardiac dysrhythmias occur.

Hypotension

Hypotension following the administration of D-tubocurarine and occasionally after metocurine is most likely due to the release of histamine (Fig

1).[1,3] Autonomic ganglion-blocking effects contribute minimally to BP lowering effects of these drugs.

Cardiac Output

A decrease in cardiac output following the administration of D-tubocurarine is due to a reduction in systemic vascular resistance that is not offset by an increase in heart rate or stroke volume. This decrease in cardiac output is more prominent in the presence of a volatile anesthetic than in the presence of balanced anesthesia. Increases in cardiac output produced by pancuronium and gallamine are similar despite the greater increase in heart rate produced by gallamine (Fig 1).[1,2] This similarity may reflect a greater indirect sympathomimetic effect of pancuronium.

Cardiac Dysrhythmias

Because of its agonist activity on the peripheral autonomic nervous system, succinylcholine is probably the muscle relaxant most likely to produce cardiac dysrhythmias.[12,13] Succinylcholine stimulates cholinergic (nicotinic) receptors in both sympathetic and parasympathetic ganglia and muscarinic receptors in the sinus node of the heart. Bradycardia following administration of succinylcholine reflects stimulation of cardiac muscarinic receptors.[14] Junctional rhythm probably reflects relatively greater stimulation of cholinergic receptors in the sinus node, the result being suppression of the sinus mechanism and emergence of the atrioventricular node as a pacemaker. Succinylcholine lowers the threshold of the ventricle to catecholamine-induced ventricular dysrhythmias. The occurrence of ventricular dysrhythmias is further encouraged by the release of potassium from skeletal muscle as a consequence of the depolarizing action of the drug. Finally, ventricular escape beats may also occur as a result of severe sinus and atrioventricular nodal slowing secondary to succinylcholine administration.

MUSCLE RELAXANT CHOICE IN THE PATIENT WITH CORONARY ARTERY DISEASE

The basic challenge during anesthesia in the patient with coronary artery disease is to prevent myocardial ischemia. This goal is best achieved by maintaining the balance between myocardial oxygen requirements and myocardial oxygen delivery (Fig 5). Muscle relaxant-induced increases in BP, heart rate, or myocardial contractility may increase myocardial oxygen requirements, while decreases in systemic vascular resistance with associated diastolic hypotension can decrease coronary blood flow and jeopardize myo-

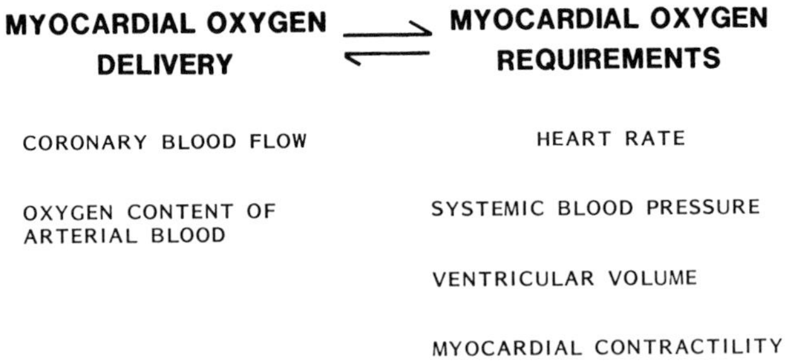

Figure 5. Schematic depiction of the determinants of the balance between myocardial oxygen delivery and myocardial oxygen requirements.

cardial oxygen delivery. Ultimately, the choice of muscle relaxant for the patient with coronary artery disease is determined by the likely circulatory effects of these drugs on myocardial oxygen requirements and delivery.

D-Tubocurarine

D-Tubocurarine would be unlikely to increase myocardial oxygen requirements since it does not alter heart rate or myocardial contractility. Persistent hypotension, however, may impair myocardial oxygen delivery and offset the beneficial effects of reduced myocardial oxygen requirements.

Pancuronium

BP is increased by pancuronium such that myocardial oxygen delivery should be maintained. The occasional marked increase in heart rate with pancuronium, however, may be undesirable from the standpoint of increased myocardial oxygen requirements. Nevertheless, circulatory changes after pancuronium are usually moderate and may serve to offset the negative chronotropic and/or inotropic effects of the anesthetic drugs.

Metocurine

Minimal reductions in BP and no significant change in heart rate are characteristic circulatory responses associated with this drug. Therefore, alterations in myocardial oxygen requirements and delivery are minimal, and metocurine is often selected for administration to the patient with coronary artery disease.

Atracurium

Heart rate or BP changes are unlikely following the administration of up to twice the ED_{95} dose (eg, 0.4 mg/kg) of atracurium (Fig 3).[8] Therefore, atracurium is an attractive muscle relaxant selection when the primary goal is to avoid heart rate and/or BP changes that could alter the favorable balance between myocardial oxygen requirements and delivery. It is recommended, however, that atracurium be administered over one minute to reduce the likelihood of histamine-induced BP changes in patients with coronary artery disease.[15]

Vecuronium

Vecuronium, like atracurium, is an intermediate-acting muscle relaxant devoid of circulatory effects. In contrast to atracurium, even doses far above three times the ED_{95} do not evoke the release of histamine.[16] In patients undergoing elective coronary artery bypass graft operations, vecuronium in doses sufficient to provide ideal conditions for intubation of the trachea failed to produce any circulatory changes (Fig 6).[17] For these reasons, vecuronium,

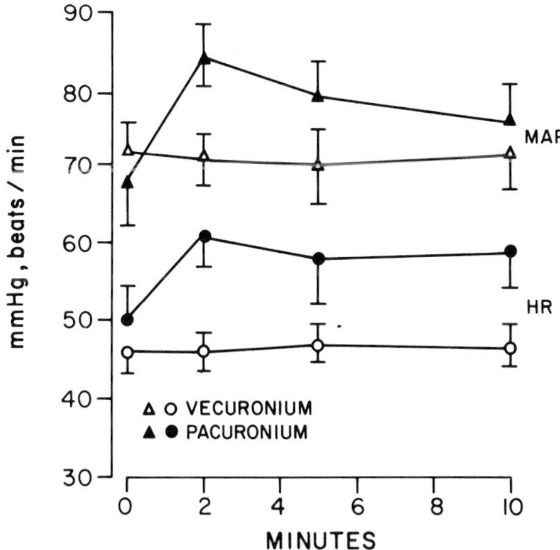

Figure 6. Administration of vecuronium 0.28 mg/kg to seven patients scheduled for elective coronary artery bypass graft surgery did not alter MAP or HR. Pancuronium 0.1 mg/kg administered to five similar patients increased MAP and HR above control values ($P < 0.05$). Data are mean ± SD. (Data adapted from Morris et al.[17])

like atracurium, is an appropriate drug to consider for administration to patients with coronary artery disease. Conversely, these intermediate-acting muscle relaxants, unlike pancuronium, are unlikely to offset circulatory effects of the anesthetic such as fentanyl-induced bradycardia.

Succinylcholine

Succinylcholine produces a variety of circulatory changes that may be difficult to distinguish from effects secondary to anesthetic drugs. Typically, the heart rate increases about 10 beats/min when succinylcholine is administered with a barbiturate. Furthermore, BP reductions are similar following an intravenous (IV) barbiturate with or without succinylcholine, suggesting that succinylcholine-produced autonomic ganglion stimulation is not a significant consideration. Cardiac rhythm disturbances are reliably prevented by small doses of nondepolarizers administered one to three minutes before succinylcholine.[18] Conceivably, cholinergic stimulation from succinylcholine would accentuate heart rate slowing in patients receiving propranolol, but this speculation has not been documented.

MUSCLE RELAXANT CHOICE IN THE PATIENT WITH VALVULAR HEART DISEASE

All drug selections for the patient with valvular heart disease depend on an understanding of the pathophysiology of the underlying heart disease.[19] As in the patient with coronary artery disease, knowing the likely circulatory effects produced by the neuromuscular blockers provides the basis for a logical muscle relaxant choice.

Aortic Stenosis

Obstruction to left ventricular emptying makes maintenance of an adequate stroke volume dependent on heart rate and BP. Furthermore, the hypertrophied left ventricle is vulnerable to ischemia from increased myocardial oxygen requirements or decreased oxygen delivery. Moderate increases in heart rate and BP (pancuronium) are acceptable, but the implications in terms of myocardial ischemia must be remembered. Peripheral vasodilation with reductions in BP (D-tubocurarine) may greatly reduce coronary blood flow. In the final analysis, minimal changes in heart rate and BP as provided by atracurium or vecuronium (succinylcholine for tracheal intubation) would make this drug a logical choice in the patient with severe aortic stenosis. Metocurine would be an alternative selection to the newer intermediate-acting muscle relaxants (atracurium, vecuronium).

Aortic Regurgitation

Theoretically, peripheral vasodilation with reductions in diastolic BP as produced by D-tubocurarine would reduce regurgitant flow and improve forward left ventricular stroke volume. Sudden or persistent vasodilation and reductions in BP, however, may dangerously decrease coronary blood flow. In contrast, moderate increases in heart rate following administration of pancuronium would promote forward left ventricular stroke volume, making this drug an attractive choice for the patient with aortic regurgitation. Alternatively, atracurium or vecuronium would be acceptable selections if the goal is to avoid any drug-induced changes.

Mitral Stenosis

The small mitral valve orifice impairs left ventricular filling such that heart rate responses must be considered with any drug (especially pancuronium) administered to patients with mitral stenosis. Diuretics and digitalis are frequently administered to these patients. Chronic diuresis, in addition to potassium depletion, may reduce blood volume, which becomes manifest as hypotension with peripheral vasodilation particularly after administration of D-tubocurarine. An increased incidence of ventricular dysrhythmias with succinylcholine and digitalis has not been a consistent observation.[20] Atracurium or vecuronium with minimal to no circulatory effects is the best selection in the presence of severe mitral stenosis. Metocurine would be a better selection than pancuronium or D-tubocurarine if a long-acting rather than intermediate-acting muscle relaxant is selected.

Mitral Regurgitation

Mitral regurgitation produces volume overload of the left ventricle. Forward left ventricular stroke volume may be improved by moderate increases in heart rate due to pancuronium or peripheral vasodilation following administration of D-tubocurarine. Since the magnitude of circulatory changes after these drugs is often unpredictable, however, the best choice may again be the muscle relaxant associated with the least hemodynamic effects—atracurium or vecuronium. Metocurine is the best selection if a long-acting muscle relaxant is selected.

Mitral Valve Prolapse

Mitral valve prolapse is probably due to an abnormality of the mitral valve support structure that results in prolapse of the mitral valve into the left atrium during ventricular systole.[21] The auscultatory finding of this abnormality (a nonejection click followed by a high-pitched systolic murmur best heard at the apex) is present in 5% to 10% of the adult population, which makes mitral valve prolapse one of the most common of all the cardiac abnormalities.

The important principle in the management of anesthesia for patients known to have mitral valve prolapse is the recognition that increased cardiac emptying can accentuate the prolapse. Events that can increase cardiac emptying include sympathetic nervous system stimulation and reductions in systemic vascular resistance. For these reasons, pancuronium would be an unlikely selection in view of its potential effects on myocardial contractility and heart rate. Likewise, peripheral vasodilation following D-tubocurarine would be undesirable. Metocurine, atracurium, or vecuronium are ideal choices since these muscle relaxants lack significant effects on the circulation. Succinylcholine is acceptable when the rapid onset of short-duration neuromuscular blockade is desired.

HYPERTROPHIC CARDIOMYOPATHY

Hypertrophic cardiomyopathy is also known as idiopathic hypertrophic subaortic stenosis or asymmetric septal hypertrophy. The major problem associated with hypertrophic cardiomyopathy is an obstruction to left ventricular outflow produced by an asymmetric hypertrophy of the intraventricular septal muscle.

The management of anesthesia in patients with hypertrophic cardiomyopathy is directed toward minimizing the pressure gradient across the left ventricular outflow obstruction.[22] Intraoperative events that will increase left ventricular obstruction include drug-induced activation of the sympathetic nervous system or peripheral vasodilation resulting in reductions in BP. A nondepolarizing muscle relaxant with minimal (metocurine) to absent (atracurium, vecuronium) circulatory effects is the best choice for production of prolonged skeletal muscle paralysis. Pancuronium is not a good selection because of its ability to increase heart rate and myocardial contractility. Likewise, sudden reductions in systemic vascular resistance produced by D-tubocurarine are unacceptable.

CONGENITAL HEART DISEASE

Cyanotic congenital heart disease characterized by right-to-left intracardiac shunting of blood is most often due to tetralogy of Fallot. Drug-induced reductions in systemic vascular resistance and BP can increase the magnitude of the shunt and further exaggerate arterial hypoxemia.[23] Intraoperative skeletal muscle paralysis is best provided by pancuronium as this drug maintains systemic vascular resistance and BP. The mild increase in heart rate associated with its administration is also helpful in maintaining the left ventricular cardiac output. Atracurium or vecuronium would be equally acceptable, although these drugs, being devoid of circulatory effects, would be less likely than pancuronium to reduce the magnitude of right-to-left intracardiac shunt. D-Tubocurarine would not be a logical choice as this drug could increase the magnitude of the right-to-left intracardiac shunt, by virtue of its ability to decrease systemic vascular resistance secondary to histamine release and blockade of impulse transmission through peripheral autonomic ganglia. Metocurine would be a better selection than D-tubocurarine but less ideal than pancuronium or the intermediate-acting nondepolarizing muscle relaxants.

SUMMARY

The logical selection of a muscle relaxant for administration to a patient with heart disease is based on an understanding of the pathophysiology of the cardiac dysfunction. When the pathophysiology of the heart disease is considered, it may be appropriate to select a muscle relaxant with predictable circulatory effects so as to produce changes that reduce the adverse effects produced by the heart disease. More often, however, the best approach is selection of a muscle relaxant with minimal to absent circulatory effects so as to minimize the likelihood of any drug-induced changes in the circulation.

REFERENCES

1. Stoelting RK: The hemodynamic effects of pancuronium and d-tubocurarine in anesthetized patients. Anesthesiology 36:612–615, 1972
2. Stoelting RK: Hemodynamic effects of gallamine during halothane-nitrous oxide anesthesia. Anesthesiology 39:645–647, 1973
3. Stoelting RK: Hemodynamic effects of dimethyl-tubocurarine during nitrous oxide-halothane anesthesia. Anesth Analg 53:513–515, 1974
4. Bonta IL, Goorissen WM, Derkx FH: Inhibition of vagal receptors in the heart of pancuronium. Eur J Pharmacol 4:83–90, 1968
5. Savarese JJ: The autonomic margin of safety of metocurine and d-tubocurarine. Anesthesiology 50:40–46, 1979
6. Gardier RW, Tsevdos EJ, Jackson DB: Effects of gallamine and pancuronium on inhibitory transmission in cat sympathetic ganglia. J Pharmacol Exp Ther 204:46–53, 1978
7. Segarra Domenech J, Carlos Garcia R, Rodriquez Sasiain JM, et al: Pancuronium bromide: An indirect sympathomimetic agent. Br J Anaesth 48:1143–1148, 1976
8. Basta SJ, Ali HH, Savarese JJ, et al: Clinical pharmacology of atracurium besylate (BW 33A): A new nondepolarizing muscle relaxant. Anesth Analg 61:723–729, 1982
9. Moss J, Rosow CE, Savarese JJ, et al: Role of histamine in the hypotensive action of d-tubocurarine in humans. Anesthesiology 55:19–25, 1981

10. Stoelting RK, McCammon RL, Hilgenberg JC: Changes in blood pressure with varying rates of administration of d-tubocurarine. Anesth Analg 59:697–699, 1980
11. Booij LHDJ, Edwards RP, Sohn YJ, et al: Cardiovascular and neuromuscular effects of Org NC 45, pancuronium, metocurine, a d-tubocurarine in dogs. Anesth Analg 59:26–30, 1980
12. Galindo AHF, Davis TB: Succinylcholine and cardiac excitability. Anesthesiology 23:32–40, 1962
13. Schoenstadt DA, Whitcher CE: Observations on the mechanism of succinylcholine-induced cardiac arrhythmias. Anesthesiology 24:358–362, 1963
14. Stoelting RK, Peterson C: Heart-rate slowing and junctional rhythm following intravenous succinylcholine with and without intramuscular atropine preanesthetic medication. Anesth Analg 54:705–709, 1975
15. Philbin DM, Machaj VR, Tomichek RC, et al: Haemodynamic effects of bolus injections of atracurium in patients with coronary artery disease. Br J Anaesth 55:131S, 1983
16. Fahey MR, Morris RB, Miller RD, et al: Clinical pharmacology of ORG NC 45 (Norcuron™): A new nondepolarizing relaxant. Anesthesiology 55:6–11, 1981
17. Morris RB, Cahalan MK, Miller RD, et al: The cardiovascular effects of vecuronium (ORG NC 45) and pancuronium in patients undergoing coronary artery bypass grafting. Anesthesiology 58:438–440, 1983
18. Stoelting RK, Peterson C: Adverse effects of increased succinylcholine dose following d-tubocurarine pretreatment. Anesth Analg 54:282–288, 1975
19. Hilgenberg JC: Valvular heart disease, in Stoelting RK, Dierdorf SF (eds): Anesthesia and Co-Existing Disease. New York, Churchill Livingstone, 1983, pp 27–45
20. Perez HR: Cardiac arrhythmias after succinylcholine. Anesth Analg 49:33–38, 1970
21. Cheitlin MD, Byrd RC: The click-murmur syndrome. A clinical problem in diagnosis and treatment. JAMA 245:1357–1361, 1981
22. Hilgenberg JC: Cardiomyopathies, in Stoelting RK, Dierdorf SF (eds): Anesthesia and Co-Existing Disease. New York, Churchill Livingstone, 1983, pp 129–133
23. Haselby KA: Congenital heart disease, in Stoelting RK, Dierdorf SF (eds): Anesthesia and Co-Existing Disease. New York, Churchill Livingstone, 1983, pp 47–70

Henry Rosenberg

10

Neuromuscular Blockade in the Patient With Neuromuscular Disorders

Neuromuscular blocking drugs are used daily in the operating room with minimal problems. As might be anticipated, however, patients with myopathies or disorders of the neuromuscular apparatus may not respond normally to these agents. Therefore, an understanding of the basic pathophysiology of myopathies and a knowledge of the pharmacology of neuromuscular blocking drugs are essential for rational and safe use of these agents in such patients. This is especially true because the response to anesthesia and surgery is poorly documented in patients affected by myopathies and neuromuscular diseases.

Because of the large number of myopathies this article can only cover the more frequent problems of the more common disorders.

PHYSIOLOGY OF SKELETAL MUSCLE CONTRACTION

The essential steps in activation and contraction of skeletal muscle have been understood for the past decade and further clarification is growing rapidly. The process is summarized and portrayed in Fig 1. The nerve impulse arriving at the nerve terminal releases acetylcholine from "packets" contained within the nerve. Acetylcholine, after release, crosses the neuromuscular junction and attaches to specific receptor sites at the muscle end of the neuromuscular junction. Channels are opened, leading to influx of sodium and efflux of potassium; this results in a brief depolarization of the membrane at the endplate, which then spreads throughout the muscle membrane.

MUSCLE RELAXANTS
ISBN 0-8089-1784-6

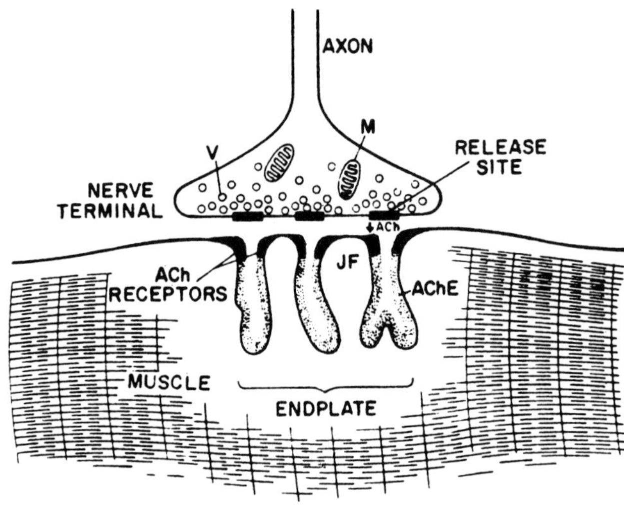

Figure 1. Schematic diagram of the neuromuscular junction showing vesicles (V) containing acetylcholine. Junctional folds (JF), acetylcholine receptors (ACh Receptors), and acetylcholinesterase (AchE) are depicted on the postjunctional membrane. (Reprinted with permission.[13])

Through invaginations of the membrane, the depolarization is transmitted to the sarcoplasmic reticulum of the muscle cell, which then releases calcium ion into the myoplasm. Calcium attaches to troponin, a protein located on the actin filament. This event disinhibits actin and myosin interaction, and muscle contraction occurs. However, following calcium release the ion is rapidly taken back up into the sarcoplasmic reticulum, muscle relaxation occurs, and the contraction phase is over. In the meantime, acetylcholine has been degraded by the enzyme acetylcholinesterase located at the neuromuscular junction. Acetate ion and choline are then resequestered into the prejunctional membrane and resynthetized into acetylcholine. Each step in this complicated process can go awry and lead to clinical problems.

DISORDERS OF PREJUNCTIONAL ACETYLCHOLINE RELEASE

Two disorders of acetylcholine release that affect the action of neuromuscular blocking agents are myasthenic syndrome (the Eaton-Lambert syndrome) and botulism.

Eaton-Lambert syndrome is a disorder of impaired aceteylcholine release characterized by proximal muscle weakness, usually slowly progressive, and almost always associated with small cell carcinoma of the lung.[1] Paresthesias may be present as well. The characteristic feature of myasthenic syndrome is muscle weakness that improves transiently with exercise and is most easily demonstrated on electromyogram (EMG). Unlike patients with myasthenia gravis (MG), patients suffering from myasthenic syndrome are not helped by anticholinesterases. However, striking functional improvement and remissions may occur following chemotherapy or excision of the primary tumor.[2] Myasthenic syndrome is felt to result from the production of antibodies to the sites in the prejunctional membrane responsible for acetylcholine release. Indeed, transfer of muscle weakness may be induced in mice by innoculation of the IgG fraction of plasma from patients with Eaton-Lambert syndrome.

Patients with myasthenic syndrome are exquisitely sensitive to nondepolarizing as well as depolarizing muscle relaxants.[3] Therefore, patients who, for example, undergo diagnostic bronchoscopy for a lung tumor and then fail to regain muscle strength after the use of muscle relaxants should be thought of as having myasthenic syndrome until proven otherwise. Mechanical ventilation for a number of hours is the best therapy since anticholinesterases do not improve clinical conditions. The patients may also show significant muscle weakness with the use of aminoglycoside antibiotics. They are frequently treated with guanidine hydrochloride.

At the other end of the age spectrum is infant botulism, a disorder that has only been recognized in recent years.[4] All cases of botulism are related to failure of acetycholine release from the prejunctional membrane. In adults, botulism results from the ingestion of botulinum toxin from contaminated foodstuffs. In infants, however, symptoms result from absorption of the toxin produced in the gut by ingestion of spores of *Clostridium botulinum*. Susceptible patients range from of 2 to 8 months. They present with symptoms of failure to thrive, constipation, hypotonia, ptosis, loss of head control, and poor feeding. In some cases, sudden infant death syndrome has also been associated with this disorder. Because many of these patients present in a nonspecific manner, they may be treated empirically with antibiotics. If aminoglycoside antibiotics are used, respiratory arrest may result. Treatment is supportive, consisting of respiratory support and gavage feeding, with response occurring over the course of weeks. Sensitivity to all neuromuscular blocking drugs is likely.

PSEUDOCHOLINESTERASE DISORDERS

Although strictly speaking not a problem of the neuromuscular junction itself, atypical or markedly depressed levels of the enzyme pseudocholinesterase will lead to prolonged neuromuscular blockade following succinylcholine. Pseudocholinesterase is found in the serum and in most cells of the body.

It is related to but different from acetylcholinesterase, which is found only at the neuromuscular junction and in red cells. Typically, patients with pseudocholinesterase abnormalities will be apneic for four to eight hours after 1 mg/kg of succinylcholine. Most patients who develop such a response to succinylcholine have an atypical pseudocholinesterase enzyme rather than a deficient amount of pseudocholinesterase.[5] Viby-Mogensen[6] has recently shown that in order for there to be a marked increase in duration of neuromuscular blockade following succinylcholine, a 75% to 80% decrease in levels of the normal enzyme is necesary. A decrease of this magnitude is rare even in pregnancy, where a typical decrease may be 25% to 30%. Three clinical situations where significant decreases in normal pseudocholinesterase enzyme can be expected are severe hepatic dysfunction, use of echothiophate eyedrops, and patients who have recently undergone plasmapheresis.

There are four separate alleles that determine the phenotype and production of pseudocholinesterase enzyme.[5] They are labeled U for usual enzyme, S for silent (nonproduction of the enzyme), A for atypical, and F for fluoride resistant. Individuals with a combination of a normal and an abnormal gene for the pseudocholinesterase enzyme will generally have a normal response to succinylcholine. Heterozygotes with a combination of an atypical gene plus either a silent gene or a fluoride gene show a prolonged blockade with succinylcholine.[7] Homozygotes, with two atypical genes, two fluoride or two silent, show a duration of neuromuscular blockade of at least three hours. The most common reason for prolonged response to succinylcholine is the homozygote atypical condition that occurs in approximately 1 in 2,500 patients. Thus, if a group of anesthesiologists use succinylcholine in 5,000 cases per year, they can expect to encounter two patients with a prolonged response. When confronted with a patient with prolonged apnea from succinylcholine there is a temptation to reverse the blockade with edrophonium or neostigmine. However, when given too early this can worsen the blockade. Fresh frozen plasma or whole blood can be used to hasten the recovery from this neuromuscular blockade. However, because of the problems of blood products, it is wisest merely to ventilate the patient during the period of paralysis. It should be remembered, however, that the patient is likely to be fully awake, and therefore the transient nature of the blockade should be explained and the patient reassured. Follow-up investigation should consist of determining the genotype of the patient and his or her family members since the inheritance of pseudocholinesterase enzyme abnormalities follows classical mendelian genetics. The evaluation should consist of a determination of the pseudocholinesterase activity, dibucaine number, fluoride number, and succinylcholine or urea number for completion. Even though atracruium is degraded in part by pseudocholinesterases, patients with atypical pseudocholinesterase do not have an atypical response to this drug. An identifying bracelet should be obtained for those with atypical pseudocholinesterase.

DISORDERS OF THE POSTJUNCTIONAL MEMBRANE: MYASTHENIA GRAVIS

For many years, MG was considered a disorder of acetylcholine release from prejunctional sites. Over the past 15 years, definitive studies have shown MG to be a disorder of the postjunctional acetylcholine receptor.[8] Autoantibodies are formed to the acetylcholine receptor leading to a reduction in the number of receptors and their functional state. Microscopic examination of the neuromuscular junction reveals a loss of the normal architecture and variation in depth and integrity of the membrane invaginations. This syndrome may also be transferred by the serum of the affected patient when given in sufficient quantities. Babies of myasthenic mothers may therefore display several days of muscle weakness until the antibodies are cleared (neonatal myasthenia).

The characteristic symptom of MG is muscle weakness that increases with exercise. The disorder usually effects younger individuals and is not associated with underlying carcinoma. Ocular findings, particularly ptosis, are common. The muscle weakness may be mild and slowly progressive or rapidly progressive and affect the respiratory muscles. Most myasthenics are helped by anticholinesterases and are usually taking pyridostigmine, although some may be taking neostigmine. Steroids have also been found to be helpful, and it is therefore important to ascertain whether the patient has been or is currently taking steroid medication. Another characteristic feature of MG is transient improvement by plasmapheresis. Remissions of weeks to months may be noted. However, this therapy is usually reserved for the acute management of rapidly progressive myasthenia in an attempt to stabilize the patient prior to optimization of drug therapy or thymectomy.

The diagnosis of MG is usually made on the basis of the characteristic history of muscle weakness, ptosis, responsiveness to edrophonium injection, typical changes on EMG, and the detection of acetylcholine receptor antibodies in the serum. The curare test, either a systemic or regional injection of a small amount of curare with measurement of muscle weakness, is sometimes used in the less clear-cut cases to diagnose this syndrome.[9,10]

Most patients with MG present for surgery for thymectomy. The thymus gland is felt to be the site of the autoantibody production that results in the clinical syndrome. Thymectoy is now recommended very soon after the diagnosis of the syndrome.

Anesthetic problems with the patient with MG center on the use of the relaxants, continuation of anticholinesterase medication, and advisability of extubation postoperatively. Myasthenics are sensitive to nondepolarizers and sometimes (rarely) show resistance to depolarizing relaxants. It is, therefore, generally advised to avoid all muscle relaxants. However, variability in response to the relaxants is characteristic. Some patients with mild forms of the disorder may have a close to normal response to nondepolarizing relaxants. Although there may be resistance to succinylcholine initially, if the patient is on pyridostigmine or has recently undergone plasmapheresis there may be a prolonged response to succinylcholine because of the reduction of the activity amount of pseudocholinesterase enzyme. Induction and maintenance of the anesthetic with halogenated agents is usually sufficient for intubation and muscle relaxation.

More controversial is the preoperative preparation of the patients for thymectomy. Some authorities taper or decrease the anticholinesterase medication prior to surgery, the concern being that there will be an altered response after thymectomy that may lead to myasthenic crisis. Others continue the medication until the time of surgery so as to insure optimum neuromuscular strength. However, all agree that tracheostomy is usually not necessary and that all myasthenics require intensive care postoperatively. In one study that evaluated the factors that could predict the need for continued ventilation following transternal thymectomy, four significant predictors were found to determine the need for prolonged postoperative ventilation: (1) the duration of the disease greater than 6 years; (2) concomitant respiratory disease, (3) dosage of pyridostigmine of over 750 mg/d and (4) a vital capacity of less than 2.9 L.[11] A point scale was devised with a possible total of 32 points. Patients with scores below 9 did well enough to be extubated routinely; those with scores of 10 to 12 usually required some ventilation postoperatively; those with scores over 14 usually required lengthy ventilation. All patients, however, required close observation postoperatively, because even those with low scores occasionally required ventilation if there were complicating respiratory problems or if they went into cholinergic crisis on reinstitution of anticholinesterase therapy. In the management of the pyridostigmine dosage postthymectomy, 1 mg of inravenous neostigmine is taken as the equivalent of 120 mg of oral pyridostigmine. In a separate study, the criteria for extubation was not found to apply to myasthenics undergoing surgery other than transternal thymectomy.[12]

DENERVATION HYPERSENSITIVITY

Following spinal cord transection, it is well known that hyperkalemia may follow the use of succinycholine.[13] In other patients with denervated muscle, focal muscle contractures may develop after succinylcholine. A spread of neuromuscular junction receptors from the normally well-localized endplate regions to the entire muscle membrane has been demonstrated following denervation.[14] Therefore, on depolarization there is an increase in the normal ion flux leading to marked increase of potassium efflux into the serum, which can lead to cardiac arrest. Problems may also arise with nondepolarizing relaxants. When monitoring neuromuscular blockade in patients following nerve transection, it is important to monitor the unaffected side since denervated muscle may be unusually resistant to nondepolarizors. If the anesthesiologist is unaware of this phenomenon, an inadvertant overdose of neuromuscular blocking agents may occur.[15]

MYOPATHIES

Disorders of muscle itself are numerous. The muscular dystrophies are a group of disorders characterized by dysfunctional muscle or muscle destruction occurring in the muscle elements themselves. Very little is known about the pathophysiology of most muscular dystrophies. The most common and most important of the human muscular dystrophies is Duchenne's muscular dystrophy (DMD).[16] In this disorder muscle destruction followed by replacement with fibrous tissue and fat occurs. Clinically, the most important finding is muscle weakness. Since DMD is an X-linked disorder, women are asymptomatic carriers. The usual onset is at approximately age 3 to 5 years. Psesudohypertrophy of the calf muscles and muscle weakness are characteristic. The disorder progresses rapidly and patients are generally wheelchair bound by their teen years or earlier and die of respiratory failure often complicated by cardiomyopathy by age 20. The creatine phosphokinase (CPK) enzymes are characteristically elevated into the many thousands.

Cardiomyopathy is a frequent feature of DMD, involving the left ventricle most often.[17] Tachycardia with large R waves in the right precordium is characteristic. These findings may be unaccompanied by evidence of congestive failure or overt symptoms until the patient also has concomitant respiratory muscle dysfunction. The extent of cardiac and respiratory failure is often not apparent on history because the patient is wheelchair bound and inactive. However, cardiomyopathy and respiratory failure should be suspected in all patients with DMD.

Patients with DMD usually present for muscle biopsy or minor orthopedic procedures to enhance mobility, or more recently, for the placement of Luqui rods (like Harrington rods) to enhance mobility. The DMD patient should be carefully evaluated for myocardial and respiratory compromise. Increased sensitivity to muscle relaxants is predictable based on the decrease in muscle bulk. Unexpected and unpredictable, however, has been the recent finding that when given in the presence of halothane, succinylcholine is associated with increased destruction of muscle tissues. Even in patients with an apparently normal response to succinylcholine, there may be myoglobinuria in the postoperative period.[18] In addition, a number of cases of malignant hyperthermia (MH) have been noted in DMD patients. The relationship between MH and DMD has been further strengthened by the finding of typical changes for MH on muscle biopsy contracture testing.[19] It is my feeling, therefore, that although not all patients with DMD are at risk to MH, a suficient number are and the trigger agents for MH should be avoided in such patients.

OTHER MUSCULAR DYSTROPHIES

Of the many other muscular dystrophies, the most common are the facioscapulohumeral and limb-girdle dystrophies. The inheritance of these dystrophies is autosomal rather than X-linked. Fortunately, they do not make their appearance until adolescence, progression is slower, and concomitant cardiomyopathy and respiratory disturbances are not as severe or as common as in DMD.[16] When muscle relaxants are used, the doses of nondepolarizing agents must be reduced. Little information is available regarding the use of depolarizing relaxants. It is my opinion that depolarizing relaxants are best avoided because of expected muscle destruction.

MYOTONIAS

The myotonias are disorders of the muscle membrane. Their characteristic feature is a delayed relaxation after muscle contraction and a prolonged contracture following stimulation such as striking the muscle with a reflex hammer. After stimulation the muscle stays shortened and contracted for several seconds. Animal models of the myotonias implicate a disorder of chloride fluxes across the membrane associated with membrane depolarization. The relationship to human myotonias is not as clear.[16]

There are several forms of myotonia: myotonia dystrophica, myotonia congenita, and paramyotonia. Of the three, myotonic dystrophy is the most devastating since it is a systemic disease. Inheritance is usually autosomal dominant, and therefore both sexes are affected. The onset is usually in the teens or early twenties with slow progression usually first involving the distal musculature. The patient characteristically displays the myotonic phenomenon in association with progressive muscle wasting, hatchet-jaw appearance, frontal balding, cataracts, and mild endocrine abnormalities. Cardiomyopathies and rhythm disturbances such as Stokes-Adams attack and ventricular irritability are common along with premature ventricular contractions (PVCs) and intraventricular conduction delays.[20] Decreases in static pulmonary function, vital capacity, and inspiratory reserve volume are common in patients with myotonic dystrophy. Many also have an abnormal response to carbon dioxide challenge, and their response to hypoxia may be blunted. Speculation that the CNS is affected in the disease has been implicated to explain this abnormal response to carbon dioxide and to oxygen.

All respiratory depressants should be used with caution in patients with decreased respiratory volumes and decreased sensitivity to carbon dioxide and hypoxia. The anesthesia literature has specifically recommended that thiopental be avoided in myotonics,[21] but there is no evidence to suggest that it is any more harmful than any of the other respiratory depressants. Occasionally, smooth muscle is involved in myotonia dystrophica, leading to abnormalities in swallowing and digestion. A stormy postoperative course is characteristic of patients with severe myotonic dystrophy, usually related to respiratory complications such as atalectasis and pneumonia and requirements for postoperative ventilation.[22]

In myotonia congenita the myotonic phenomenon is observed but without the associated cardiomyopathy and muscle atrophy. An increase in muscle bulk is noted. Several reports indicate that these patients are more likely to develop MH. When succinylcholine is given to a myotonic patient, a prolonged contracture response occurs. This is similar to the response seen in MH, but what is not consistent with MH is the lack of metabolic changes. Whether myotonia increases the risk for MH is an unsettled issue (it does not in myotonic goats).

Paramyotonia is a rare disorder characterized by a myotonic phenomenon elicited on exposure to cold.

All the myotonias present problems with the use of succinylcholine.[23] The characteristic contracture to succinylcholine (in myotonics) results in difficulty in ventilating the patient for two to five minutes. The myotonic phenomenon is not abolished by nondepolarizing relaxants, spinal anesthesia, or regional anesthesia because the problem derives from the intrinsic membrane disorder of the muscle itself. The only strategy that has been suggested to overcome the muscle rigidity in myotonia such as may occur on direct manipulation of the muscle is by injection of procainamide into the muscle.

Depending on the extent of muscle wasting, patients with myotonia may be more prone to developing musle weakness with nondepolarizing relaxants. Succinylcholine should not be used in myotonics at all. It is important to establish baseline pulmonary functions and cardiac evaluation prior to surgery in patients with myotonias.[24]

OTHER MYOPATHIES

Most other myopathies have been poorly described with regard to the response patients have to neuromuscular blocking drugs. It should be borne in mind, however, that patients with muscle disorders may have an increased sensitivity to nondepolarizing relaxants because of decreased muscle bulk and a decrease in pulmonary reserve. Many patients with myopathies are also treated empirically with steroids. Some have associated arthritis and smooth muscle abnormalities affecting esophageal motility, and these patients may be at risk for aspiration pneumonia.

The more that patients affected by muscle diseases are studied, the more often is it found that the myocardium may be affected in subtle manners.[25] For example, patients with polymyositis not uncommonly have mitral valve prolapse and arrhythmias. The same has been noted in some patients with MH susceptibility.[26]

MALIGNANT HYPERTHERMIA

The other disorder of skeletal muscle that is of vital importance to anesthesiologists and is linked to problems with depolarizing muscle relaxants is MH. MH is said to be a pharmacogenetic disease of skeletal muscle because the disorder is inherited and is triggered by exposure to certain pharmacologic agents. The basic pathophysiology of MH is not well understood but is felt to be related to an abnormal release from and reuptake of calcium into the sarcoplasmic reticulum.[27] Calcium activates those metabolic processes that sustain muscle contraction. As a consequence heat is generated, and acidosis may occur. MH can be rapid in onset or slowly progressive. Patients with MH susceptibility are usually asymptomatic though many will have a history of muscle cramps, muscle imbalance such as kyphoscoliosis, ptosis, strabismus, and chronic subluxation of shoulder or knee joint.[28] Several distinct myopathies have been linked to MH including DMD as mentioned previously; an unusual disorder characterized by muscle weakness called central core disease (so termed because on microscopic examination of the muscle there are hollowed-out areas within each muscle cell); and a syndrome characterized by slow developmental milestones, hypotonia, cryptorchidism, web neck, and pectus deformity termed the King-Denborough syndrome. Other unusual disorders associated with MH are the Schwartz-Jampal syndrome, some cases of myotonia congenita, neuromyotonia (cramp fasciculation syndrome), sudden infant death syndrome, and neuroleptic malignant syndrome.[28]

Although MH can be triggered by the inhalation anesthetics alone, the most aggressive forms of the syndrome are usually triggered in conjunction with the use of succinylcholine. Instead of muscle relaxation occurring after succinylcholine, gross fasciculations are noted and muscle rigidity occurs. Jaw muscle rigidity is a particularly common finding. Commonly, the jaw muscle rigidity resolves over a number of minutes but the syndrome of MH ensues if anesthesia is continued with a halogenated hydrocarbon anesthetic. Since, by laboratory tests, over 50% of patients who dislay paradoxical muscle rigidity after succinylcholine will be MH susceptible, it is advised to discontinue anesthesia and surgery after trismus or muscle rigidity. The patient should be observed for a number of hours for evidence of myoglobinuria, elevated CPK, and the early signs of MH.

Other symptoms and signs of MH are tachycardia, tachypnea, ventricular arrhythmias, muscle breakdown (myoglobinuria and massive elevation of CPK), acidosis, DIC in extreme cases, and of course, marked temperature elevation. A more complete description of MH, the management of susceptible patients, and the therapy of MH is given in reviews by Gronert[28] by Nelson and Flewellyn,[29] and by Britt,[30] among other sources.

Patients who are MH susceptible do not have a problem with the nondepolarizing relaxant pancuronium. However, there is indirect evidence that curare may be a trigger for MH. Experience with the use of gallamine, metocurine, and atracurium is lacking. However, complete neuromuscular paralysis with metocurine has shown to delay or prevent the onset of halothane-induced MH in susceptible swine.

Therefore, the safest anesthetic regimen (aside from regional anesthesia) for MH susceptibles consists of barbiturate, nitrous oxide–narcotic, and pancuronium. Another controversy surrounds the use of reversal of the nondepolarizing relaxants with edrophonium or neostigmine in the MH susceptible who has not triggered. Although it has been theorized that anticholinesterases may lead to activation of the neuromuscular junction in a manner similar to administering succinylcholine, which may result in an episode of MH, this has not proven to be the case clinically.

The neuroleptic malignant syndrome is an unusual disorder resembling MH in that skeletal muscle rigidity, muscle destruction, acidosis, and fever develop in patients receiving antipsychotic medication such as the phenothiazines or haloperidol over a period of days.[31] Some, but not all, neuroleptic malignant syndrome patients are also MH susceptible.[32] Should such patients require surgery or electroconvulsive therapy, it is best to avoid succinylcholine and to have dantrolene available since they too may be at risk of developing MH.

Although the disorders of the neuromuscular junction and skeletal muscle are numerous and present in different ways, neuromuscular blocking agents can be used effectively and rationally provided that the pathophysiology of the disorders are understood and the pharmacology of the neuromuscular blocking agents are appreciated.

REFERENCES

1. Jablecki C: Lambert Eaton myasthenic syndrome. Muscle Nerve 7:250–257, 1984
2. Calmon GH, Evans WK, Shepherd FA, et al: Myasthenic syndrome and small cell carcinoma of the lung. Arch Intern Med 144:999–1000, 1984

3. Wise RP: A myasthenic syndrome complicating bronchial carcinoma. Anaesthesia 17:488–504, 1967
4. Dowell VR: Infant botulism: New guise for an old disease. Hosp Pract 13:67–72, 1978
5. Whittaker M: Plasma cholinesterase variants and the anaesthetist. Anesthesia 35:174–197, 1980
6. Viby-Mogensen J: Correlation of succinylcholine duration of action with plasma cholinesterase activity in subjects with genotypically normal enzyme. Anesthesiology 53:517–520, 1980
7. Viby-Mogensen J: Succinylcholine neueromuscular blockade in subjects heterozygous for abnormal plasma cholinesterase. Anesthesiology 55:231–235, 1981
8. Lisak PP: Myasthenia gravis: Mechanisms and management. Hosp Pract 18:101–109, 1983
9. Horowitz SH, Genkins G, Kornfeld P,et al: Electrophysiologic diagnosis of myasthenia gravis and the regional curare test. Neurology 26:410–417, 1976
10. Balestrerri FJ, Prough D: Diagnostic value of systemic curare testing. Anesthesiology 57:226–227, 1982
11. Leventhal S, Orkin FK, Hirsh RA: Prediction of the need for postoperative mechanical ventilation in myasthenia gravis. Anesthesiology 53:26–30, 1980
12. Grant RP, Jenkins LC: Prediction of the need for postoperative mechanical ventilation in myasthenia gravis: Thymectomy compared to other surgical procedures. Can Anaesth Soc J 29:112–116, 1982
13. Gronert GA, Theye RA: Pathophysiology of hyperkalemia induced by succinylcholine. Anesthesiology 43:89–99, 1975
14. Carter JG, Sokoll MD, Gergis S: Effect of spinal cord transection on neuromuscular function in the rat. Anesthesiology 55:542–546, 1981
15. Graham DH: Monitoring neuromuscular block may be unreliable in patients with upper-motor-neuron lesions. Anesthesiology 52:74–75, 1980
16. Walton JN, Gardner-Medwin D: Progressive muscular dystrophy and the myotonic disorders, in Walton JN (ed): Disorders of Voluntary Muscle. Edinburgh/London, Churchill Livingstone, 1974, pp 561–613
17. Sanyal S, Johnson W, Thopar M, et al: An ultrastructural basis for electrocardiographic alterations associated with Duchenne's progressive muscular dystrophy. Circulation 57:1122–1128, 1978
18. Miller ED, Sanders DB, Rowlingson JC, et al: Anesthesia-induced rhabdomyolysis in a patient with duchenne's muscular dystrophy. Anesthesiology 48:146–148, 1978
19. Rosenberg H, Heiman-Patterson T: Duchenne's muscular dystrophy and malignant hyperthermia: Another warning. Anesthesiology 59:362, 1983
20. Ludatscher SM, Kerner H, Amikam S, et al: Myotonia dystrophica with heart involvement: An electron microscopic study of skeletal, cardiac, and smooth muscle. J Clin Pathol 31:1057–1064, 1978
21. Dundee JW: Thiopentone in dystrophia myotonia. Anesth Analg 31:257–262, 1952
22. Ravin M, Newmark Z, Saviello G: Myotonia dystrophica. An anesthetic hazard: Two case reports. Anesth Analg 54:216–218, 1975
23. Mitchell MM, Ali HM, Savarese JJ: Myotonia and neuromuscular blocking agents. Anesthesiology 49:44–48, 1978
24. Kaufman L: Anesthesia in dystrophica myotonia. Proc Roy Soc Med 53:183, 1960
25. Strasberg B, Karakis C, Dhingna R, et al: Myotonia dystrophia and mitral valve prolapse. Chest 78:845–848, 1980
26. Huckell VP, Staniloff HM, Britt BA, et al: Electrocardiographic abnormalities associated with malignant hyperthermia susceptibility. J Electrocardiol 15:137–141, 1982
27. Rosenberg H: Malignant Hyperthermia: Etiology. Annual Refresher Course Lectures, American Society of Anesthesiologists, vol 29, 1978, pp 1–7
28. Gronert GA, Malignant hyperthermia. Anesthesiology 53:395–423, 1980

29. Nelson TE, Flewellen EH: The malignant hyperthermia syndrome. N Engl J Med 309:416–418, 1983
30. Britt BA (ed): Malignant Hyperthermia. International Anesthesiology Clinics, vol 17. Boston, Little Brown, 1979
31. Caroff S: The neuroleptic malignant syndrome. J Clin Psych 41:79–83, 1980
32. Caroff S, Rosenberg H, Gerber JC: Neuroleptic malignant syndrome and malignant hyperthermia. Lancet 1:244, 1983
33. Drachman DB: Myasthenia Gravis. N Engl J Med 298:136, 1978

Colin A. Shanks

11

Muscle Relaxants in Renal Failure Patients

The kidneys are less than 0.5% of the body weight, yet they receive 25% of the cardiac output. The adult kidneys produce approximately 180 L of glomerular filtrate daily, at filtration rates that vary between 10 and 200 mL/min, and most of this is reabsorbed. Many of the neuromuscular blocking drugs are excreted largely by the kidney; their highly polarized molecular structure make it unlikely that tubular function plays a role in their excretion.

While there are many factors that can reduce the glomerular filtration rate during anesthesia, patient management problems with the muscle relaxants are likely to arise only when chronic disease has markedly diminished glomerular function. With end-stage renal disease, more than half the nephron mass has been lost. The disease spectrum ranges from renal insufficiency with mild azotemia, anemia, and inability to concentrate urine to the virtually anephric, with hyponatremia, hyperkalemia, uremia, etc. Patients with severe renal failure seldom present for major surgery before undergoing hemodialysis; the creation of arteriovenous shunts or fistulas rarely includes the mandatory use of muscle relaxants as part of the anesthetic technique.

Many anesthesiologists use muscle relaxants in patients scheduled for renal transplant surgery. While these patients probably are not hyperkalemic, they usually have received many drugs in the treatment of their hypertension, heart failure, arrhythmia, diabetes actual or potential infectious, psychotherapy, and for immunosuppression. With this polypharmacy it is possible for several drug interactions to occur simultaneously.

DEPOLARIZING RELAXANTS

The muscular relaxation essential for short procedures is usually provided by a depolarizing agent in common use. In the weeks following burns,

MUSCLE RELAXANTS
ISBN 0-8089-1784-6

neural damage, etc, the administration of succinylcholine can be followed by a rapid increase in serum potassium, sufficiently large in some patients to induce cardiac arrest. It is unlikely that these hyperkalemic episodes will occur in treated conditions associated with abnormalities in potassium excretion; use of succinylcholine in patients with renal failure is followed by minimal rises of serum potassium.[1–3]

NONDEPOLARIZING RELAXANTS

For the nondepolarizing agents, knowledge of structure-function relationships has made possible the design of drug molecules that produce adequate muscular relaxation yet have minimal unwanted effects, allowing the anesthesiologist a choice of agents according to the needs of the particular patient. When the patient has renal failure, there may not only be reduced elimination of drugs in the urine, but also concurrent pathophysiology in other systems, such as hypertension. Desirable features in a muscle relaxant might then include minimal possibility of producing a further rise in BP.

In patients with renal failure the problem most likely to be encountered with the nondepolarizing muscle relaxants is continuing unwanted postoperative paralysis. Prolonged block can follow either altered disposition of the drug in a patient or changes in effects observable with a given drug concentration. Pharmacokinetics characterize what the body does to the drug, whereas pharmacodynamics describe what the drug does to the body. Sheiner et al[4] have shown by sophisticated modeling that the response of the neuromuscular junction to D-tubocurarine is largely unaffected by renal disease. This is in contrast to conditions such as myasthenia gravis, where sensitivity to a given relaxant concentration is more marked.

Pharmacodynamics

Drug Interactions

Many drugs used during anesthesia and surgery have been shown to intensify neuromuscular blockade; the powerful inhalation agents can augment waining paralysis and then be removed by ventilation during and after the surgical closure. Azathioprine can produce partial antagonism.[5] Administration of mannitol does not increase the excretion of tubocurarine.[6] Treatment (eg, of arrhythmias) with intravenous (IV) lidocaine intensifies partial neuromuscular block.[7]

Probably of greatest clinical significance is the interaction between the relaxants and antibotics.[8] Agents that do not require dosage modification, such as clindamycin and lincomycin, are frequently used in patients with chronic renal failure. Others, including the aminoglycosides, should be used either in reduced dosage or with dosage-interval extension. Neostigmine may provide partial antagonism; with polymyxin B it augments the block.[9] These problems appear to be minimal with atracurium.[10]

Reversal

An overdose of relaxants, whether absolute or relative, is probably the most important single factor that predisposes to the so-called neostigmine-resistant curarization.[11] Physiologic factors such as acid-base and electrolyte imbalance can interfere with the reversibility of blockade. Both respiratory acidosis and metabolic alkalosis impair the ability of neostigmine to reverse curarization,[12] although hypothermia does not.[13] The pharmacokinetics of both edrophonium and neostigmine in patients undergoing renal transplantation are not different from those in patients with normal renal function but show a prolonged serum half-life in the anephric.[14,15] Recurarization does not seem to occur following adequate antagonism of pancuronium in renal failure.[16] In two patients, persistence of the anticholinesterase has been implicated in prolonged neuromuscular blockade from succinylcholine when it was administered several hours after previous surgery.[17]

Neuromuscular Junction

The amount of drug reaching the neuromuscular junction from the plasma should not change in the presence of renal disease; the binding of nondepolarizers by plasma proteins is unaltered for both tubocurarine[18,19] and pancuronium.[20] The relationship between the plasma concentration and the intensity of neuromuscular blockade is not entirely consistent. The plasma concentration of metocurine associated with 90% block in patients with renal failure averaged more than twice that found in normal patients.[21] Patients with and without renal failure had similar plasma concentrations of relaxant for comparable intensities of blockade with tubocurarine,[22] pancuronium,[23] gallamine,[24] and atracurium.[25] With the exception of metocurine, therefore, it would seem that the sensitivity of the neuromuscular junction to nondepolarizing agents is unaffected by renal disease.

Pharmacokinetics

The rate of spontaneous recovery from established neuromuscular blockade parallels the decline in plasma concentrations of the nondepolarizing relaxant. Following a single dose of relaxant, its plasma concentrations initially fall rapidly as the drug disperses into its apparent volume of distribution. In the later elimination phase, the rate of decline in plasma concentrations is proportional to the clearance from the body. Clearance is the irreversible loss of drug by metabolism, excretion, or inactivation. If a drug is almost entirely eliminated by the kidney, then renal failure would be predicted to prolong its elimination half-life. The relationship between the half-life of such drugs and creatinine clearance is discussed in an excellent review by Nancarrow and Mather.[26]

Gallamine, although a relaxant now seldom used clinically, allows us to explore the worst possible case of changed kinetics in renal failure, as its elimination is almost entirely by urinary excretion.[27] When plasma concentration-time curves for gallamine are compared at two dose levels, 2 mg/kg and 6 mg/kg, the elimination half-lives are similar[28] (Fig 1), the 6 mg/kg curve replicating the lower curve in a higher concentration range. However, the scale is log-linear, and after the 6 mg/kg dose, plasma concentrations of gallamine above that producing 95% blockade persist for a much longer time than three times that of the 2 mg/kg dose. Figure 1 also shows the curve

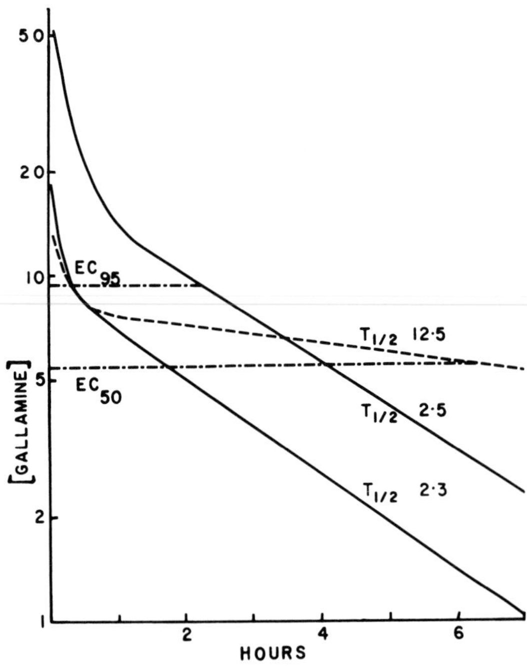

Figure 1. Plasma gallamine-time curves derived from pooled data. The solid lines represent normal patients to whom gallamine was administered in doses of 6 mg/kg (upper) and 2 mg/kg (lower).[28] The dotted curve represents patients in renal failure who received a dose of 2 mg/kg.[24] The horizontal lines indicate the mean effective plasma concentrations of gallamine associated with 50% and 95% paralysis.

obtained from patients in renal failure to whom gallamine 2 mg/kg was administered. For most of these patients in chronic renal failure, redistribution enabled normal neuromuscular response patterns; the patient with the lowest volumes of distribution showed complete paralysis for three hours. When large, multiple, or infused doses of gallamine nullify the effects of redistribution, then slow decline of plasma concentrations through the range producing paralysis will result in prolonged relaxation. Had a larger dose of gallamine transposed upward the curve with a half-life of 12.5 hours, then these patients may have needed dialysis to recover from the paralysis.[29] Similarly, the drug excreted in both urine and bile shows prolonged effect in the presence of combined renal and hepatic dysfunction; such a patient required hemodialysis when her pancuronium blockade could not be reversed.[30]

When the pharmacokinetic profiles of the nondepolarizing relaxants are contrasted between normal patients and those in renal failure, the most striking feature is the diminution of their clearance from the plasma (Table 1). Due to its reliance on renal excretion, gallamine is the drug that shows the greatest change. Pancuronium, metocurine, and tubocurarine are also excreted in the bile, so that this alternate pathway becomes the major route of excretion in the anephric. The usual two- to three-hour half-life of these agents is increased, but not as markedly as for gallamine. As the volumes of distribution are not greatly affected by renal failure, the effects of an initial small dose of any of the nondepolarizing agents would not be expected to differ from normal. This is in contrast to patients with cirrhosis of the liver, where the increased volume of distribution of pancuronium[31] would be associated with an initial resistance. The usual initial dose would produce a plasma concentration inadequate for intubation or surgery.

In contrast, atracurium and vecuronium have little reliance on renal function for their clearance. Atracurium undergoes rapid biodegradation in the mild alkaline conditions of the body. Vecuronium is taken up by the liver and much of it is excreted unchanged in the bile. The onset, duration, and recovery rate times of neuromuscular blockade do not change in the presence

Table 1
Decrease in Plasma Clearance With Renal Failure

Decrease in Plasma Clearance	Drug	Reference
More than 5 times	Gallamine	24
1.5 to 5 times	Pancuronium	23, 37, 38
	Metocurine	21
	Tubocurarine	22
Unchanged	Atracurium	34
	Vecuronium	33, 35

of renal failure,[32,33] with little differences in the pharmacokinetic profiles.[34,35] These two agents must now be seen as the relaxants of choice when neuromuscular blockade is required for patients with renal failure. As clearance of atracurium (by Hofmann elimination) is independent of organ function, it is easy to understand the reason for a report that neither its pharmacokinetics nor its pharmacodynamics were altered in patients with combined renal and hepatic failure.[25]

CONCLUSION

If there is a need for neuromuscular blockade in the patient with renal failure, then it would seem easiest to choose one of these two agents whose intermediate duration of action is unaffected by the disease. The decision would then rest with the anesthesiologist in opting for atracurium, when a large dose might produce hypotension,[36] or for vecuronium, when concurrent hepatic dysfunction might alter its clearance.

REFERENCES

1. Miller RD, Way WL, Hamilton WK, et al: Succinylcholine-induced hyperkalemia in patients with renal failure? Anesthesiology 36:138–141, 1972
2. Koide M, Waud BE: Serum potassium concentrations after succinylcholine in patients with renal failure. Anesthesiology 36:142–145, 1972
3. Walton JD, Farman JV: Suxamethonium, potassium and renal failure. Anaesthesia 28:626–630, 1973
4. Sheiner LB, Stanski DR, Vozeh S, et al: Simultaneous modelling of pharmacokinetics and pharmacodynamics: Application to d-tubocurarine. Clinical Pharmacol Ther 25:358–371, 1979
5. Dretchen KL, Morgenroth VH, Standaert FG, et al: Azathioprine: Effects on neuromuscular transmission. Anesthesiology 45:442–445, 1976
6. Matteo RS, Nishitateno K, Pua EK, et al: Pharmacokinetics of d-tubocurarine in man: Effect of an osmotic diuretic on urinary excretion. Anesthesiology 52:335–338, 1980
7. Telivuo L, Katz RL: The effects of modern intravenous local analgesics on respiration during partial neuromuscular block in man. Anaesthesia 25:30–35, 1970
8. Cronnelly R, Morris RB: Antagonism of neuromuscular blockade. Br J Anaesth 54:183–194, 1982
9. Van Nyhuis LS, Miller RD, Fogdall RP: The interaction between d-tubocurarine, pancuronium, polymyxin B, and neostigmine on neuromuscular function. Anesth Analg 55:224–228, 1976
10. Chappel DJ, Clark JS, Hughes R: Interaction between atracurium and drugs used in anaesthesia. Br J Anaesth 55:17S–22S, 1983
11. Baraka A: Irreversible curarization. Anaesth Intensive Care 5:244–246, 1977
12. Miller RD, Van Nyhuis LS, Eger EI, II, et al: The effect of acid-base balance on neostigmine antagonism of d-tubocurarine-induced neuromuscular blockade. Anesthesiology: 42:377–383, 1975
13. Miller RD, Van Nyhuis LS, Eger EI, II: The effect of temperature on a tubocurarine neuromuscular blockade and its antagonism by neostigmine. J Pharmacol Exp Ther 195:237–241, 1975

14. Morris RB, Cronnelly R, Miller RD, et al: Pharmacokinetics of edrophonium in anephric and renal transplant patients. Br J Anaesth 53:1311–1314, 1981
15. Cronnelly R, Stanski DR, Miller RD, et al: Renal function and the pharmacokinetics of neostigmine in anesthetized man. Anesthesiology 51:222–226, 1979
16. Bevan DR, Archer D, Donati F, et al: Antagonism of pancuronium in renal failure: No recurarization. Br J Anaesth 54:63–68, 1982
17. Bishop MJ, Hornbein TF: Prolonged effect of succinylcholine after neostigmine and pyridostigmine administration in patients with renal failure. Anesthesiology 58:384–386, 1983
18. Ghoneim MM, Kramer E, Bannow R, et al: Binding of d-tubocurarine to plasma proteins in normal man and in patients with hepatic or renal disease. Anesthesiology 39:410–415, 1973
19. Walker JS, Shanks CA, Brown KF: Determinants of d-tubocurarine plasma protein binding in health and disease. Anesth Analg 62:870–874, 1983
20. Wood M, Stone WJ, Wood AJJ: Plasma binding of pancuronium: Effects of age, sex, and disease. Anesth Analg 62:29–32, 1983
21. Brotherton WP, Matteo RS: Pharmacokinetics and pharmacodynamics of metocurine in humans with and without renal failure. Anesthesiology 55:273–276, 1981
22. Miller RD, Matteo RD, Benet LZ, et al: The pharmacokinetics of d-tubocurarine in man with and without renal failure. J Pharmacol Exp Ther 202:1–7, 1977
23. Somogyi AA, Shanks CA, Triggs EJ: The effect of renal failure on the disposition and neuromuscular blocking action of pancuronium bromide. Eur J Clin Pharmacol 12:23–29, 1977
24. Ramzan MI, Shanks CA, Triggs EJ: Gallamine disposition in surgical patients with chronic renal failure. Br J Clin Pharmacol 12:141–147, 1981
25. Ward S, Wright D, Corall I, et al: Combined pharmacokinetic and pharmacodynamic studies with atracurium besylate (in normal patients and patients with hepatic and renal failure). Can Anaesth Soc J 30:S81, 1983
26. Nancarrow C, Mather LE: Pharmacokinetics in renal failure. Anaesth Intensive Care 11:350–360, 1983
27. Agoston S, Vermeer GA, Kersten UW, et al: A preliminary investigation of the renal and hepatic elimination of gallamine triethiodide in man. Br J Anaesth 50:345–351, 1978
28. Ramzan MI, Triggs EJ, Shanks CA: Pharmacokinetic studies in man with gallamine triethiodide. Eur J Clin Pharmacol 17:145–152, 1980
29. Lowenstein E, Goldfine C, Flacke WE: Administration of gallamine in the presence of renal failure—Reversal of neuromuscular blockade by peritoneal dialysis. Anesthesiology 33: 556–558, 1970
30. Abrams RE, Hornbein TF: Inability to reverse pancuronium blockade in a patient with renal failure and hepatic disease. Anesthesiology 42:362–364, 1975
31. Duvaldestin P, Agoston S, Henzel D, et al: Pancuronium pharmacokinetics in patients with liver cirrhosis. Br J Anaes 50:1131–1136, 1978
32. Hunter JM, Jones RS, Utting JE: Use of atracurium in patients with no renal function. Br J Anaesthesia 54:1251–1258, 1982
33. Fahey MR, Rupp SM, Fisher DM, et al: Pharmacokinetics and pharmacodynamics of atracurium in normal and renal failure patients. Anesthesiology 59:A263, 1983
34. Fahey MR, Morris RB, Miller RD, et al: Pharmacokinetics of ORG NC45 (Norcuron) in patients with and without renal failure. Br J Anaesth 53:1049–1053, 1981
35. Meistelman C, Lienhart A, Leveque C, et al: Pharmacology of vecuronium with end stage renal failure. Anesthesiology 59:A293, 1983
36. Basta SJ, Savarese JJ, Ali HH, et al: Histamine-releasing potencies of atracurium, dimethyl tubocurarine and tubocurarine. Br J Anaesth 55:105S–106S, 1983
37. McLeod K, Watson MJ, Rawlins MD: Pharmacokinetics of pancuronium in patients with normal and impaired renal function. Br J Anesth 48:341–345, 1976
38. Buzello W, Agoston S: Pharmacokinetics of pancuronium in patients with normal and impaired renal function. Anaesthesist 27:291–297, 1978

Pim J. Hennis
Donald R. Stanski

12

Pharmacokinetic and Pharmacodynamic Factors That Govern the Clinical Use of Muscle Relaxants

When an anesthesiologist administers an adequate dose of a nondepolarizing muscle relaxant, a drug response occurs: muscle paralysis. The drug response may be measured using stimulation of a peripheral motor nerve or the paralysis may be clinically assessed by the surgical operating conditions. This dose-paralysis relationship consists of two parts: pharmacokinetic component, which describes the relationship between dose and muscle relaxant blood concentrations (what the body does to the drug), and a pharmacodynamic component, which describes the relationship between the muscle relaxant blood concentrations and the degree of paralysis (what the drug does to the body). The muscle relaxant pharmacokinetics and pharmacodynamics and, therefore, the dose-paralysis relationship may be influenced by many physiologic and pathologic factors. By understanding the basic principles of pharmacokinetics and pharmacodynamics, the anesthesiologist can obtain better insight into the factors that can alter the muscle relaxant dose-paralysis relationship.

In this review article the basic concepts of pharmacokinetics and pharmacodynamics will be discussed in general terms that are applicable to most drugs used in anesthetic practice. These concepts will then be used to indicate the factors that govern the onset, degree, and recovery of paralysis induced by nondepolarizing muscle relaxants (Fig. 1). When appropriate, examples of how disease or altered physiology affect the pharmacokinetics or pharmacodynamics will be indicated. Computer simulations (using data from d-tubocurarine [dTc]) will be extensively used to visually display the basic concepts and applications of pharmacokinetics and pharmacodynamics to the muscle

MUSCLE RELAXANTS
ISBN 0-8089-1784-6

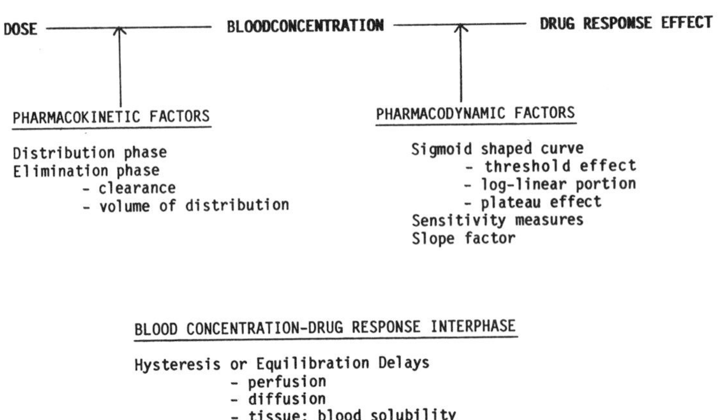

Figure 1. The compoments of the dose-response relationship.

relaxants. For a more detailed discussion of this topic the reader is urged to examine several recent textbooks written specifically for anesthesiologists.[1-3]

PHARMACOKINETIC FACTORS

Figure 2 displays the blood concentration *v* time curve after an intravenous (IV) bolus dose of dTc. Immediately after the IV bolus injection there is almost instantaneous mixing of the drug into blood and certain tissues that have high perfusion (vessel-rich group). This phase occurs within one or two circulations of the drug in the body and is so rapid that it is generally not detectable with conventional venous blood sampling at one- or two-minute intervals. This very rapid mixing phase defines the peak drug concentrations seen in blood one-half to one minute after the IV injection. After the peak blood concentrations are achieved, two distinct phases are visible, a distribution phase where the blood concentrations decline rapidly and an elimination phase where the blood concentrations decline at a slower rate.

The distribution phase is the equilibration of the blood concentration (after the immediate mixing phase that defines the peak concentration) with tissues that are less well perfused. During this phase there is not an equilibrium between the blood concentration and the drug concentrations in most of the tissues of the body. Drug is being distributed and redistributed between various tissues, with several factors governing the rate at which the tissue concentrations equilibrate with the blood concentration. These include the perfusion of the tissues (high perfusion causes rapid equilibration) and the partitioning or solubility of the drug in the tissues (low partitioning causes

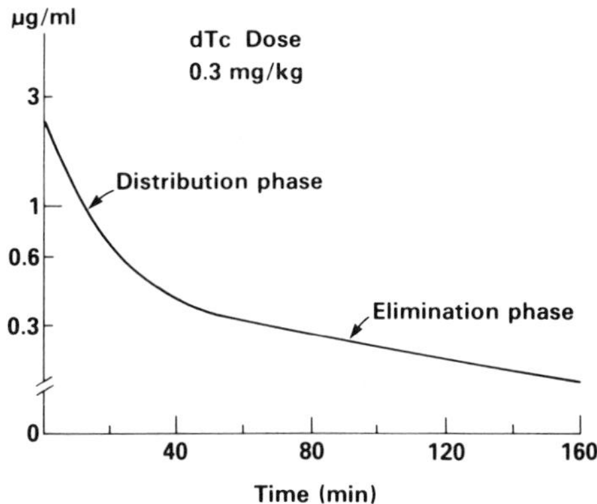

Figure 2. A computer simulation of the blood concentration v time curve after an IV bolus dose of dTc 0.3 mg · kg. The following pharmacokinetic data were used: distribution half-life = 6.8 minutes; elimination half-life = 115 minutes, initial distribution volume = 0.090 L · kg^{-1}; Vdss = 0.36 L · kg^{-1}; total body clearance = 3 mL^{-1} · kg^{-1} · min^{-1}. (dTc data adapted from Stanski et al.[8])

rapid equilibration). If the drug has very limited ability to penetrate membranes (low lipid solubility, high degree of ionization, large molecular weight), diffusion factors can also become rate limiting in the equilibration of the blood concentration with the tissues.

Distribution and redistribution are terms that describe the same process: transfer of drug to and from various organs of the body. These terms are interchangeable, the only difference being a temporal component (drug has to be distributed before it can be redistributed).

After the drug has distributed/redistributed throughout the body, the elimination phase becomes obvious. During this phase the decline of the blood concentration is slower relative to the distribution phase. The decline of the drug concentration is due to the irreversible elimination of the drug from the body. This can be due to metabolism in the liver (blood or other tissues can also metabolize drug) to generally less active compounds and/or excretion of the unchanged drug via the kidney or bile. Because the change of the blood concentration is relatively slow in the elimination phase compared with the distribution phase, a pseudoequilibrium is said to exist between the blood concentration and the drug concentrations in the various tissues.

The magnitude of the distribution and elimination phases can be quantitated by taking the slope of the natural log of the blood concentration *v* time curve. This slope is termed a rate constant, with a large value indicating a rapid process and a small value a slow process. These rate constants can be converted into the term half-life (half-life = natural log of 2/rate constant, or

0.693/rate constant). The half-life defines the time needed for the blood concentration to decline by a factor of 2, or 50%. The half-life also defines the time needed to complete the distribution or elimination process (50% of the process is completed in one half-life, 75% in two half-lives, 87% in three half-lives). After four to five half-lives a distribution or elimination process is virtually complete.

The distribution and elimination phases can be conceptualized as a two-compartment pharmacokinetic model. A compartment may be thought of as a group of tissues that are kinetically indistinguishable. In the two-compartment pharmacokinetic model there is one central compartment into which the drug is administered and from which blood is sampled. From the central compartment the drug distributes to a peripheral compartment or tissues in which one cannot measure the drug concentration. This results in the distribution phase that was previously discussed. From the peripheral compartment the drug can redistribute back to the central compartment. All of the drug elimination occurs from the central compartment.

The volume of distribution is a measure of the extent of drug distribution in the body. There are several distribution volumes. The initial volume of distribution, also called the central compartment distribution volume, or V_1, indicates the apparent space needed to explain the relationship between a given dose and the resulting peak drug concentrations occurring immediately after the bolus IV injection. This initial volume of distribution is a reflection of the distribution space of the vessel-rich or rapidly equilibrating organs that have extremely high perfusion and are responsible for the initial mixing phase that was previously described. The size of this space can sometimes exceed the blood volume since it can include drug partitioning into tissues that have extensive perfusion (lungs, heart, liver, kidneys). The volume of distribution at steady state (Vdss) indicates the apparent space needed to explain the relationship between dose and drug concentration when there is a (pseudo) equilibrium between blood and all of the various tissue concentrations, assuming that the partitioning coefficient between blood and all tissues is one. If a drug partitions extensively into tissues, the Vdss state will be large, often exceeding total body mass. This large distribution volume indicates that most of the drug is not in blood, but in the tissues. When blood concentrations are low, a relatively small amount of drug is available in the blood for delivery to the eliminating organs.

All of the drug that is administered is ultimately cleared or removed from the body. Drug clearance can be due to metabolism of the drug to inactive or less pharmacologically active products or the irreversible elimination of the unchanged drug from the body. Clearance is defined as the volume of blood that is completely removed of drug per unit time. Drug clearance is analogous to the concept of creatinine clearance, the only difference being that the drug is an exogenous compound administered to the body and creatinine is an endogenous body product. Drug clearance occurs mainly in the liver or kidney, although the blood can act as the clearing organ, as is the case for succinylcholine. If the drug is eliminated by metabolism and the liver is the only eliminating organ, drug clearance becomes a measure of the efficiency of the liver. If the liver is very efficient (high hepatic extraction ratio), clearance will approach liver blood flow (21 $mL \cdot kg^{-1} \cdot min^{-1}$). Note that clearance (volume per unit time) is independent of drug concentration. At high concentrations of drug a greater amount is removed or cleared than at low concentrations — a characteristic of first-order kinetics.

The pharmacokinetic terms clearance and steady-state distribution volume are the primary pharmacokinetic parameters that describe the rate of elimination (clearance) and the extent of drug distribution (volume of distribution). The terminal elimination half-life of a drug is related to the steady-state distribution volume and clearance in the following manner:

$$\text{terminal elimination half-life} = \frac{0.693 \times \text{distribution volume}}{\text{clearance}}$$

One can see that the terminal elimination half-life is a derived parameter from clearance and steady-state distribution volume. As the distribution volume increases, the terminal elimination half-life becomes longer. As drug clearance increases, the terminal elimination half-life becomes shorter. If the terminal elimination half-life of a drug changes, one must examine both clearance and steady-state distribution volume to determine which factor has altered the elimination half-life.

The pharmacokinetics of the nondepolarizing muscle relaxants have been extensively reviewed elsewhere.[1-4] For the longer-acting relaxants (pancuronium, dTc, gallamine, metocurine) a general pattern of pharmacokinetic properties can be described. The distribution half-life is between two to ten minutes whereas the terminal elimination half-life is between 2 to 6 hours. The variability in the terminal elimination half-life in different studies of the same relaxant can be due to the duration of blood sampling—the longer blood samples are obtained after administration, the greater will the terminal elimination half-life be. The steady-state distribution volumes range from 0.2 to 0.5 $L \cdot kg^{-1}$. These distribution volumes are relatively small compared with 2 to 4 $L \cdot kg^{-1}$ for barbiturates and narcotics, indicating very limited tissue distribution of the relaxants. The ionized, polar nature of the relaxant molecule limits the tissue uptake and therefore the magnitude of the distribution volume. The clearance of the relaxants is approximately 2 to 5 $mL \cdot kg^{-1} \cdot min^{-1}$. This suggests that the hepatic and renal elimination mechanisms are relatively inefficient in removing the relaxant drugs when compared with other drugs used in anesthetic practice. The clearance of most narcotics is 10 to 20 $mL \cdot kg^{-1} \cdot min^{-1}$.

PHARMACODYNAMIC FACTORS

The relationship between steady-state blood concentration and the magnitude of drug response is indicated in Fig. 3. One sees a sigmoid-type shape, with threshold concentrations needed to achieve 10% to 20% of the drug effect, a log-linear increase of the concentration causing a linear increase of effect from 20% to 80%, and finally a plateau beyond which increasing concentrations cause no additional increase of drug effect.[5,6] A measure of the sensitivity of the subject to the drug can be determined from the blood concentration that causes 50% of the maximal response ($Cpss_{50}$). An important factor is the steepness of the sigmoid curve, or the change in concentration needed to go from 20% to 80% of the response (slope of the concentration-response curve). If the slope factor is small, a relatively large change of the blood concentration is needed to produce a given change of the drug response. If the slope factor is large, then a small change of the blood concentration can cause a marked change in the drug response. A sigmoid-shaped concentration *v* response curve will be defined only if it is possible to measure the drug response in a reasonably accurate manner and when there is a measurable maximal drug effect.

The range of drug concentrations that give a desired effect is the therapeutic window. For the muscle relaxants, this therapeutic window generally would be concentrations that cause 90% to 95% paralysis ($Cpss_{90}$ and $Cpss_{95}$, respectively). This range of paralysis is generally optimal for intra-abdominal surgery.

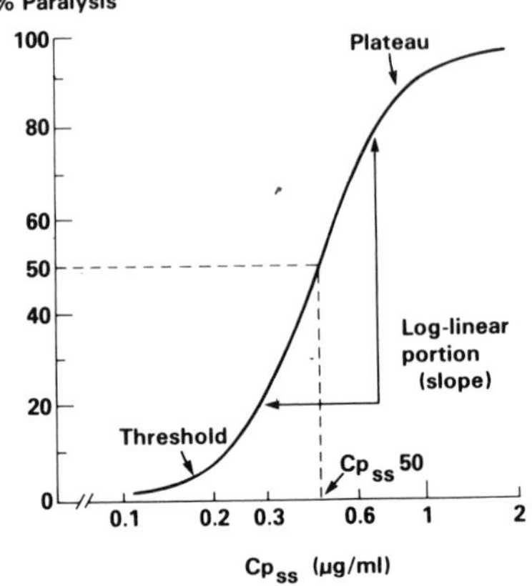

Figure 3. A computer simulation of the sigmoid-shaped relationship between steady-state blood concentrations of dTc and paralysis. Note the threshold concentrations, log-linear phase, and plateau concentrations. The Cp_{ss}^{50} (blood concentration that causes 50% of the maximum response) is 0.45 $\mu g \cdot mL^{-1}$. (dTc data adapted from Stanski et al.[8])

BLOOD CONCENTRATION–DRUG RESPONSE INTERPHASE

In the previous section, drug response was related to the steady-state blood concentrations. Steady state is defined as a situation in which the blood concentration is constant because the rate of drug elimination is equaled by the rate of drug administration. Since the steady-state blood concentration is in equilibrium with all of the tissue drug concentrations, the biophase, or site of action, concentrations will also be constant (an exception will be in any organ that eliminates the drug). Since the drug effect occurs in the tissues, at steady state the drug concentration at the site of action (biophase) will also be constant.

After a bolus IV injection of a drug, a true steady state is never achieved because the drug is constantly being distributed, redistributed, and eliminated. During the drug distribution phase there can be a great deal of disequilibrium between the blood concentrations and the drug concentrations in the tissues or biophase of drug effect. This will translate into a time delay between the blood concentration and the drug effect.[5–7] Only during the elimination phase is a pseudoequilibrium said to exist. During this phase the drug has been distributed to the tissues and the slow decline of the blood concentration will be paralleled by an equally slow decline of the tissue and biophase concentration (pseudo–equilibrium), causing a minimal time delay between the blood concentration and drug effect.

Four factors can cause a time delay between the blood concentration and the drug effect.

Perfusion or delivery of drug to the biophase. If the perfusion to the biophase is high, drug delivery will be enhanced, and therefore the rate of equilibration between the blood concentration and the biophase concentration will be enhanced.

Diffusion of drug from the capillary lumen to the biophase. Once in the capillary lumen of the biophase, the drug must diffuse into the tissue where it can act. If physiochemical factors (ionization, molecular size) significantly limit the rate of membrane penetration (diffusion) into the biophase, this can translate into a time delay between the blood concentration and the drug effect.

Partitioning of the drug between the blood and the biophase. Once the drug has reached the biophase, several processes can occur. The drug can reach the receptor sites within the biophase and induce the drug effect. The drug can also be nonspecifically bound to various (nonreceptor) proteins within the biophase analogous to the drug-protein binding that occurs in blood. If the drug is bound to proteins that are not relevant in creating the drug effect, the drug is effectively "unavailable" to induce a pharmacologic effect. One measure of these processes is the drug partition coefficient between blood and the biophase. A relatively high solubility of the drug in a tissue suggests exclusive "nonspecific tissue binding" such that the rate of equilibration between blood and the free, pharmacologically active concentrations in the tissue will be prolonged. A relevant analogy in anesthesia is the difference in air: blood solubility for nitrous oxide and ether. The equilibration between the lung and blood is very slow for ether because of the high solubility of ether in blood, therefore the induction of anesthesia with ether is slow. The opposite is true for nitrous oxide, where induction is fast because of the low air:blood solubility. This analogy also applies to the equilibration of a drug between the blood and tissue (biophase) where the drug effect occurs.

Time to achieve receptor events and create the drug effect. Once the drug has reached the biophase (receptors, membranes), the actual time of receptor association/dissociation and translation of the receptor events into a pharmacologic effect become important. If the time to achieve receptor events is very slow, then a significant delay between the blood concentration and drug effect will be obvious.

Of these four factors, the time delay that occurs between peak relaxant blood concentrations and the achievement of paralysis is due mainly to perfusion (muscle blood flow) and the partitioning of the relaxant between blood and muscle.[7–9] Diffusion and receptor events do not appear to be rate limit-

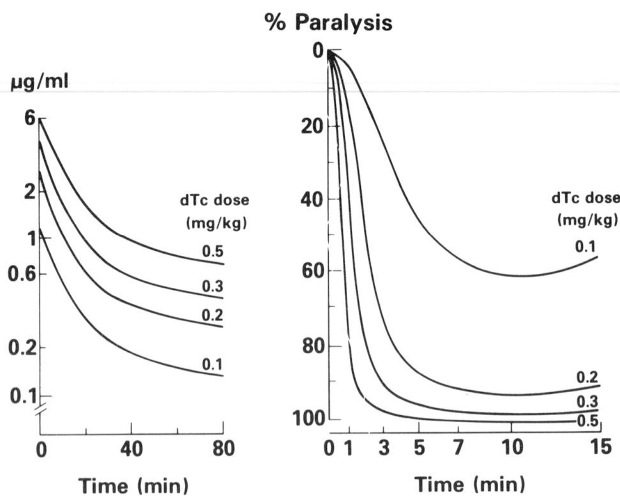

Figure 4. A computer simulation of how increasing dTc dose affects the blood concentrations (left panel) and the onset of paralysis (right panel). The onset of paralysis is more rapid as the dose is increased. The more rapid onset of paralysis is due to the higher peak dTc blood concentrations from the increased dose.

ing.[6,10] The half-life of muscle-blood equilibration is approximately five to eight minutes. This explains the delay in the onset of paralysis after a bolus IV injection of a relaxant. The low perfusion of muscle (3 $mL \cdot 100\ g^{-1} \cdot min^{-1}$) is the main factor that causes the relatively long blood concentration–paralysis equilibration delay. If muscle blood flow were as high as cerebral blood flow (50 $mL \cdot 100\ g^{-1} \cdot min^{-1}$), then the nondepolarizing muscle relaxants would have a much more rapid onset of effect.

WHAT GOVERNS THE ONSET OF PARALYSIS?

The onset of paralysis is defined as the time from bolus IV injection of the muscle relaxant until the degree of paralysis is maximal (no change in the degree of paralysis). With the nondepolarizing muscle relaxants, the onset time of five to ten minutes is relatively slow when compared with the one- to two-minute onset time of succinylcholine or the IV anesthetics (thiopental). The onset of paralysis is governed by the dose, distribution/redistribution pharmacokinetics, the blood concentration–paralysis relationship, and pharmacodynamic factors.

Dose

Figure 4 is a computer simulation of the relationship between different IV bolus doses of (dTc), the resulting blood concentrations, and the degree of paralysis over time. If the dose of dTc is such that less than 100% paralysis occurs, one sees an onset time of five to ten minutes. This relatively long onset time is due to the blood concentration–response interphase factors discussed previously. As the dose of dTc is progressively increased, the onset time appears to become shorter. Larger doses cause higher peak blood concentrations, which result in more relaxant being delivered to the neuromuscular junction in the first few circulation times. The larger amount of relaxant delivered to the neuromuscular junction causes the more rapid onset of paralysis. While a relatively rapid onset of paralysis occurs with large doses, the underlying blood concentration–paralysis equilibration time still remains at six to seven minutes because the plateau of maximal paralysis has been achieved with the large dose of relaxant. Large doses of the relaxant may cause a rapid onset of paralysis; however, the time for recovery of paralysis also becomes longer, as will be shown later.

Distribution/Redistribution Kinetics

If the initial and/or the steady-state distribution volume (V_1 or Vdss) of the muscle relaxant is changed and/or the rate of redistribution (distribution half-life) is altered, the onset of paralysis can be affected. An increase in the initial distribution volume will result in lower peak blood concentrations after an IV bolus injection. The lower blood concentrations will result in less relaxant being delivered to the neuromuscular junction per unit time and therefore an apparent delay in the onset of paralysis. Figure 5 indicates the effect of changing the initial and steady-state distribution volumes on the blood concentration and the onset of paralysis. A clinical example of this occurs in patients with hepatic cirrhosis receiving pancuronium.[11]

Blood Concentration–Paralysis Interphase

The rate of equilibration between the blood concentration and paralysis is governed mainly by muscle perfusion and blood: muscle partitioning. Muscle perfusion has the greatest potential to be affected by altered pathophysiology. Enhanced muscle blood flow should increase the onset of paralysis, with decreased muscle perfusion delaying the onset of paralysis. Figure 6 indicates how the onset of paralysis is affected by a change in the rate of blood–paralysis equilibration. A delayed rate of blood concentration–paralysis equilibration has been quantitated in patients having a moderate degree of

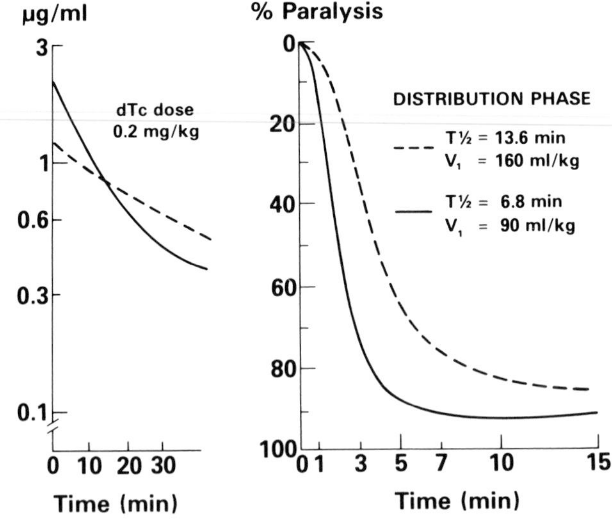

Figure 5. A computer simulation of how altered distribution pharmacokinetics (left panel) influence the blood concentrations and the onset of paralysis after an IV bolus dose of dTc 0.2 mg · kg^{-1}. As the distribution volume increases and the distribution half-life becomes longer, the onset of paralysis also becomes longer. (Data adapted from Duvaldestin et al.[11])

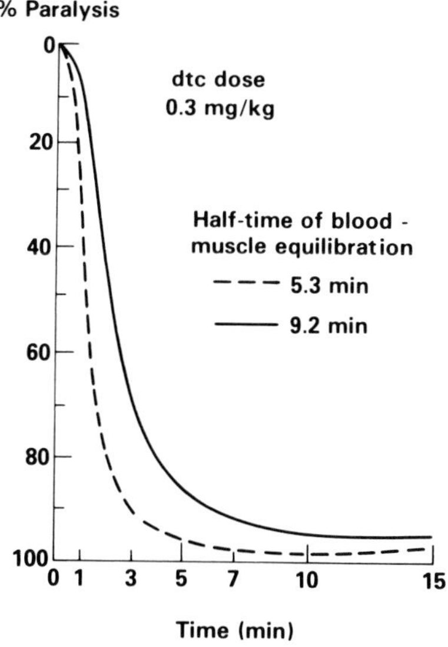

Figure 6. A computer simulation of how an altered blood-paralysis equilibration delay influences the onset of paralysis after an IV bolus dose of dTc 0.3 mg · kg^{-1}. As the half-life of muscle:blood equilibration increases, the onset of paralysis becomes longer. (Data adapted from Ham et al.[12])

hypothermia, presumably due to decreased muscle perfusion.[12] In patients with a low cardiac output, the onset of succinylcholine paralysis has been shown to be delayed.[13]

Pharmacodynamics

Just as the administered dose can change the apparent onset of paralysis, so can a change in the tissue responsiveness alter the onset of paralysis. If the patient is "sensitive" (blood concentration–paralysis relationship is shifted to the left with a lower $Cpss_{50}$), then the onset of paralysis will appear more rapid. In the sensitive patient a smaller amount of drug is needed at the neuromuscular junction to achieve the same degree of paralysis. For a given dose of relaxant, this amount of drug will be achieved at an earlier point in time after the bolus IV injection. Examples of an increased sensitivity (lower $Cpss_{50}$) are found in myasthenia gravis patients and when nondepolarizing muscle relaxants are administered concomitantly with inhalational anesthestic agents such as halothane.[8] Figure 7 is a simulation of the influence of increasing $Cpss_{50}$ (secondary to halothane) on the onset of paralysis. With a low $Cpss_{50}$ there is a relatively rapid onset of paralysis. The opposite occurs if the patient is "resistant" (concentration-paralysis relationship or $Cpss_{50}$ shifted to the right). An example of resistance occurs in patients with thermal burns.[14] The slope of the concentration-paralysis relationship also governs the onset of paralysis. When the slope is very steep the onset of paralysis will occur earlier

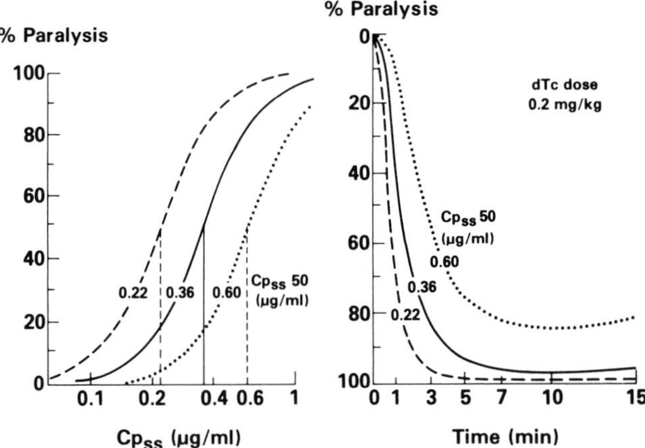

Figure 7. A computer simulation of how altered muscle sensitivity (left panel) changes the onset of paralysis after an IV bolus dose of dTc 0.2 mg · kg^{-1} (right panel). As the Cp_{ss}^{50} becomes higher, the onset of paralysis becomes slower. (Data adapted from Stanski et al.[8])

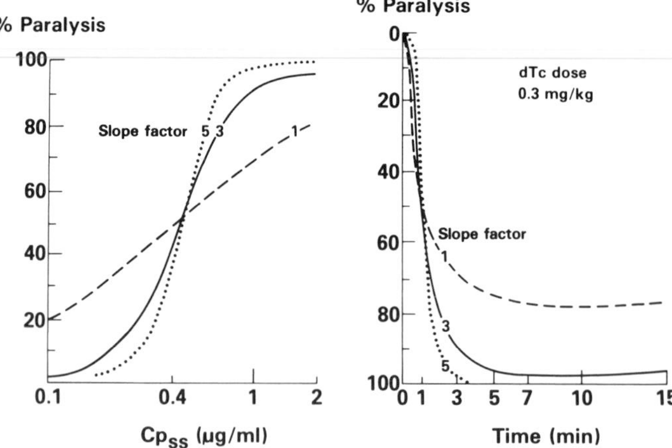

Figure 8. A computer simulation of how an alteration of the slope of the concentration-paralysis relationship changes the onset of paralysis after an IV bolus dose of dTc 0.3 mg · kg^{-1}. The steady-state blood concentration *v* paralysis curves are in the left panel, and the paralysis v time curves are in the right panel. As the slope factor of the concentration-paralysis relationship increases, the onset of paralysis becomes more rapid. (Data adapted from Hull et al.[15])

than when the slope is shallow (Fig. 8). Pancuronium and fazadinium have a significantly different slope factor, which explains in part the clinical differences in onset of effect between these relaxants.[15]

WHAT GOVERNS THE DEGREE OF PARALYSIS?

The degree of paralysis for a given bolus dose of relaxant is best assessed at the time when the maximal effect is present. If the dose is large enough to cause complete (100%) paralysis, then it becomes difficult to accurately assess the true degree of drug response. Analogous to the onset of paralysis, many factors can change the degree of paralysis including the dose, pharmacokinetics, and pharmacodynamics.

As the magnitude of the bolus dose is increased, the peak blood concentrations will also increase and cause a greater degree of paralysis (Fig. 4).

Pharmacokinetic factors that cause lower initial blood concentration for a given dose will result in a decreased degree of paralysis. The altered distribution/redistribution factors discussed previously would be relevant here (Fig. 5).

A major factor in determining the degree of paralysis is the neuromuscular junction sensitivity, or pharmacodynamics. For a given dose of relaxant, if

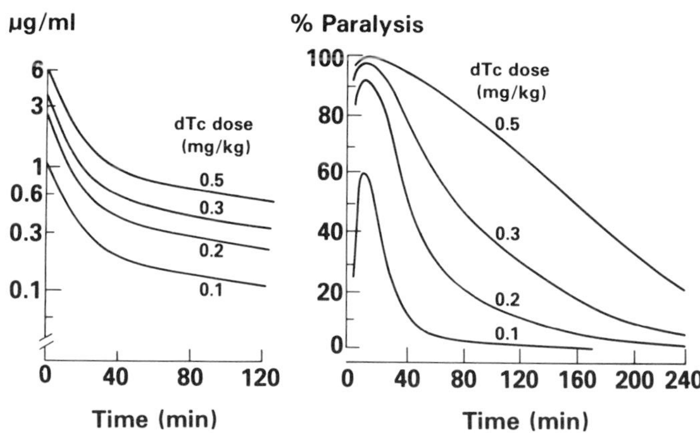

Figure 9. A computer simulation of how increasing dTc dose affects the blood concentrations (left panel) and the recovery of paralysis (right panel). Note that the paralysis axis has been inverted from the previous simulations to allow better visualization of the recovery process. With low doses of dTc, recovery occurs during the distribution/redistribution phase and therefore is very rapid. With larger doses of dTc, recovery occurs during the elimination phase and therefore is slower.

a patient is sensitive (low $Cpss_{50}$) then a greater degree of paralysis will be present than if a patient is resistant (high $Cpss_{50}$) (Fig. 7).

WHAT GOVERNS THE RECOVERY OF PARALYSIS?

The recovery of paralysis can be quantitated by the time needed to recover from the peak effect to a given degree of paralysis or the rate of recovery (time needed to recover from 75% to 25% paralysis). As before, dose, pharmacokinetics, and pharmacodynamics govern the recovery of paralysis.

Pharmacokinetic Factors

If a small dose of relaxant is given that causes a submaximal (60% to 80%) degree of paralysis, recovery will commence immediately. Recovery will occur during the distribution/redistribution phase and will be relatively rapid in this situation since the relaxant is being redistributed from the neuromuscular junction to other tissues. Given that most relaxants have a distribution half-life of five minutes, this distribution/redistribution phase would be completed in three to four half-lives, or 15 to 20 minutes. An example of the

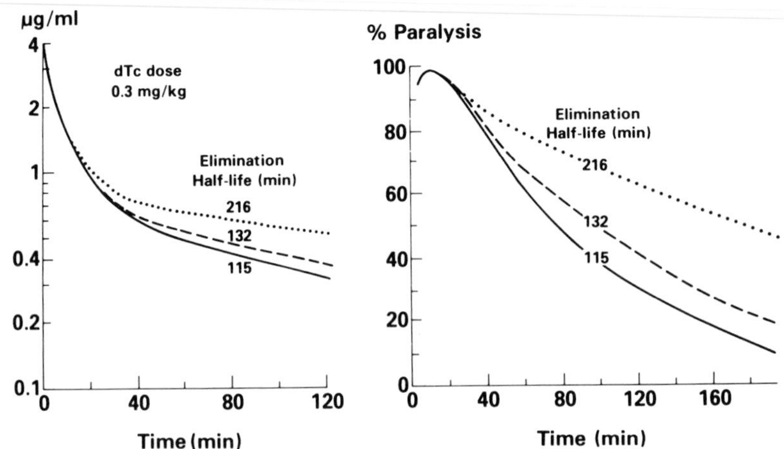

Figure 10. A computer simulation of how an alteration of the elimination half-life (left panel) changes the blood concentration and the recovery of paralysis after an IV bolus dose of dTc 0.3 mg · kg^{-1} (right panel). When the elimination half-life increases, the time for recovery of paralysis increases. (Data adapted from Sheiner et al.[7])

recovery occurring in the distribution/redistribution phase is given in Fig. 9 for the dTc dose of 0.1 mg · kg^{-1}.

If larger doses of relaxant are given that cause more than 90% paralysis, recovery will occur during the elimination phase (Fig. 9). The time needed for recovery of paralysis will be longer for two reasons. First, the relaxant concentrations have to fall low enough so that the plateau of the concentration-paralysis relationship is reached (Fig. 3). Only at this plateau will visible recovery (90% to 95% paralysis) of the paralysis be present. As the dose of relaxant is increased, the time for the relaxant concentrations to decline to the plateau levels will be longer. Thus, the duration of maximal paralysis will increase and the recovery of paralysis will be prolonged. Second, once visible recovery of paralysis has occurred (95% to 97% paralysis), complete recovery involves decending the concentration-paralysis relationship (Fig. 3). This will generally occur during the pharmacokinetic elimination phase. Shanks et al[16] have shown that the rate of recovery of paralysis (from 80% to 20%) is linearly related to the rate constant of drug elimination. The elimination half-life will determine the rate of decrease of the tissue (neuromuscular junction) concentrations, which will parallel the blood concentrations because of the pseudo-equilibrium present during this phase. Since the elimination half-life is determined by the Vdss and clearance, a change in one of these variables can change the elimination half-life and therefore the recovery time. Since most of the nondepolarizing relaxants are eliminated in part by the kidney, renal failure will decrease the clearance and therefore the elimination half-life. This will result in a prolonged period of time for recovery of paralysis.[17] Figure 10 is a simulation of the influence of an increased elimination half-life on the blood concentrations and paralysis *v* time relationship.

Pharmacodynamic Factors

If a patient is relatively sensitive to the relaxant (low $Cpss_{50}$), recovery of paralysis will be longer relative to a patient who is resistant (high $Cpss_{50}$). In the sensitive patient, lower blood concentrations must be achieved before recovery of paralysis will occur. If the pharmacokinetics are unchanged, then a longer period of time is needed to achieve these lower blood concentrations (Fig. 11). The slope of the blood concentration-paralysis curve can also affect the rate of recovery of paralysis. If the concentration-paralysis curve is steep, a small change of the blood concentration could result in a relatively rapid recovery of paralysis (Fig. 12). If the concentration-paralysis curve is relatively shallow, then a greater change of the blood concentration will be necessary to go from complete paralysis to minimal paralysis. Assuming that the elimination half-life is similar, it will require a longer period of time to lower the blood concentrations to threshold concentrations. Consequently, the recovery time will be prolonged.

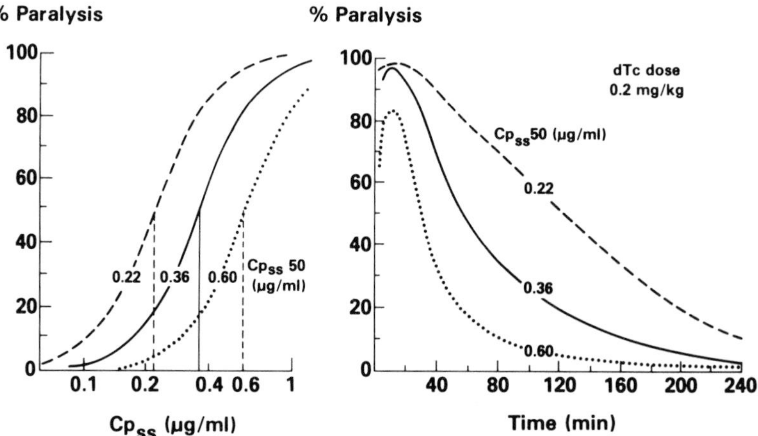

Figure 11. A computer simulation of how a change of muscle sensitivity (left panel) alters the recovery of paralysis after an intravenous bolus dose of dTc 0.2 mg · kg^{-1}. The time for recovery of paralysis increases when Cp_{ss}^{50} decreases. (Data adapted from reference[8]).

SUMMARY

Many factors affect the relationship between a given dose of a nondepolarizing relaxant, the time for onset, and the degree of and time for recovery of paralysis. It is not possible for the clinical anesthesiologist to know the exact muscle relaxant pharmacokinetics or pharmacodynamics for a given patient

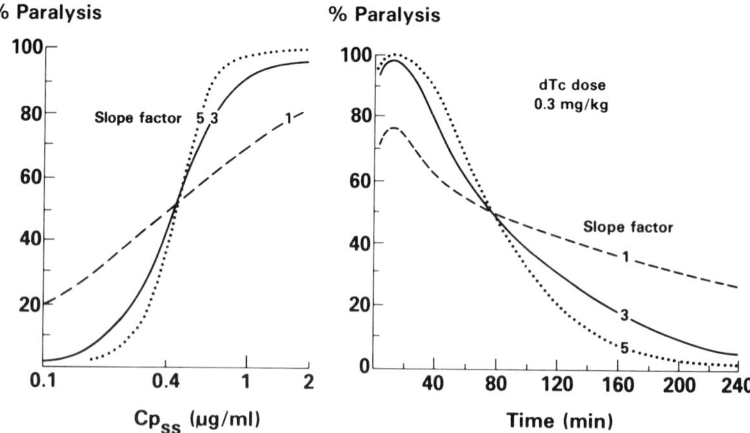

Figure 12. A computer simulation of how an alteration of the slope of the concentration-paralysis relationship changes after an IV bolus dose of dTc 0.3 mg · kg^{-1}. Recovery is most rapid when the slope factor is the largest.

and to therefore accurately predict the degree of paralysis for a given dose of relaxant. Pharmacokinetic and pharmacodynamic research has, however, identified diseases, concurrent drugs, and anesthetic states that can cause a relatively profound change in the muscle relaxant pharmacokinetics and pharmacodynamics. By understanding the principles that govern the relationship between the relaxant dose and paralysis, one can interpret this knowledge and better understand when and why the relaxant dosage needs be altered in certain groups of patients. Hopefully this will translate into the safer use of relaxants in clinical anesthetic practice.

REFERENCES

1. Stanski DR, Watkins WD: Drug Disposition in Anesthesia. New York, Grune & Stratton, 1982
2. Prys-Roberts C, Hug CC Jr: Pharmacokinetics of Anaesthesia. London, Blackwell Scientific, 1984
3. Wood M, Wood AAJ: Drugs and Anesthesia-Pharmacology for Anesthesiologists. Baltimore, Williams & Wilkins, 1982
4. Ramizan MI, Somogyi AA, Shanks CA, et al: Clinical pharmacokinetics of the non-depolarizing muscle relaxants. Clin Pharmacokinet 6:25–60, 1981
5. Holford NGH, Sheiner LB: Understanding the dose-effect relationship: Clinical application of pharmacokinetic-pharmacodynamic models. Clin Pharmacokinet 6:429–453, 1981
6. Hull CJ: Pharmacodynamics of non-depolarizing neuromuscular blocking agents. Br J Anaesth 54:169–182, 1982
7. Sheiner LB, Stanski DR, Vozeh S, et al: Simultaneous modeling of pharmacokinetics and pharmacodynamics: Application to d-tubocurarine. Clin Pharmacol Ther 25:358–371, 1979
8. Stanski DR, Ham J, Miller RD, et al: Pharmacokinetics and pharmacodynamics of d-tubocurarine during nitrous oxide-narcotic and halothane anesthesia in man. Anesthesiology 51:235–241, 1979
9. Stanski DR, Sheiner LB: Pharmacokinetics and dynamics of muscle relaxants. Anesthesiology 51:103–105, 1979
10. Armstrong DL, Lester HA: The kinetics of tubocurarine action and restricted diffusion within the synaptic cleft. J Physiol 294:365, 1979
11. Duvaldestin P, Agoston S, Henzel E, et al: Pancuronium pharmacokinetics in patients with liver cirrhosis. Br J Anaesth 50:1131–1135, 1978
12. Ham J, Stanski DR, Neufield P, et al: Pharmacokinetics and dynamics of d-tubocurarine during hypothermia in humans. Anesthesiology 55:631–635, 1981
13. Harrison GA, Janis F: Effect of circulation time on the neuromuscular action of suxamethonium. Anaesth Intensive Care 1:33–40, 1972
14. Martin JAJ, Szynfelbein K, Ali HH, et al: Increased d-tubocurarine requirement following major thermal injury. Anesthesiology 52:352–355, 1980
15. Hull CJ, English MJM, Sibbald A. Fazadinium and pancuronium: A pharmacodynamic study. Br J Anaesth 52:1209–1221, 1980
16. Shanks CA, Somogyi AA, Triggs EJ: Dose-response and plasma concentration-response relationships of pancuronium in man. Anesthesiology 51:111–118, 1979
17. Miller RD, Matteo RS, Benet LZ, et al: The pharmacokinetics of d-tubocurarine in man with and without renal failure. J Pharmacol Exp Ther 202:1–7, 1977

Roy Cronnelly

13

Muscle Relaxant Antagonists

The pharmacologic approach to antagonism or reversal of neuromuscular blockade induced by muscle relaxants has been directed at one goal: increasing the concentration of the neurotransmitter at the neuromuscular junction to favor the interactions between cholinergic (nicotinic) receptors and acetylcholine rather than those between receptors and muscle relaxants. This is accomplished through the use of drugs that inhibit the enzyme acetylcholinesterase ("true," or red-cell, cholinesterase), thereby preventing the normal destruction of acetylcholine and promoting its accumulation. If the resulting concentration of acetylcholine is in sufficient excess relative to the muscle relaxant, acetylcholine-receptor interactions will be favored, neuromuscular blockade will be antagonized, and normal neuromuscular transmission will be restored. However, since this is a competitive concentration-dependent event, all degrees (ie, none to complete) of antagonism are possible. Although this is the classic explanation of reversal, it is probably overly simplistic.

Historically, drugs that inhibit acetylcholinesterase stem from the compound eserine (also called physostigmine), which is an alkaloid derived from the Calabar bean. This bean was once used as a poison by African tribes during witchcraft trials. When the pharmacologic properties of physostigmine were investigated in the 1840s, the drugs ability to inhibit acetylcholinesterase was discovered. After elucidation of the chemical structure of physostigmine in 1925, structure-activity studies determined the active portion of the molecule. This discovery resulted in the synthesis of many related compounds among which were neostigmine, pyridostigmine, and edrophonium (Fig 1).

MUSCLE RELAXANTS
ISBN 0-8089-1784-6

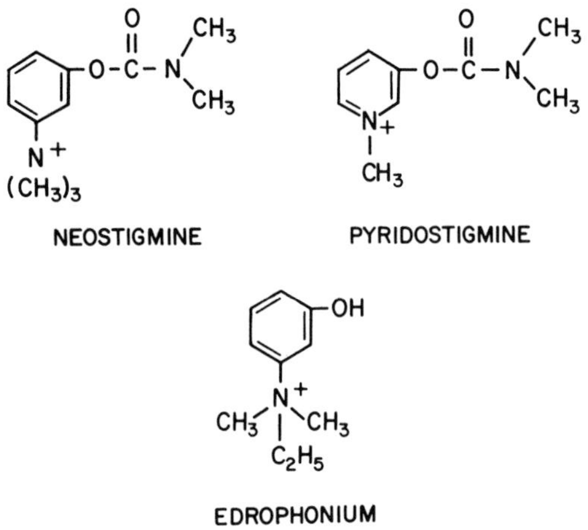

Figure 1. Chemical structures for neostigmine, pyridostigmine, and edrophonium.

DO REVERSAL DRUGS INHIBIT ACETYLCHOLINESTERASE THROUGH THE SAME MECHANISM?

Although all of these drugs inhibit acetylcholinesterase, they differ in their mechanism of inhibition (Fig 2). The active site of acetylcholinesterase at which acetylcholine is hydrolyzed is composed of two subsites. Edrophonium forms an electrostatic bond between the quaternary nitrogen and the negatively charged subsite on the enzyme, the anionic site. This binding is further stabilized by hydrogen bonding at the esteratic subsite. When attached in this manner, edrophonium inhibits enzyme activity by preventing hydrolysis of acetylcholine. Since no real chemical bond is formed (between edrophonium and the enzyme), acetylcholine can easily compete with edrophonium in a concentration-dependent manner for access to the active site. Thus, inhibition by edrophonium is easily reversible and short lived. In contrast, both neostigmine and pyridostigmine produce a longer-lasting inhibition. These inhibitors also form electrostatic attachments at the anionic site; in addition, their ester group is hydrolyzed by the esteratic site. As a result, the dimethylcarbamyl group is transferred and chemically bonded to the esteratic site. Once this occurs, acetylcholine can no longer compete with these inhibitors for access to the active site on the enzyme until the carbamyl group is removed by hydrolysis. This reaction occurs spontaneously and has a half-time of about 30 minutes. Both neostigmine and pyridostigmine form the same carbamylated enzyme; thus, the duration of enzyme inhibition produced

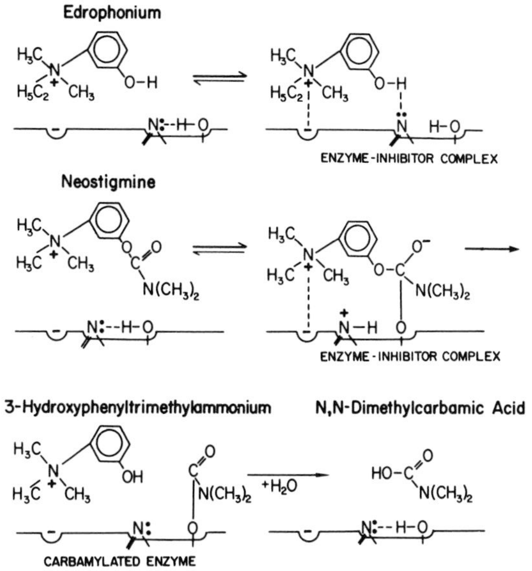

Edrophonium

ENZYME-INHIBITOR COMPLEX

Neostigmine

ENZYME-INHIBITOR COMPLEX

3-Hydroxyphenyltrimethylammonium

N,N-Dimethylcarbamic Acid

CARBAMYLATED ENZYME

Figure 2. Steps involved in binding of edrophonium and neostigmine to acetylcholinesterase.

by these drugs is the same and exceeds that produced by edrophonium. Another difference with respect to enzyme inhibition is that both neostigmine and pyridostigmine are inactivated (metabolized) through their interaction with the cholinesterase enzyme, whereas edrophonium is not chemically altered during inhibition of the enzyme.

DOES REVERSAL INVOLVE MORE THAN JUST ENZYME INHIBITION?

In addition to inhibition of acetylcholinesterase, several other mechanisms may be involved in the antagonism of neuromuscular blockade. The anticholinesterase drugs are able to induce repetitive firing in the motor nerve terminal in response to a single action potential. This repetitive firing contributes to antagonism by converting a single twitch response into a brief tetanic contracture, thereby increasing the strength of muscle contraction. Repetitive firing can spread back up the axon of the motor nerve to involve other nerve terminals in the same motor unit, resulting in depolarization of these terminals and increasing the amount of transmitter released. Anticholinesterase drugs can directly depolarize the motor nerve terminals and the nicotinic cholinergic receptors on the postsynaptic membrane. In this way, they directly compete with the muscle relaxant. In addition, they improve mobilization and release of transmitter within the nerve terminal and thereby oppose the effects of muscle relaxants on these structures. It is important to realize that, like the muscle relaxants, these drugs have presynaptic and postsynaptic effects in addition to the inhibition of acetylcholinesterase. What is seen clinically as antagonism is probably a combination of all these effects plus those resulting from accumulation of acetylcholine.[1]

HOW DO THE DRUGS COMPARE IN POTENCY, ONSET, AND DURATION OF ACTION?

This question is particularly relevant to edrophonium since this drug has not been used clinically as an antagonist for many years. Fears of inadequate effect and short duration of action leading to recurarization prevented its use. However, these fears were based on inadequate data. Dose-response relationships for the reversal drugs have been determined in anesthetized patients using two methods. The first method is to administer the antagonist at the end of anesthesia and surgery as occurs clinically. This approach, however, cannot separate the effect of the antagonist from the effects of other events occurring at the same time, ie, a decrease in the concentration of anesthetic or of muscle relaxant at the neuromuscular junction. Since removal of the anesthetic and muscle relaxant improves neuromuscular function, it is difficult to quantitate the effect of the antagonist. Although this is the usual clinical procedure, it does not lead to accurate determinations of dose-response relationships. The second method involves the use of constant levels of anesthesia and neuromuscular blockade, so that when the antagonist is given, its effect will be solely responsible for the reversal produced. Although this technique does not mimic the clinical situation, it allows for comparisons of drugs under identical conditions and for clinically applicable results. When the second method was used, neostigmine (3 mg/70 kg) was found to produce antagonism equal to that achieved with pyridostigmine (15 mg/70 kg) or edrophonium (35 mg/70 kg) (Fig 3).[2]

The dose-response curve for edrophonium does not parallel the curves for neostigmine and pyridostigmine, a fact that suggests differing mechanisms of action. In animals and perhaps in humans, edrophonium seems to have predominantly presynaptic (nerve terminal) effects compared with the other drugs. However, attempts to demonstrate differing mechanisms in humans have produced conflicting results. When twitch tension was less than 70% of control, the train-of-four ratio was greater with edrophonium than with neostigmine, and greater with neostigmine than with pyridostigmine (Fig 4).[3] If the train-of-four ratio reflects only presynaptic effects, then these results would support a presynaptic predominance for edrophonium and a postsynaptic predominance for pyridostigmine. If this were true, inhibition or potentia-

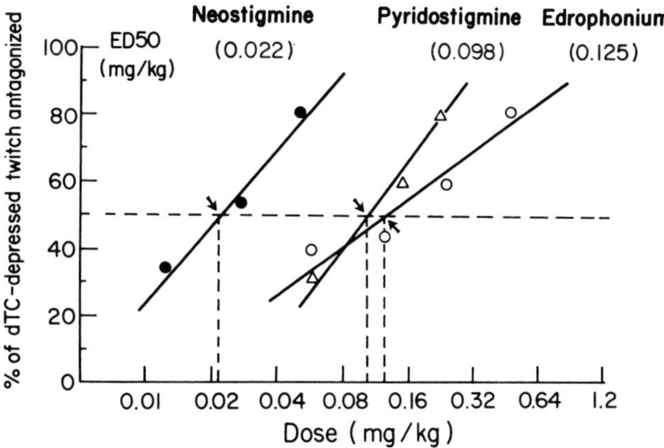

Figure 3. Dose-response curves for neostigmine (●), pyridostigmine (△), and edrophonium (○) in anesthetized patients. (Reproduced with permission from Cronnelly et al.[2])

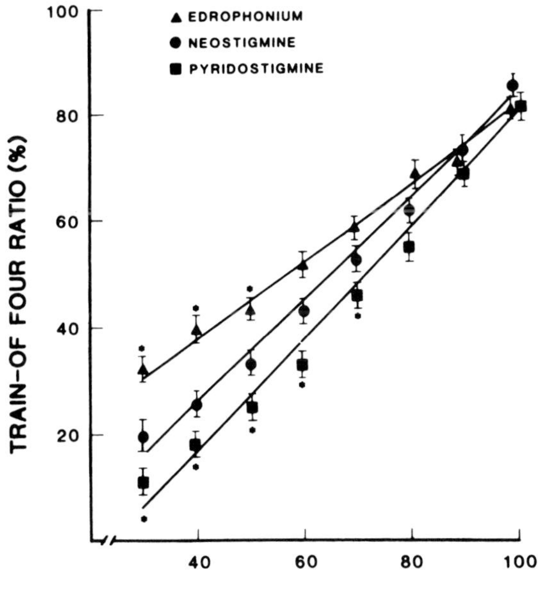

Figure 4. Train-of-four ration *v* first twitch height after reversal of a pancuronium-induced neuromuscular blockade with edrophonium (▲), neostigmine (●), or pyridostigmine (■). (Reproduced with permission from Donati et al.[3])

tion of the reversal effect might be expected upon combining or mixing the antagonist drugs. However, combining edrophonium with pyridostigmine or neostigmine resulted in strictly additive effects with respect to the amount of reversal achieved. These findings do not support the concept of different mechanisms of action. The mixtures also did not result in faster onset or longer duration of effects. In addition, use of mixtures demonstrated no clinical advantage over use of the individual agents themselves.[4]

When equipotent doses of the drugs are compared for onset of action (ie, time from IV administration until peak effect), pyridostigmine has the slowest onset. From a stable 90% D-tubocurarine–induced neuromuscular blockade, pyridostigmine required 12 to 16 minutes to produce its peak effect on muscle twitch height, whereas neostigmine required seven to ten minutes. Edrophonium was the most rapid, producing peak antagonism in 1.2 minutes (Fig 5).[2] Onset of action with edrophonium is also rapid when neuromuscular blockade is antagonized during spontaneous recovery. However, differences among the drugs in the magnitude of reversal produced (measured by muscle twitch height or train-of-four) are no longer apparent after ten to 15 minutes (Fig 6).[5]

In the past, concern about the use of edrophonium as an antagonist of long-acting muscle relaxants related to its supposed short duration of action and possibility of recurarization. However, carefully controlled studies in

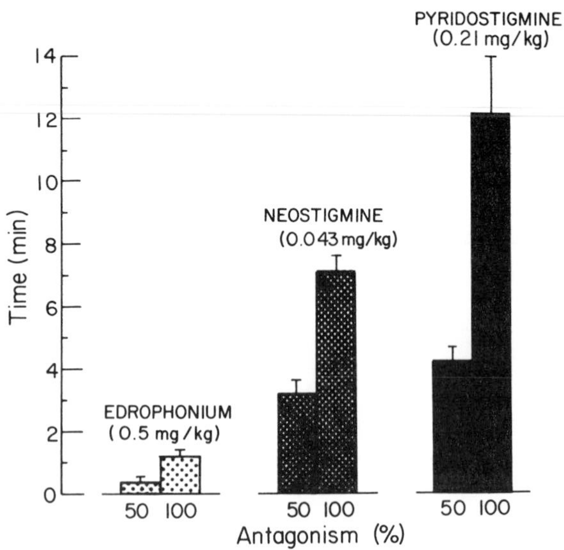

Figure 5. Onset of action for equipotent doses of neostigmine, pyridostigmine, and edrophonium during steady-state neuromuscular blockade. (Reproduced with permission from Cronnelly et al.[2])

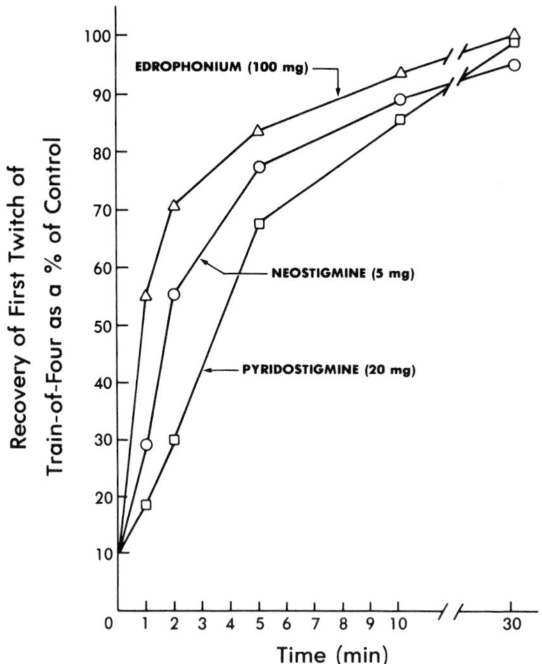

Figure 6. Onset of neostigmine (○), edrophonium (△), and pyridostigmine (□) when administered during spontaneous recovery from neuromuscular blockade. Values plotted from the data of Ferguson et al.[5]

anesthetized patients have demonstrated that the duration of antagonism produced by edrophonium does not differ from that seen with neostigmine (Fig 7). Therefore, edrophonium can produce effective and sustained antagonism of long-acting muscle relaxants.

Antagonism of neuromuscular blockade induced by the new intermediate-acting nondepolarizing relaxants is also easily accomplished. Dose-response relationships for neostigmine are the same for metocurine and pancuronium as for atracurium and vecuronium. Also, the duration of antagonism produced by neostigmine does not differ for either a vecuronium- or pancuronium-induced neuromuscular blockade.[6] Therefore, the same dose of antagonist drug should be used to antagonize a long- or intermediate-acting muscle relaxant. In contrast to the long-acting muscle relaxants, antagonism will not always be necessary for neuromuscular blockade induced by atracurium and vecuronium. However, spontaneous recovery from these new drugs should not be relied upon for termination of neuromuscular blockade unless a sustained response to tetanic stimulation (100 Hz for 5 seconds) or a normal train-of-four response is present.

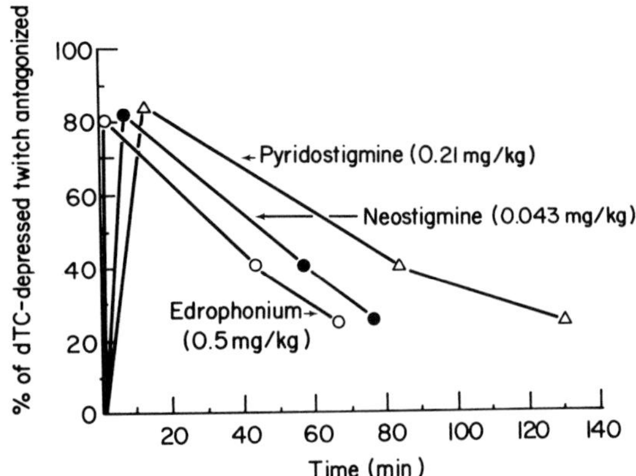

Figure 7. Duration of action for equipotent doses of neostigmine, pyridostigmine, and edrophonium in anesthetized patients. (Reproduced with permission from Cronnelly et al.[2])

Physostigmine has also been evaluated as an antagonist of nondepolarizing neuromuscular blockade in anesthetized patients.[7] Two milligrams of physostigmine did not antagonize neuromuscular block induced by 10 mg of D-tubocurarine. A dose of 4 to 8 mg of physostigmine was necessary to initiate antagonism. Although higher doses produced antagonism, the reversal achieved was slow in onset and did not restore muscle twitch height to control levels. It is, of course, possible that increasing the dose of physostigmine even more would have produced antagonism similar in magnitude to that produced by the other drugs. However, because physostigmine is a tertiary amine, it can penetrate the blood-brain barrier and inhibit CNS cholinesterase, thereby causing unwanted excitant effects. The quality of antagonism produced by physostigmine is interesting because this compound is thought to act only through inhibition of acetylcholinesterase. This emphasizes the importance of mechanisms other than enzyme inhibition during reversal of neuromuscular blockade.

IS THE DOSE OF ANTICHOLINESTERASE DRUG OR THE DURATION OF REVERSAL ALTERED BY PATIENT AGE?

In the past, pediatric patients were believed to need more neostigmine than adults for reversal of neuromuscular blockade. However, studies performed during steady-state neuromuscular block did not confirm this. In fact, the dose-response curves for neostigmine in infants (age 3 to 48 weeks) and in children (1 to 8 years) shifted to the left of the curve for adults. Pediatric patients actually required one half to two thirds less neostigmine than adults. In contrast, the dose-response relationship for edrophonium did not differ between pediatric and adult patients. The variability of response following edrophonium, however, was greater in pediatric patients than in adults. Therefore, the effect of the reversal drug should be monitored in pediatric patients and the adequacy of reversal documented. As will be discussed later, differences in dose requirements did not result from age-related changes in anticholinesterase pharmacokinetics. These differences may have been related to differences in the number of receptors, amount of acetylcholine reserves, or enzyme activity between pediatric and adult patients. The onset and duration of antagonism produced by both neostigmine and edrophonium in pediatric patients was the same as in adults patients.[8,9] The differing effects of age on the dose-response relationships for neostigmine and edrophonium again suggest differences in the mechanism of their reversal.

For the elderly, information is not yet complete. The dose-response relationship and the duration of antagonism did not differ between elderly patients and younger adults given edrophonium. Therefore, elderly patients require the same dose of edrophonium for reversal of neuromuscular blockade as do younger adults and pediatric patients. The onset of action of edrophonium, however, was longer in elderly patients. Therefore, more time should be allowed for adequate reversal in these patients.[10]

WHAT ARE THE DOSE REQUIREMENTS FOR ANTICHOLINERGIC DRUGS?

An anticholinergic agent (eg, atropine or glycopyrrolate) must be administered with the anticholinesterase agent. This is necessary to block side effects (muscarinic) resulting from acetylcholine accumulation of sites other than the neuromuscular junction. The most troublesome side effect is bradycardia. Equivalent doses of neostigmine (3 mg/70 kg) and pyridostigmine (15 mg/70 kg) require the same amount of atropine (15 μg/kg) to prevent bradycardia. When administered together, this combination results in an initial tachycardia due to the more rapid onset of action of atropine. After six to eight minutes, heart rate decreases toward baseline values. In contrast, an equivalent amount of edrophonium (35 mg/70 kg) required less atropine (7 μg/kg) to prevent bradycardia in patients anesthetized with nitrous oxide and halothane. This combination of edrophonium and atropine resulted in minimal changes in heart rate during antagonism of neuromuscular blockade because the onset of these two drugs are more closely matched. Since the onset of anticholinergic action from glycopyrrolate is much slower than atropine, the combination of glycopyrrolate with either neostigmine or pyridostigmine also results in fewer changes in heart rate. Because of differences in onset, glycopyrrolate should be administered several minutes prior to edrophonium.[2,11]

WHAT IS THE EFFECT OF THE REVERSAL DRUGS ON THE DURATION OF ACTION OF SUCCINYLCHOLINE?

Neostigmine, pyridostigmine, and edrophonium inhibit not only acetylcholinesterase but also pseudocholinesterase (or butyrylcholinesterase). Butyrylcholinesterase hydrolyzes succinylcholine to succinylmonocholine and finally to succinic acid and choline. If succinylcholine is given after an anticholinesterase drug, the neuromuscular blockade for succinylcholine is prolonged. Presumably, inhibition of butyrylcholinesterase (eg, by neostigmine) prevents hydrolysis of succinylcholine, thereby prolonging its effect. This explanation may not be entirely correct. Edrophonium is a weaker inhibitor of butyrylcholinesterase (Ic_{50}, the concentration producing 50% inhibition = 1.4×10^{-3} mol/L) than is neostigmine ($Ic_{50} = 1.0 \times 10^{-8}$ mol/L) or pyridostigmine ($Ic_{50} = 1.9 \times 10^{-7}$ mol/L), and the mechanism of inhibition is the same as for acetylcholinesterase (Fig 2). Because of carbamylation of the esteratic site, the duration of inhibition produced by neostigmine and pyridostigmine is longer than that produced by edrophonium. After administration of either neostigmine or pyridostigmine in equivalent doses, butyrylcholinesterase activity is still significantly inhibited (approximately 50% of control) after 30 minutes but returns to normal by 180 minutes. One minute after administration of edrophonium (0.5 mg/kg), butyrylcholinesterase activity is only 50% of control and recovers to normal in one half hour. Neostigmine and pyridostigmine can prolong a succinylcholine-induced neuromuscular blockade two to three times its normal duration, whereas edrophonium prolongs it 1.6 times. The duration of enzyme inhibition does not correlate with the effect on duration of neuromuscular blockade. Several explanations can be offered for these data. If enzyme inhibition and prolongation of neuromuscular blockade are related, then a significant amount of butyrylcholinesterase must be inhibited before the hydrolysis of succinylcholine is impaired. Thus, neuromuscular blockade could recover at a time when enzyme inhibition was still present. If true, the mount of inhibition produced by edrophonium may be inadequate to result in a prolongation of response on the basis of impaired succinylcholine hydrolysis. In addition, if succinylcholine is given 30 minutes after the edrophonium, when enzyme inhibition is no longer measurable, neuromuscular blockade is still prolonged. A prolonged succinylcholine response can also be demonstrated 40 to 60 minutes after the administration of pyridostigmine. Alternatively, inhibition of butyrylcholinesterase activity and the prolongation of succinylcholine-induced neuromuscular blockade may be unrelated. Perhaps combined effects of the anticholinesterase drugs and succinylcholine at the neuromuscular junction are responsible for the altered duration of action. Although the site and mechanism of this interaction remain unclear, administration of succinylcholine after a reversal drug results in prolongation of paralysis that probably does not exceed 30 minutes.[12–14]

INADEQUATE ANTAGONISM

If adequate doses of anticholinesterase drugs (edrophonium 0.5 to 1.0 mg/kg, neostigmine 0.035 to 0.07 mg/kg, or pyridostigmine 0.175 to 0.35 mg/kg) fail to antagonize neuromuscular blockade, the cause should be sought. The following questions may be helpful in defining the problem.

WAS ENOUGH TIME ALLOWED FOR THE REVERSAL DRUG TO WORK?

The speed of antagonism can be influenced by the magnitude of neuromuscular blockade, the antagonist administered, and the dose given. When twitch height depressed by either pancuronium or D-tubocurarine spontaneously recovers to more than 20% of control, the time for administration of neostigmine (2.5 mg) until control twitch height is restored can vary from three to 14 minutes. When twitch height is less than 20% of control, recovery can take 30 to 40 minutes or even longer for a sustained contraction in response to stimulation at 50 to 100 Hz. The time for reversal also depends on the drug administered, since edrophonium has a more rapid onset of action than neostigmine or pyridostigmine. However, like neostigmine, more time is required with edrophonium to completely reverse muscle twitch height when intense neuromuscular blockade is present. When twitch height depressed by either pancuronium or D-tubocurarine had recovered to 1% to 10% of control, complete recovery was not achieved for 30 minutes or more after edrophonium (0.5 mg/kg).[5] With all the antagonist drugs, speed of reversal is also directly proportional to the dose administered. Another factor influencing the onset of action may be age: the peak effect of edrophonium was achieved more slowly in elderly patients than in younger patients.

IS THE NEUROMUSCULAR BLOCKADE TOO INTENSE TO BE REVERSED?

In the average adult patient, any of the anticholinesterase drugs in adequate dosage will antagonize most neuromuscular blockades. However, studies defining dosage were not attempting to antagonize a block in which muscle twitch was depressed 100% at the time of antagonism, ie, muscle relaxant overdosage. If no response can be elicited by the peripheral nerve stimulator before administration of the anticholinesterase drug, reversal will probably be inadequate. If no response can be elicited after administration of the anticholinesterase drug, more should not be given. Controlled ventilation should be continued until muscle twitch can be evoked, at which time more reversal drug may be given.

IS THE ACID-BASE AND ELECTROLYTE STATUS NORMAL?

In anesthetized patients, respiratory acidosis will decrease muscle twitch height in the presence or absence of neuromuscular blockade. Respiratory alkalosis produces the opposite effect. In animals, respiratory acidosis impairs antagonism by neostigmine. If, however, reversal occurred prior to respiratory acidosis, neuromuscular blockade did not reappear. Several clinical conclusions may be drawn if these data are extrapolated to humans. If a patient in the recovery room has a residual neuromuscular blockade, the respiratory depression that can result could be augmented by administering narcotic analgesics. Under these circumstances, attempts to antagonize the residual neuromuscular blockade may fail unless the respiratory acidosis is corrected by ventilation prior to the administration of anticholinesterase drug. If neuromuscular blockade is completely antagonized intraoperatively, postoperative respiratory acidosis should not result in reappearance of the blockade.

Potassium, calcium, and magnesium levels should be checked if suspected of being abnormal. Nondepolarizing neuromuscular blockade may be augmented by elevated levels of magnesium or low levels of potassium or calcium. Diuretic-induced hypokalemia was found to potentiate a pancuronium neuromuscular blockade and to increase the requirement of anticholinesterase. However, complete reversal could be achieved.

HAVE DRUGS BEEN ADMINISTERED THAT COULD MAKE ANTAGONISM DIFFICULT?

Many drugs such as local anesthetics, antiarrhythmics, ganglionic-blocking agents, calcium-channel blockers, and diuretics can potentiate nondepolarizing neuromuscular blockade. The influence of these drugs on the ability of anticholinesterase agents to reverse the resulting neuromuscular blockade is in most cases unknown. In animals, lidocaine will potentiate a pancuronium-induced neuromuscular blockade; however, the combined blockade requires the same dose of edrophonium for reversal as one of equal magnitude produced by pancuronium alone. The neuromuscular blockade produced by antibiotics resembles that produced by the nondepolarizing relaxants, ie, fade of muscle contraction in response to tetanic stimulation and posttetanic potentiation. Therefore, the proportion of residual blockade caused by the antibiotic and that due to the relaxant cannot be determined. The antagonism of these combined blockades is problematic in that neostigmine (to 5 mg/70 kg) provides inconsistent or partial reversal and in some cases may augment the block. Calcium (to 1 gm/70 kg) is equally inconsistent. Therefore, ventilation must be supported until the neuromuscular blockade has terminated spontaneously.[11]

PHARMACOKINETICS

In the past, research involving antagonism of neuromuscular blockade was limited to observation of responses without knowledge of the influence of drug distribution, metabolism, or excretion. Pharmacokinetic determinations are now possible because of the development of analytical techniques for measuring of anticholinesterase drugs in biologic fluids. The remaining questions address the pharmacokinetics of anticholinesterase drugs.

ARE THERE PHARMACOKINETIC DIFFERENCES BETWEEN THE REVERSAL DRUGS WHEN RENAL AND HEPATIC FUNCTION ARE NORMAL?

The pharmacokinetics of neostigmine, edrophonium, and pyridostigmine are similar in anesthetized patients (Fig 8). The central compartment (V_1) and steady-state (Vd_{ss}) volumes of distribution for the reversal drugs exceed plasma and extracellular fluid volume. They also exceed the distribution volumes for the nondepolarizing muscle relaxants. This is remarkable since quaternary amines would not be expected to cross lipoid membranes easily. Presumably, extensive tissue localization occurs (eg, in liver and kidney), resulting in magnification of the volumes of distribution. Since the distribution volumes for the reversal drugs are similar, differences in potency between the drugs do not appear to have a pharmacokinetic basis. In addition, onset of action does not appear to depend on pharmacokinetic properties. Pyridostigmine and edrophonium have similar distribution half-lives but are markedly different on onset of action. Perhaps differences in affinity for acetylcholinesterase and in site of action account for the lack of similarity in potency and onset.[15–17]

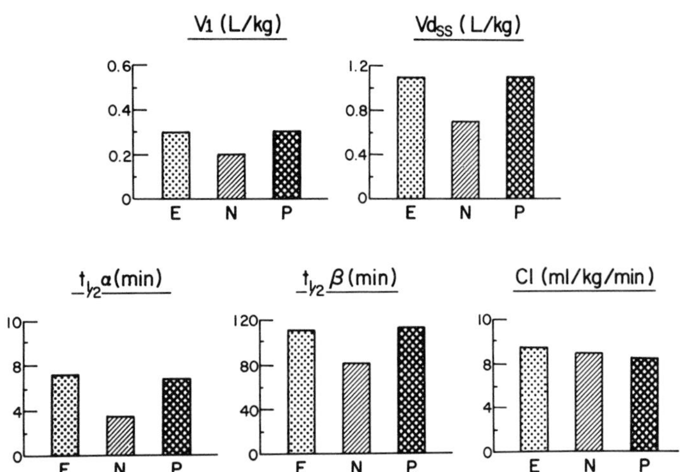

Figure 8. Pharmacokinetics of edrophonium (E), pyridostigmine (P), and neostigmine (N) in patients with normal renal and hepatic function.

ARE REVERSAL DRUGS METABOLIZED

In the absence of renal function, nonrenal or metabolic clearance accounts for 50% of a dose of neostigmine, 25% of a dose of pyridostigmine, and 30% of a dose of edrophonium in anesthetized patient's metabolism of anticholinesterase drugs. In humans, the primary metabolites for neostigmine, pyridostigmine, and edrophonium are 3-hydroxyphenyltrimethylammonium (PTA), 3-hydroxy-N-methylpyridinium (NMP), and edrophonium glucuronide. For neostigmine and pyridostigmine, the primary metabolites are formed in the liver and also at the neuromuscular junction through interaction with acetylcholinesterase. Since metabolites are formed in the area of the postsynaptic receptors, they may contribute to antagonism of neuromuscular blockade. In animals, edrophonium glucuronide and NMP are inactive as antagonists, whereas PTA was eight to ten times less potent than neostigmine. If this is also true in humans, the contribution of the metabolites of neostigmine and pyridostigmine to antagonism is probably minimal.[15–19]

ARE REVERSAL DRUGS EXCRETED BY THE KIDNEYS?

The anticholinesterase drugs are highly dependent on the kidney for excretion. Renal excretion accounts for 75% of the clearance of pyridostigmine, 70% of the clearance of edrophonium, and 50% of the clearance of

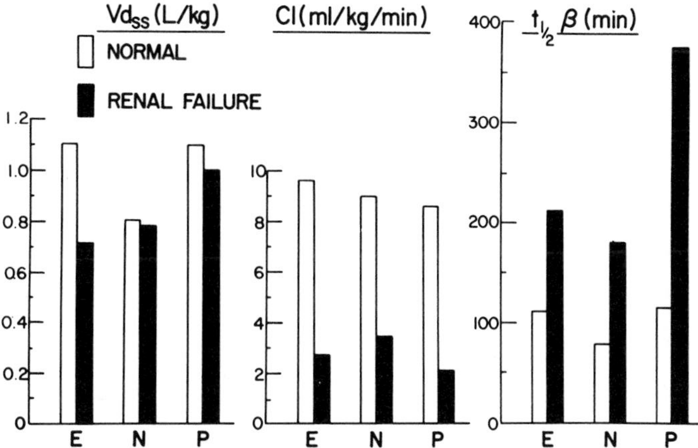

Figure 9. Pharmacokinetics of edrophonium (E), neostigmine (N), and pyridostigmine (P) in patients with and without renal failure.

neostigmine (Fig 9). The proportion of the clearance that is dependent on renal mechanisms exceeds that expected from glomerular filtration alone, suggesting the involvement of tubular secretory processes in the clearance of these drugs.

WHAT IS THE INFLUENCE OF RENAL FAILURE AND KIDNEY TRANSPLANTATION?

Pharmacokinetics of the reversal drugs and D-tubocurarine are similar for patients having a functioning renal transplant and for those having normal renal function (Fig 10). However, if renal function is severly impaired or absent, elimination of reversal drugs decreases and half-lives increase (Fig 9). The decrease in anticholinesterase clearance from plasma in anephric patients exceeds that reported for pancuronium and tubocurarine. Therefore, the muscle relaxant will probably not outlast the antagonist drug. Supporting data demonstrate that reversal of a pancuronium-induced neuromuscular blockade is sustained by neostigmine in anephric patients. However, interactions between drugs such as antibiotics or diuretics and residual neuromuscular blockade can occur. Such interactions are not well antagonized by anticholinesterase drugs and could result in muscle weakness in spite of adequate concentrations of the reversal drugs in blood. If this occurs, ventilation should be supported, and other factors that impair antagonism (eg, electrolytes, acid-base abnormalities, intensity of neuromuscular blockade,) should be investigated and corrected before administration of additional anticholinesterase drugs.[15–18]

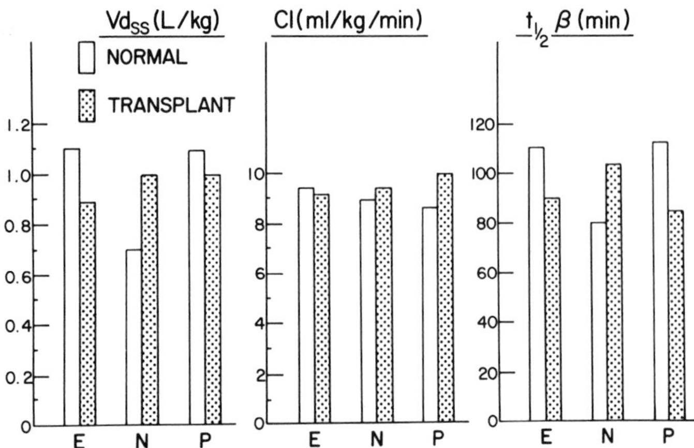

Figure 10. Pharmacokinetics of edrophonium (E), neostigmine (N), and pyridostigmine (P) in patients with a renal transplant compared to normal patients.

DOES AGE ALTER THE PHARMACOKINETICS OF THE REVERSAL DRUGS?

At present, information is only available for pediatric patients, where the kinetics of neostigmine and edrophonium are similar but differ significantly from data for adults. In infants and children, the elimination half-lives for edrophonium and neostigmine are shorter and clearance is more rapid than in adults. The values for Vd_{ss} for both drugs were the same for all ages. Since the Vd_{ss} did not change, the age-related differences in dose-response relationships (discussed previously) do not have a pharmacokinetic basis. Although pediatric patients tend to excrete the drugs at a faster rate than adults, the duration of antagonism produced by edrophonium and neostigmine was similar in pediatric and adult patients.[8,9]

Pharmacokinetic similarities between neostigmine, pyridostigmine, and edrophonium greatly outweigh any differences. This is not only true in normal patients but also in patients having physiologic or pathologic conditions that alter pharmacokinetics variables. Effective and sustained reversal or neuromuscular blockade can be achieved with any of these drugs. However, fewer similarities exist with respect to their pharmacodynamic properties. Differences in enzyme inhibition, predominant mechanism, potency, onset, and duration of action exist among the drugs. In addition, changes in pharmacodynamics appear to occur independent of changes in pharmacokinetics.

REFERENCES

1. Riker WF, Okamoto MO: Pharmacology of motor nerve terminals. Ann Rev Pharmacol 9:173–208, 1969

2. Cronnelly R, Morris R, Miller RD: Edrophonium: Duration of action and atropine requirement in humans during halothane anesthesia. Anesthesiology 57:261–266, 1982
3. Donati F, Ferguson A, Bevan DR: Twitch, depression and train-of-four ratio after antagonism of pancuronium with edrophonium, neostigmine or pyridostigmine. Anesth Analg 62:314–316, 1983
4. Cronnelly R, Miller RD: Onset and duration of edrophonium pyridostigmine mixtures. Anesthesiology 61:A301, 1984
5. Ferguson A, Egerszegi P, Bevan DR: Neostigmine, pyridostigmine, and edrophonium as antagonists of pancuronium. Anesthesiology 53:390–394, 1980
6. Gencarelli PJ, Miller RD: Antagonism of ORG NC 45 (vecuronium) and pancuronium neuromuscular blockade by neostigmine. Br J Anaesth 54:53–56, 1982
7. Baraka A: Antagonism of neuromuscular block by physostigmine in man. Br J Anaesth 50:1075–1077, 1978
8. Fisher DM, Cronnelly R, Miller RD: The neuromuscular pharmacology of neostigmine in infants and children. Anesthesiology 59:220–225, 1983
9. Fisher DM, Cronnelly R, Miller RD: Clinical pharmacology of edrophonium in infants and children. Anesthesiology (in press)
10. Cronnelly R, Miller RD: Edrophonium: Dose-response, onset and duration of antagonism in elderly patients. Anesthesiology (in press)
11. Cronnelly R, Morris R: Antagonism of neuromuscular blockade. Br J Anaesth 54:183–194, 1982
12. Sunew KY, Hicks RG: The effects of neostigmine and pyridostigmine on duration of succinylcholine action and pseudocholinesterase activity. Anesthesiology 49:188–191, 1978
13. Sohn YJ: Use of succinylcholine following reversal of pancuronium paralysis with pyridostigmine. Anesthesiology 46:A477, 1977
14. Sohn YJ, Cronnelly R, Sharma M: Is the duration of action of succinylcholine prolonged following antagonism of neuromuscular blockade by edrophonium? Anesthesiology 61:A302, 1984
15. Cronnelly R, Stanski DR, Miller RD: Renal function and the pharmacokinetics of neostigmine in anesthetized man. Anesthesiology 51:222–226, 1979
16. Cronnelly R, Stanski DR, Miller RD: Pyridostigmine kinetics with and without renal function. Clin Pharmacol Ther 28:78–81, 1980
17. Morris R, Cronnelly R, Miller RD: Pharmacokinetics of edrophonium and neostigmine when antagonizing d-tubocurarine neuromuscular blockade in man. Anesthesiology 54:399–402, 1981
18. Morris R, Cronnelly R, Miller PD: Pharmacokinetics of edrophonium in anephric and renal transplant patients. Br J Anaesth 53:1311–1314, 1981
19. Hennis PJ, Cronnelly R, Sharman M, et al: Metabolites of neostigmine and pyridostigmine do not contribute to antagonism of neuromuscular blockade. Anesthesiology 61:534–539, 1984

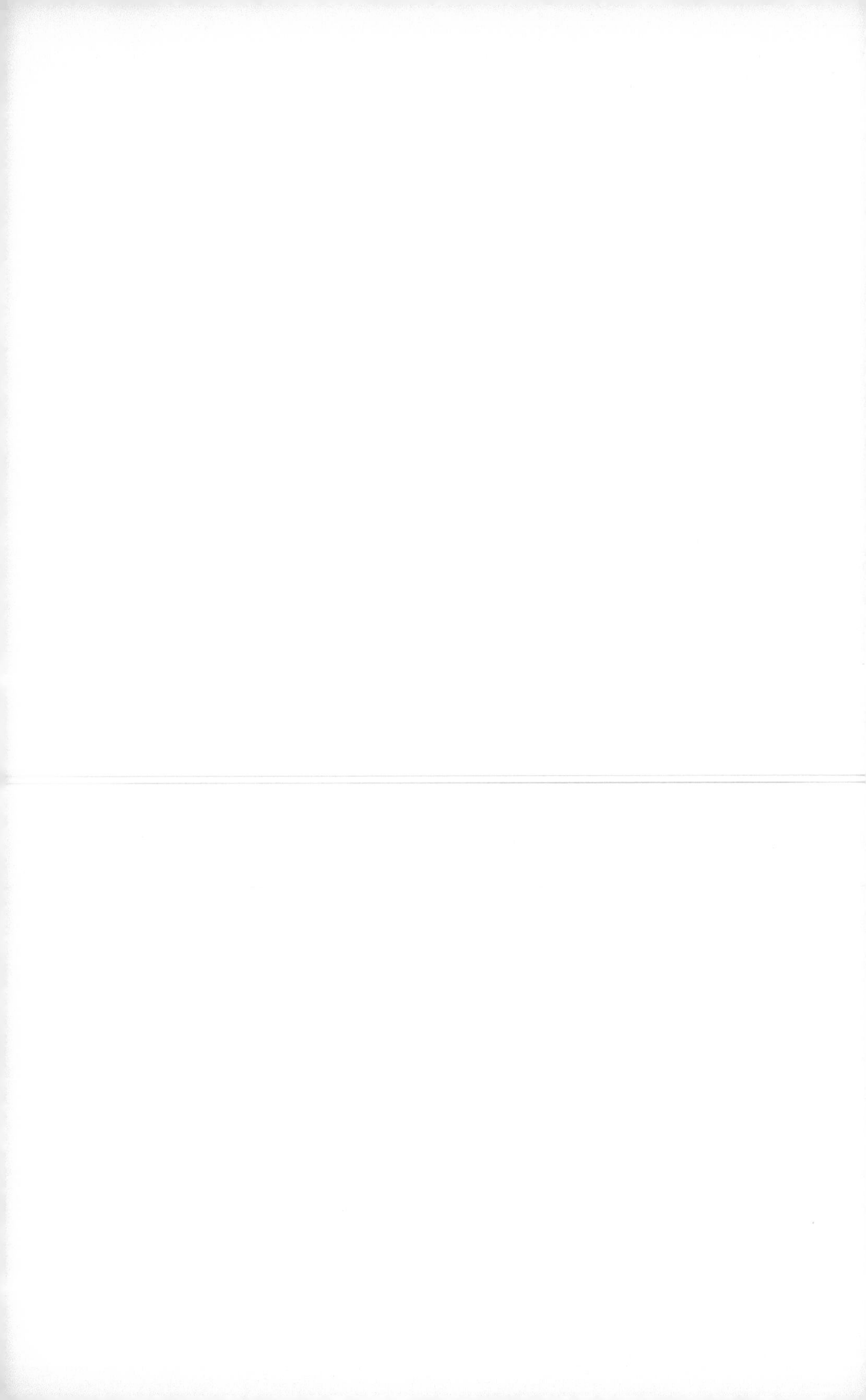

Barbara W. Brandom
D. Ryan Cook

14

Muscle Relaxants in Children

Muscle relaxants are useful in pediatric anesthesia to facilitate endotracheal intubation, to provide surgical relaxation and thus eliminate or reduce the need for high concentrations of potent inhalation anesthetics, and as adjuncts to nitrous oxide-oxygen-narcotic anesthesia. There are significant differences in the pharmacokinetics and pharmacodynamics of muscle relaxants between infants, children, and adults. These differences are attributable to age-related differences in the apparent volume of distribution of relaxants, possible changes in the rate of metabolism of relaxants, and changes in redistribution and excretion (clearance) of relaxants. In addition, throughout childhood there is physical and biochemical maturation of the neuromuscular junction, change in the contractile properties of skeletal muscle, increase in the relative amount of muscle as a proportion of body weight, and a change in the sensitivity of the neuromuscular junction to relaxants. These differences may affect the optimal initial dose and timing of subsequent repeat drug administration.

Whenever the quantitative effects of a relaxant differ from one patient to another, the differences in observed effect following a given dose could be due to differences in the distribution of the drug through the patient's body (ie, pharmacokinetic differences), so that a different concentration of drug reaches the relevant receptors. An alteration in observed effect could also be due to an altered sensitivity of the receptor (ie, pharmacodynamic difference). Simultaneous studies of drug concentration in the plasma and of drug effect are necessary to separate pharmacokinetic from pharmacodynamic differences. Few studies of this sort have been completed for the muscle relaxants in

MUSCLE RELAXANTS
ISBN 0-8089-1784-6

infants, children, and adults. There have been, however, many clinical studies of neuromuscular function and the effects of muscle relaxant drugs that suggest there are significant differences in the pharmacokinetics and pharmacodynamics of these drugs in the pediatric population. This review will discuss the evidence that pediatric patients, particularly infants, respond differently to relaxants and present clinical recommendations for the use of muscle relaxants in pediatric patients.

STRUCTURAL AND FUNCTIONAL DEVELOPMENT OF THE NEUROMUSCULAR SYSTEM

The structural and functional development of the neuromuscular system is incomplete at birth.[1–5] The conduction velocity of motor nerves increases throughout gestation as myelination of nerve fibers occurs. Conversion of myotubules to mature muscle fibers takes place in the latter part of intrauterine life and in the first several weeks after birth. Some slow-contracting muscle (eg, intrinsic muscles of the hand) is progressively converted to fast-contracting muscle with a concomitant change in the force-velocity relationship. Both the diaphragm and intercostal muscles in infants increase the percentage of slow muscle fibers in the first months of life. Synaptic transmission is relatively slow at birth; more important, the rate at which acetylcholine is made available for release during repetitive nerve stimulation is limited in the infant. This reduced margin of safety of neurotransmission is demonstrable between infants and adults.

The immaturity of the neonate's neuromuscular function can be demonstrated by different methods. Crumrine and Yodlowski[6] noted a decrease in the amplitude of the frequency sweep electromyogram (FS-EMG) at frequencies of 50 to 100 Hz in infants under 12 weeks of age. The FS-EMG is produced by recording the action potential from an electrical stimulus rate that increases exponentially from 1 pulse per second to 100 Hz over a stimulation period of 10 seconds. The exponential increase in frequency allows assessment of neuromuscular transmission at tetanic rates but without inducing fatigue. In older infants and children they found that there was little or no decrement in the response recorded by the FS-EMG at the higher frequencies of stimulation. Similarly the FS-EMG response of full-term infants less than 12 weeks old was depressed after administration of 70% nitrous oxide while that of the older patients had not changed.

Earlier investigators also found less neuromuscular reserve in unanesthetized infants. In neonates there was essentially no decrease in the height of the evoked electromyogram at stimulus frequencies of 1 and 2 Hz. But at stimulus frequencies of 20 Hz for 15 seconds, Koenigsberger[7] found a decrement in twitch height in 12 of 17 infants. This change was particularly marked in infants of less than 36 weeks postconceptual age. At 50 Hz, all infants showed a fade in twitch height. Unanesthetized adults do not demonstrate fade at tetanic rates of 50 Hz. The youngest infants were the most affected, the average decrement in the four youngest infants being 77% while the average for the entire group was 51%.

In full-term infants one to 30 days of age anesthetized with halothane, Goudsouzian[8] noted slower contraction times of the thumb following both slow and rapid rates of stimulation. With a tetanic stimulus applied for only 5 seconds there was no difference in the percent fade at 20, 50, or 100 Hz between these infants and older children up to 9 years of age. In this study the average fade after 5 seconds of stimulation was 5% at 20 Hz, 9% at 50 Hz, and 17% at 100 Hz. However, the train-of-four ratio and degree of posttetanic facilitation increased with age. This suggests that the immediately available stores of acetylcholine and the enhanced mobilization and synthesis seen with tetanic stimulation are less in the neonate than in the older infant or child. Similar conclusions were reached by others from rat data.

Studies of neuromuscular function in anesthetized subjects must be considered in concert with the effect of the anesthetic, per se, on neuromuscular function. Potent inhalation anesthetics are also potent depressants of neuromuscular function. Thus, the same kinetic and dynamic considerations apply to the effects of inhalation anesthetics as apply to an intravenously (IV) administered drug. There are substantive differences in the rate of anesthetic uptake between infants, children, and adults. This is reflected in time-related differences in the ratio of the expired anesthetic (end-tidal) concentration to the inspired anesthetic concentration, the FE/FI ratio, and, more important, in the tissue anesthetic concentration. Early in an anesthetic induction the FE/FI ratio will be higher in infants than in older patients and the muscle concentration of anesthetic may be higher.[9] It may be that cardiac output and muscle blood flow do not always change in a predictable fashion in infants exposed to potent inhalation agents. If so, one would expect variability in the anesthetic concentration in muscle to help explain the variability in depression of neuromuscular function seen in the young infant anesthetized with halothane and also given muscle relaxants. It is also possible that at the same concentration of anesthetic in muscle, neuromuscular function will be more depressed in the younger infant. The studies cited are consistent with these hypotheses.

AGE-RELATED DIFFERENCES IN SENSITIVITY OF THE CHOLINERGIC RECEPTOR TO RELAXANTS

The sensitivity of the postjunctional cholinergic receptor to acetylcholine may vary with age. When allowance is made for differences in volumes of distribution and for type and concentration of anesthesia, infants still appear relatively resistant to succinylcholine and relatively sensitive to nondepolarizing relaxants.

Depolarizing Muscle Relaxants

On a weight basis, infants require more succinylcholine than older children or adults to produce apnea, depress respiration, or depress neuromuscular transmission. Cook and Fischer[10] noted that in infants succinylcholine (1 mg/kg) produced neuromuscular blockade approximately equal to that produced by 0.5 mg/kg in children (6 to 8 years). At these equipotent doses there were no statistically significant differences between the times to recover to 50% neuromuscular tramsmission(T_{50}) and 90% neuromuscular transmission (T_{90}) in the two groups. Children given 1.0 mg/kg of succinylcholine develop complete neuromuscular blockade. The ED_{95} of succinylcholine (ie, the estimated dose of relaxant required to produce 95% depression of twitch height) in infants is 2.2 mg/kg.[10]

Goudsouzian and Liu[11] noted that young infants could require 3-fold higher infusion rates of succinylcholine (milligrams per kilogram per hour) to maintain 90% twitch depression than older infants or children. Phase II block occurred after a slightly larger dose of succinylcholine in infants resistant to succinylcholine than in the other infants or older children. Differences in cholinesterase activity, receptor sensitivity, or volume of distribution may explain these age-related differences in succinylcholine requirements.

The infant has about one half the pseudocholinesterase activity of the older child or adult. Thus, it is unlikely that augmented cholinesterase activity is responsible for the infant's resistance to succinylcholine. When succinylcholine was given in equal dose on a surface-area basis (40 mg/m^2), Walts and Dillon[12] found no difference between infants and adults in the times to recover to 10%, 50%, 90% neuromuscular transmission; this dose of succinylcholine produced complete neuromuscular blockade in all patients. Cook and Fischer[10] noted a linear relationship between the log dose on a milligrams per square meter basis and the maximum intensity of neuromuscular blockade for infants, children, and adults. They also noted a linear relationship between the logarithm of the dose on a milligrams per square meter basis and to either 50% or 90% recovery times for infants and children as a combined group. Because of its relatively small size, succinylcholine is rapidly distributed throughout the extracellular fluid.[13] The blood volume and extracellular fluid (ECF) volume of the infant are significantly greater than the child's or adult's on a weight basis. Therefore, on a weight basis (milligrams per kilogram) the infant requires about twice as much succinylcholine to produce 50% neuromuscular blockade as does the adult. Since ECF and surface area bear a nearly constant relationship throughout life (6 to 8 L/m^2), it is not surprising that there is a good correlation between succinylcholine dose (in milligrams per square meter) and response throughout life. The data of Goudsouzian and Lui[11] suggest that relative resistance to succinylcholine persists in some infants even when the dose is transformed to milligrams per square meter per minute. These data suggest that the acetylcholine receptor matures with age.

Nondepolarizing Muscle Relaxants

When one compensates for the wide variation in volumes of distribution and standardizes the anesthetic background, infants appear sensitive to the nondepolarizing muscle relaxants when compared with adults (eg, D-tubocurarine,[13] atracurium).[14] Unfortunately, few studies have controlled for each factor. Comparing the effects of relaxants in patients of different age anesthetized with different anesthetic techniques can be as inappropriate or as misleading as comparing apples with oranges.

On the basis of clinical criteria it has been suggested that the newborn is sensitive to D-tubocurarine. However, EMG studies demonstrated no increased sensitivity of hand muscles to D-tubocurarine in infants as compared with adults.[15] However, in infants respiratory depression parallels the neuromuscular blockade noted in the hands[15]; in adults neuromuscular blockade of the hand occurs prior to respiratory depression. This important observation suggests that the respiratory muscles of the infant may be more sensitive to D-tubocurarine than those of the adult, or that the infant has less respiratory reserve than the adult. In actuality both may be true.

In adults, Donlon et al[16] have determined cumulative dose-response curves and noted recovery times for D-tubocurarine, gallamine, pancuronium, and metocurine during nitrous oxide-oxygen-narcotic anesthesia. At equipotent doses of these relaxants the recovery time from 95% block to 50% block averaged 45 minutes. Similar studies have been performed in children during halothane and balanced anesthesia by other investigators.[17–21] The ED_{95} for these relaxants in children during balanced anesthesia tended to be higher than that in adults and the recovery times tended to be shorter. The dose requirements (ED_{95}) of pancuronium, metocurine, D-tubocurarine, and gallamine are reduced by halothane anesthesia in children as in adults (Table 1). During halothane-nitrous oxide anesthesia there was little difference between the ED_{95} on a weight basis for the longer-acting muscle relaxants in infants and children (Table 2).

Recently, we[13] estimated the dose of D-tubocurarine, on a surface-area basis, that would be required to produce 95% twitch depression in infants, children, and adults during halothane anesthesia. In this estimate, one attempts to compensate for the wide variation in ECF that appears in infants, children, and adults. The ECF volume mirrors the volume of distribution for the nondepolarizing muscle relaxants. One is also comparing like anesthe-

Table 1
Potency of Nondepolarizing Muscle Relaxants in Children With Various Anesthetics

Drug	ED_{95} (mg/kg) Halothane	Nitrous-Narcotic
D-tubocurarine	0.32	0.60
Metocurine	0.18	0.34
Pancuronium	0.05	0.08
Gallamine	1.9	3.4
Atracurium	0.26	0.350
Vecuronium	0.038	—

See text for references.

tics—halothane with halothane—to produce 95% blockade. The adult and child require about 7 to 8 mg/m^2 of D-tubocurarine;the 6- to 9-month-old infant requires 5 to 6 mg/m^2; but the neonate requires about 4 mg/m^2. This suggests that the neonate, and to a lesser degree the infant, is quite sensitive to D-tubocurarine when one compensates for the wide variation in volumes of distribution.

Fisher et al[22] documented the sensitivity of the infant to D-tubocurarine as compared with older patients during equipotent nitrous oxide-halothane anesthesia. Since the MAC of halothane is higher in infants than adults, infants received higher end-tidal concentrations of halothane. The volume of distribution for D-tubocurarine is quite high in the newborn infant as compared with

Table 2.
Potency of Nondepolarizing Muscle Relaxants in Patients of Different Ages Anesthetized With Halothane and Nitrous Oxide

Drug	ED_{95} (mg/kg) Infant	Child
D-tubocurarine	0.34	0.32
Metocurine	0.22	0.18
Pancuronium	0.05	0.05
Gallamine	—	1.9
Atracurium	0.150	0.260
Vecuronium	0.024	0.038

See text for references.

the older child or adult, but plasma clearance of D-tubocurarine does not differ with age. The volume of distribution for D-tubocurarine appears relatively constant on a liters per square meter basis. More important, the plasma concentration associated with 50% neuromuscular block (Cpss) was age related; Cpss in neonates was about one third that noted for adults. The largest variability in elimination half-life and volumes of distribution was seen in the data for the neonates. Likewise, Goudsouzian et al[20] noted wide variations in the ED_{95} for D-tubocurarine in neonates during halothane anesthesia. Some infants were paralyzed with 0.18 mg/kg, and others required 0.6 mg/kg; the mean ED_{95} was similar to that of older children. This suggests that the neonate's response to nondepolarizing relaxants is quite unpredictable. The clinician should titrate the dose of relaxant to produce the desired effect. The recovery times from all relaxants are dose related. If one were to overdose the infant by a factor of two times, one would expect that recovery time would be quite prolonged.

Recently, two intermediate-acting nondepolarizing relaxants, atracurium and vecuronium, have been introduced into clinical practice. Both are noncumulative and have minimal cardiovascular side effects. Atracurium is a bisquaternary compound that is eliminated by Hofmann degradation, a form of spontaneous self-destruction that is pH and temperature dependent, and by nonspecific ester hydrolysis. Vecuronium, a steroidal relaxant similar to pancuronium, is predominantly eliminated unchanged by hepatic excretion and is also slowly metabolized to 3-OH vecuronium.

We have studied the effect of both age[14, 23–25] and potent inhalation agents on dose-response relationships of atracurium in infants, children, and adolescents. On a weight basis (micrograms per kilogram) the ED_{95} for atracurium was similar in infants (1 to 6 months of age) and adolescents whereas children had a higher dose requirement (Table 3). On a surface-area basis (micrograms per square meter) the ED_{95} for atracurium was similar in children and adolescents; the ED_{95} (micrograms per square meter) for atracurium in the infants was much lower (Fig 1).

At equipotent doses (1 × ED_{95}) the duration of effect (time from injection to 95% recovery) was 23 minutes in infants and 29 minutes for children and adolescents compared with 44 minutes in adults. The time from injection

Table 3
Age-Related Potency of Atracurium[14,23]

	ED_{95} (μg/kg)	ED_{95} ($\mu g/m^2$)
Infant	150	3,330
Child	260	6,630
Adolescent	160	6,300

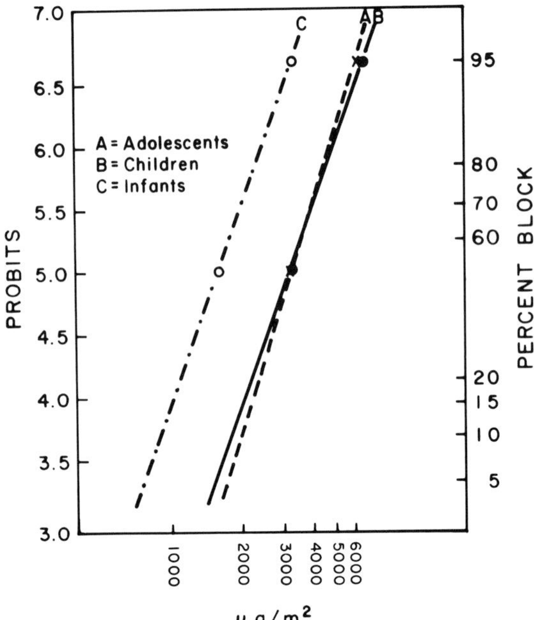

Figure 1. Mean dose-response curves (log-probit) for atracurium (μg/m^2) for (A) adolescents, (B) children and (C) infants. Data taken from Brandom et al[24] and from Cook et al.[25]

to 25% neuromuscular transmission (T_{25}) was ten minutes in infants, 15 minutes in children and adolescents, and 16 minutes in adults. At T_{25}, supplemental doses will be required to maintain surgical relaxation. At higher multiples of the ED_{95} the duration of effect will be longer but the times from T_5 to T_{25} will be the same. The shorter duration of effect in the infant may represent a difference in pharmacodynamics or pharmacokinetics.

In children, light isoflurane anesthesia (1% end-tidal) reduces the atracurium requirements by about 30% from that needed with thiopental-narcotic anesthesia. There was no statistically significant difference in the isoflurane or halothane dose-response curves (Fig 2). For clinical purposes both potent agents should be viewed as potentiating atracurium to the same degree.

Following a bolus of atracurium, we have recently used a continuous infusion of dilute atracurium (200 μg/mL) to maintain neuromuscular blockade constant at 95% ± 5% block.[25] To maintain this degree of block, infusion rates of 4 to 5 μg/kg/min were required during halothane or isoflurane anesthesia,and 8 to 10 μg/kg/min were required with thiopental-narcotic anesthesia following an initial bolus. No cumulation was seen with prolonged infusion; recovery of neuromuscular transmission was prompt. The recovery of neuro-

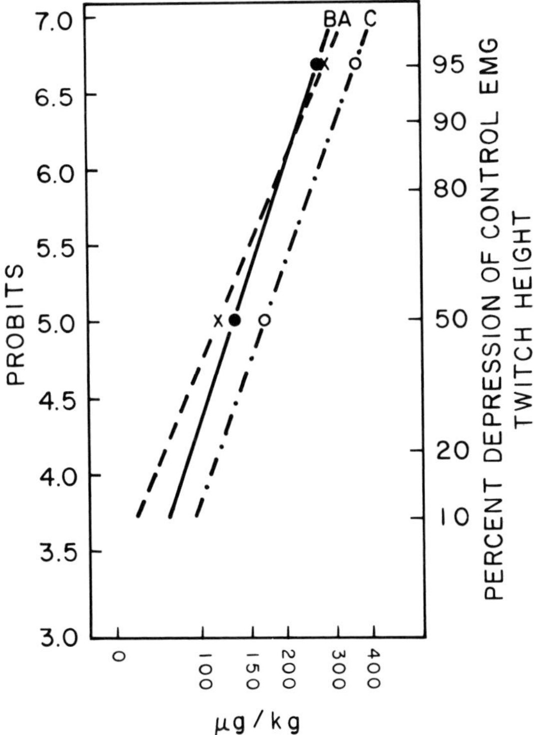

Figure 2. Mean dose-response curves (log-probit) for atracurium (micrograms per kilogram) in children anesthetized with (A) isoflurane, (B) halothane, and (C) balanced anesthesia. Data taken from Brandom et al.[24]

muscular transmission from the same degree of blockade was similar with all three anesthetics. From these infusion data one can estimate the quantity of atracurium inactivated (clearance) by ester hydrolysis, Hofmann elimination, or renal elimination. The clearance of atracurium in children on a micrograms per square meter per minute basis during nitrous-narcotic anesthesia was similar to that noted by others in adults (ie, 240 $\mu g/m^2/min$).[26]

During halothane anesthesia, children had a higher ED_{95} for vecuronium than measured in adolescents.[27] Although not of statistical significance, Fisher and Miller[28] noted a similar relationship for the dose-response curves for vecuronium in infants, children, and adults (Table 2). At equipotent doses (2 $\times$ ED_{95}) of vecuronium, the duration of effect (time from injection to 90% recovery) was longest for infants (73 minutes) compared with that for children (35 minutes) and adults (53 minutes). The duration of effect of vecuronium in infants is therefore comparable to that seen with the long-acting nondepolarizers. This prolonged duration of action of vecuronium in infants may be related to relative immaturity of the liver in infants or to a larger volume of distribution—both would be reflected in a longer elimination half-life.

SELECTION OF RELAXANTS

All muscle relaxants at an appropriate dose will produce muscle relaxation; at equipotent doses each relaxant will produce the same degree of relaxation as any other. Potency is important not only to the drug concentration in the vial but perhaps in the disparity between neuromuscular blocking effects and autonomic side effects. In selecting relaxant A over relaxant B for use in pediatric patients one should consider the onset time, duration of effect, nonneuromuscular blocking side effects including the cardiovascular side effects, and the routes of elimination (renal, liver, spontaneous) of the relaxant. Thus, one must be aware of the nonneuromuscular blocking effects of relaxants. In addition, one should consider how the age or pathologic condition of the patient may influence the kinetics of the relaxant.

NONNEUROMUSCULAR BLOCKING EFFECTS OF SUCCINYLCHOLINE

Succinylcholine can (1) have profound cardiovascular effects; (2) increase intraocular, intragastric, or intracranial pressure; and (3) be associated with hyperkalemia, myoglobinemia, and malignant hyperthermia.

Dysrhythmias

Succinylcholine exerts variable and seemingly paradoxical effects on the cardiovascular system. Typically, IV succinylcholine produces initial bradycardia and hypotension, followed after 15 to 30 seconds by tachycardia and hypertension. In the infant and small child profound sustained sinus bradycardia (rates of 50 to 60 per minute) is commonly observed[29,30]; rarely, asystole occurs. Nodal rhythm and ventricular ectopic beats are seen in about 80% of children given a single IV injection of succinylcholine; such dysrhythmias are rarely seen following intramuscular succinylcholine.

As in adults the incidence of bradycardia and other dysrhythmias is higher in children following a second dose of succinylcholine. Atropine (0.1 mg) appears to offer adequate protection against these bradyarhythmias in all age groups. In infants, vagolytic doses of atropine (0.03 mg/kg) are required for protection; in older children adequate protection is provided by doses of 0.005 mg/kg.

Pulmonary Edema and Pulmonary Hemorrhage

Recently, we have seen several young infants who developed fulminant pulmonary edema following intramuscular (IM) succinylcholine (4 mg/kg).[31] The pulmonary edema occurred within minutes of the IM injection and responded to continuous positive pressure ventilation (CPAP). Since that report we have collected additional cases of pulmonary edema and pulmonary hemorrhage following IV succinylcholine as well. In each instance the patient was lightly anesthetized. We speculate that this may represent a hemodynamic form of pulmonary edema from an acute elevation of systemic vascular resistance and an acute decrease in pulmonary vascular resistance. In addition, ''leaky'' capillaries appear to be involved. Whether these cardiovascular changes are mediated by succinylcholine itself or some other vasoactive substance (ie, histamine) is not known.

Intragastric Pressure

Succinycholine may increase intragastric pressure. The increase in intragastric pressure is directly related to the intensity of muscle fasciculations. In adults, pressures as high as 40 cm H_2O have been recorded following violent fasciculations. When the intragastric pressure exceeds 20 cm H_2O, the cardioesophageal valve (sphincter) mechanism may be rendered incompetent; regurgitation and aspiration may occur. Because of his limited muscle mass the infant or small child, in contrast to the adult, seldom has strong fasciculation. Salem et al[32] observed only a 4-cm H_2O elevation of intragastric pressure after IV succinylcholine in children. In some patients the intragastric pressure decreased.

Intraocular Pressure

IV or IM administration of succinylcholine increases intraocular pressure in both children and adults.[33] Although dilation of choroidal vessels by succinylcholine is a contributary factor, the major increase in intraocular pressure is due to contraction of extraocular muscles. Typically, after IV succinylcholine, the intraocular pressure begins to increase within 60 seconds, peaks at two to three minutes, then decreases to control levels five to seven minutes after injection. Succinylcholine-induced elevation of intraocular pressure in the presence of a penetrating wound of the eye can result in extrusion of vitreous through the site of injury and possible loss of vision. In the patient with glaucoma there may be a falsely elevated intraocular pressure, which may lead to unnecessary surgery if tonometry is performed within five to seven minutes after the administration of succinylcholine.

Hyperkalemia and Myoglobinemia

In normal adults succinylcholine increases plasma levels of potassium by 0.3 to 0.5 mEq/L.[34] Even more modest increases are seen in children.[35,36] Alarming levels of potassium, as high as 11 mEq/L, along with cardiovascular collapse, have been reported with succinylcholine in a variety of situations, some of which include burns, massive trauma, stroke, and spinal cord injury. A common denominator appears to be either massive tissue destruction or CNS injury with muscle wasting. Strong fasciculations are not necessary to produce hyperkalemia in susceptable patients. There are no data to suggest that the infant or small child is not vulnerable to massive potassium flux from the above conditions just as the adult.

Ryan et al[37] noted a high incidence of myoglobinemia (45%) following succinylcholine (1 mg/kg) in prepubertal patients anesthetized with halothane. A much lower incidence (8%) of the same degree of myoglobinemia was noted by Harrington et al,[38] although all of their children did have some myoglobin in their blood. Myoglobinuria was rare. Myoglobinemia is rarely seen in adults following succinylcholine. Likewise, significant elevation of plasma levels of creatine phosphokinase (CPK), an indicator of muscle injury, has been demonstrated following succinylcholine in children.[39, 40] Myoglobinemia and elevation of plasma levels of CPK were seen in the absence of strong fasciculations. The susceptibility of muscle in children to release myoglobin following depolarization with succinylcholine has no ready explanation. In the study by Harrington et al there was no correlation between the occurrence of fasciculations, pretreatment with gallamine, dose (1 *v* 2 mg/kg of succinylcholine), or age and the degree of myoglobinemia. However, all patients who developed myoglobinuria received 2 mg/kg of succinylcholine. This study suggests that although myoglobinemia may occur more often in children than in adults, it is of minimal clinical significance.

Malignant Hyperthermia and Masseter Spasm

Most clinicians are well aware of the association of succinylcholine with malignant hyperthermia. The typical patient with malignant hyperthermia develops profound rigidity or violent fasciculations, a rapid increase in temperature, an increase in pulse rate, and an increase in end-tidal carbon dioxide tension. These are classic signs of malignant hyperthermia. However, an occasional patient may develop trismus, a tight jaw, as the earliest or the only manifestation of malignant hyperthermia. The jaw has cogwheel-type rigidity; it can be pried open with considerable difficulty. Recent studies have documented the incidence of masseter spasm in children, but the implication of this condition are not clear. Schwartz et al[41] noted 15 cases of masseter spasm in a series of 13,160 anesthetics. Only 14% of these patients received an anesthetic induction with halothane followed by the IV administration of succinylcholine, yielded a 0.8% indicence of masseter spasm with this anesthetic technique. Thirteen of the anesthetic cases were aborted, and none of these cases nor the two short cases that were continued had evidence of hypermetabolism. More than two thirds of the cases of masseter spasm, in which urine myoglobin was obtained, had no elevation of urine myoglobin. The range of CPK was quite broad, from normal to over 40,000 units, at up to 12 hours after masseter spasm occurred. With a test of calcium uptake, all of the 12 patients who consented to study showed abnormalities that were reported as unquestionably positive for susceptibility to malignant hyperthermia. But none of these patients were evaluated with a caffeine and/or halothane contracture test, the current gold standard in the testing of MH susceptibility. When such studies are used, 50% to 70% of patients that develop trismus following malignant hyperthermia have the propensity to develop malignant hyperthermia.[42] The other patients, however, do not have this propensity. It is impossible to declare these patients susceptible to malignant hyperthermia based only on the sign of trismus. CPK measurements and muscle biopsy may be helpful in this regard. However, most centers are reluctant to do major muscle biopsies in children less than 8 to 10 years of age. Susceptibility to malignant hyperthermia then becomes an extraordinarily difficult diagnosis to make on clinical grounds.

NONNEUROMUSCULAR BLOCKING EFFECTS OF NONDEPOLARIZING RELAXANTS

The nonneuromuscular blocking properties of the nondepolarizing relaxants are primarily cardiovascular in nature. These cardiovascular effects are related to the magnitude of histamine release, ganglionic blockade, and vagolysis. In addition, the cardiovascular effects seem age related.

In infants and children, minimal cardiovascular effects are seen following atracurium, metocurine, and vecuronium at several multiples of the ED_{95}. In adults, atracurium at three times the ED_{95} causes slightly less histamine release than two times the ED_{95} of metocurine and less than half as much histamine release as one times the ED_{95} of D-tubocurarine. Vecuronium (at any multiple of ED_{95}) is not associated with histamine release. Infants and children appear less susceptible to histamine release following relaxants than adults. In a small series of infants, five times the ED_{95} of atracurium did not elicit flushing or alteration of heart rate or BP. However, when atracurium is injected directly IV in infants and children, local signs of histamine release have been described. Rarely, flushing with or without mild hypotension is seen at high multiples of the ED_{95}. At high doses, D-tubocurarine may cause hypotension and histamine release in children.

Keon and Downes (1979 unpublished data) compared changes in heart rate, changes in BP and differences in intubating conditions in infants (average age 5.6 months) "anesthetized" with nitrous oxide-oxygen following either D-tubocurarine (0.6 mg/kg) or pancuronium (0.1 mg/kg). None had received premedication. In both groups there were modest increases in pulse rate; transient episodes of bradycardia occurred in some infants in both groups during intubation. No infant given pancuronium developed significant hypotension or hypertension (greater than 10% change from control levels). In contrast, 25% of the infants given D-tubocurarine experienced decreases in BP greater than 10% from control (range 11% to 26%).

In children anesthetized with halothane and nitrous oxide, we noted that one times the ED_{95} of gallamine increases the heart rate by 42 beats per minute and that one times the ED_{95} of pancuronium increases the heart rate by 19 beats per minute. Both drugs increase mean arterial pressure under these conditions by about 10 torr. At two times the ED_{95}, further increases in heart rate were seen with pancuronium but not with gallamine. In contrast, we noted minimal effects of gallamine or pancuronium on the heart rate in infants. Unless the heart rate had slowed from halothane, neither gallamine nor pancuronium exhibited any vagolytic effects. In an occasional infant, however, gallamine or pancuronium may cause a significant increase in heart rate. Since the infant responds to a variety of stimuli with bradycardia (eg, potent inhalation agents, hypoxia, intubation) the potential vagolytic effects of pancuronium and gallamine may be *wanted* side effects. For example, in adults pancuronium is usually administered with high-dose fetanyl anesthesia to minimize the bradycardia seen with fentanyl; substitution of atracurium for pancuronium has resulted in profound bradycardia from the fentanyl—a totally predictable side effect. Whether profound bradycardia will be seen in infants anesthetized with deep halothane given atracurium or vecuronium remains to be seen. We have noted no significant change in heart rate and only a minimal (7 torr) decrease in BP in infants anesthetized with halothane 1% end-tidal and nitrous oxide given 0.3 mg/kg of atracurium.[14] No changes in heart rate or BP have been noted after 70 μg/kg of vecuronium in pediatric patients also anesthetized with halothane and nitrous oxide.[28]

REVERSAL OF RELAXANTS

Because of the increased potential for respiratory inadequacy from residual neuromuscular blockade in infants, most pediatric anesthesiologists routinely antagonize the neuromuscular blockade of nondepolarizing relaxants.

The rule is to always reverse. Large doses of neostigmine (70 μg/kg) were usually used, not because this was necessarily the right dose but to buy insurance. Perhaps this is an overzealous pragmatic approach, but it is one that usually minimized the number of "floppy" babies with poor motor tone and inadequate ventilation. In infants, as in adults, return of neurotransmission will be prompt if few receptors are blocked at the time of reversal. By proper choice of relaxants and careful timing and titration of the dose of relaxant, one can usually assure that some motor tone is present by the time reversal is attempted. One should be aware that potent inhalation anesthetics, certain antibiotics, hypotension, hypothermia, acidosis, or hypocalcemia can prolong or potentiate neuromuscular blockade from nondepolarizing relaxants. Hypothermia per se can lead to respiratory depression in infants.[13]

Use of intermediate-acting relaxants forces one to re-examine the dictum to always reverse. Clearly, the margin of safety in using relaxants is increased by documenting objective criteria for adequacy of neuromuscular transmission. These criteria include a train-of-four ratio greater than 0.7; ability to sustain tetnus at 50 Hz; a vital capacity of 15 to 20 mL/kg; ability to flex the arms and legs; and an inspiratory force greater than 25 cm H_2O.If the infant or child can meet several of these criteria without reversal, no reversal is needed. But if in doubt, reversal drug should be given.

Fisher et al[43] have recently examined the dose of neostigmine required in infants, children, and adults to reverse a 90% block from a continuous D-tubocurarine infusion. In infants and children 15.0 μg/kg of neostigmine produced a 50% antagonism of the D-tubocurarine block; in adults 23 μg/kg was required. It was claimed that the duration of antagonism was equal in all three groups although the elimination half-life was clearly shorter for infants. A larger dose than that seemingly recommended would give a higher sustained blood concentration. Whether this is of pharmacologic benefit in the absence of a continuous infuisson of relaxant is doubtful. The dissociation between the elimination half-life and the duration of antagonism may result from the carbamylation of cholinesterase by neostigmine. Edrophonium has been recommended to antagonize nondepolarizing neuromuscular blockade. In adults 300 μg/kg has been recommended. Fisher et al[44] have recently noted that the elimination half-life for edrophonium is shorter in infants and children than in adults. Since the molecular interaction between edrophonium and cholinesterase is readily reversible, they suggest that the shorter elimination half-life for edrophonium might limit the value of edrophonium in pediatric patients.

Meakin et al[45] compared the rate of recovery of pancuronium-induced neuromuscular blockade with several doses of neostigmine (0.036 or 0.07 mg/kg) or edrophonium (.7 or 1.43 mg/kg) in infants and children. In the first five minutes recovery of neuromuscular transmission was more rapid after edrophonium than neostigmine in all age groups; the speed of recovery was faster in infants and children than in adults. By ten minutes there were no differences in neuromuscular transmission achieved in infants and children with either reversal agent (at either dose); adults had lower neuromuscular transmission at the lower dose (0.036 mg/kg) of neostigmine. Thus, if speed of initial recovery is a critical issue, then edrophonium is better than neostigmine and a high dose of neostigmine is better than a low dose. At 30 minutes following injection of either reversal agent (at any dose) there were no differences in neuromuscular transmission between age groups.

SUMMARY

In the first 2 years of life of humans there is physical and biochemical maturation of the neuromuscular junction. With this maturation there is an increase in the neuromuscular reserve (margin of safety) of the infant and a change in the contractile properties of skeletal muscle. When dosage is calculated on the basis of surface area, neonates and young infants are not resistant to succinylcholine but appear sensitive to nondepolarizing relaxants. Variation in ECF volume and receptor sensitivity probably explain these differences. Awareness of the clinical response of neonates and infants to muscle relaxants and awareness of the nonneuromuscular blocking properties of relaxants in infants and children permits the use of these anesthetic adjuncts in patients of any age.

REFERENCES

1. Anggard L, Ottoson D: Observations on the functional development of the neuromuscular apparatus in fetal sheep. Exp Neurol 7:294–304, 1963
2. Close R: Dynamic properties of fast and slow skeletal muscles of the rat during development. J Physiol 173:74–95, 1964
3. Close R: Force-velocity properties of mouse muscles. Nature 206:718–719, 1965
4. Close R: Effects of cross-union of motor nerves to fast and slow skeletal muscles. Nature 206:831–832, 1965
5. Buller AJ: Developmental physiology of the neuromuscular system. Br Med Bull 22:45–48, 1966
6. Crumrine RS, Yodlowski EH: Assessment of neuromuscular function in infants. Anesthesiology 54:29–32, 1981
7. Koenigsberger MR, Patten B, Lovelace RE: Studies of neuromuscular function in the newborn—A comparison of myoneural function in the full term and premature infant. Neuropadiatrie 4:350–361, 1973
8. Goudsouzian NG: Maturation of neuromuscular transmission in the infant. Br J Anaesth 52:205–213, 1980
9. Brandom BW, Brandom RB, Cook DR: Uptake and distribution of halothane in infants: In vivo measurements and computer simulations. Anesth Analg 62:404–410, 1983

10. Cook DR, Fischer CG: Neuromuscular blocking effects of succinylcholine in infants and children. Anesthesiology 42:662–665, 1975
11. Goudsouzian NG, Liu LMP: The neuromuscular response of infants to a continuous infusion of succinylcholine. Anesthesiology 60:97–101, 1984
12. Walts LF, Dillon JB: The response of newborns to succinylcholine and d-tubocurarine. Anesthesiology 31:35–38, 1969
13. Cook DR: Muscle relaxants in infants and children. Anesth Analg 60:335–343, 1981
14. Brandom BW, Woelfel SK, Cook DR, et al: Clinical pharmacology of atracurium in infants. Anesth Analg 63:309–312, 1984
15. Churchill-Davidson HC, Wise RP: The response of the newborn infant to muscle relaxants. Can Anaesth Soc J 11:1–5, 1964
16. Donlon JV, Ali HH, Savarese JJ: A new approach to the study of four nondepolarizing relaxants in man. Anesth Analg 53: 924–939, 1974
17. Goudsouzian NG, Liu LMP, Cote CJ: Comparison of equipotent doses of nondepolarizing muscle relaxants in children. Anesth Analg 60:862–866, 1981
18. Goudsouzian NG, Liu LMP, Savarese JJ: Metocurarine in infants and children: Neuromuscular and clinical effects. Anesthesiology 49:266–269, 1978
19. Goudsouzian NG, Ryan JF, Savarese JJ: The neuromuscular effects of pancuronium in infants and children. Anesthesiology 41:95–98, 1974
20. Goudsouzian NG, Donlon JV, Savarese JJ, et al: Re-evaluation of dosage and duration of action of d-tubocurarine in the pediatric age group. Anesthesiology 43:416–425, 1975
21. Goudsouzian NG, Martyn JJA, Liu LMP: The dose response effect of long-acting non-depolarizing neuromuscular blocking agents in children. Can Anaesth Soc J 3:246–250, 1984
22. Fisher DM, O'Keefe C, Stanski DR, et al: Pharmacokinetics and pharmacodynamics of d-tubocurarine in infants, children, and adults. Anesthesiology 57:203–208, 1982
23. Brandom BW, Rudd GD, Cook DR: Clinical pharmacology of atracurium in pediatric patients. Br J Anaesth 55:117S–121S, 1983
24. Brandom BW, Woelfel SK, Cook DR, et al: Relative potency of atracurium in children during halothane, isoflurane, or thiopental-fentanyl anesthesia. Anesthesiology 59:A442, 1983
25. Cook DR, Brandom BW, Woelfel SK, et al: Atracurium infusion in children during fentanyl, halothane, and isoflurane anesthesia. Anesth Analg 64:471–476, 1985
26. D'Hollander AA, Luyckx C, Barvais L, et al: Clinical evaluation of atracurium besylate requirement for a stable muscle relaxation during surgery: Lack of age-related effects. Anesthesiology 59:237–240, 1983
27. Goudsouzian NG, Martyn J, Liu LMP, et al: Safety and efficacy of vecuronium in adolescents and children. Anesth and Analg (in press)
28. Fisher DM, Miller RD: Neuromuscular effects of vecuronium (ORG NC45) in infants and children during N_2O, halothane anesthesia. Anesthesiology 58:519–523, 1983
29. Digby-Leigh M, McLoyd D, Belton MK, et al: Bradycardia following intravenous administration of succinylcholine in anesthetized children. Anesthesiology 18:698–702, 1957
30. Craythorne NWB, Turndorf H, Dripps RD: Changes in pulse rate and rhythm associated with the use of succinylcholine in anesthetized children. Anesthesiology 21:465–471, 1960
31. Cook DR, Westman H, Rosenfeld L, et al: Pulmonary edema in infants: Possible association with intramuscular succinylcholine. Anesth Analg 60:220–223, 1981
32. Salem MR, Wong AY, Lin YH: The effect of suxamethonium on the intragastric pressure in infants and children. Br J Anaesth 44:166–170, 1972
33. Craythorne NWB, Rohenstein HS, Dripps RD: Effects of succinylcholine on intraocular pressure in adults, infants, and children during general anesthesia. Anesthesiology 21:59–65, 1960
34. Weintraub HD, Heisterkamp DV, Cooperman LH: Changes in plasma potassium concentration after depolarizing blockers in anesthetized man. Br J Anaesth 41:1048–1052, 1969

35. Henning RD, Bush GH: Plasma potassium after halothane-suxamethonium induction in children. Anaesthesia 37: 802–805, 1982
36. Dierdorf SF, McNiece WL, Wolfe TM, et al: Effect of thiopental and succinylcholine on serum potassium concentrations in children. Anesth Analg 63:1136–1138, 1984
37. Ryan JF, Kagen LJ, Hyman AI: Myoglobinemia after a single dose of succinylcholine. N Engl J Med 285:824–825, 1971
38. Harrington JF, Ford DJ, Striker TW: Myoglobinemia and myoglobinuria after succinylcholine in children. Anesthesiology 59:A439, 1983
39. Tammisto T, Airaksinen M: Increase of creatine kinase activity in serum as sign of muscular injury caused by intermittently administered suxamethonium during halothane anesthesia. Br J Anaesth 38:510–515, 1966
40. Innes RKR, Stromme JH: Rise in creatine phosphokinase associated with agents used in anaesthesia. Br J Anaesth 45:185–189, 1973
41. Schwartz L, Koka BV, Rockoff MA: Masseter spasm after halothane and succinylcholine: Incidence and implications. Anesthesiology 59:A438, 1983
42. Rosenberg H, Reed S, Heiman T: Masseter spasm, rhabdomyolysis and malignant hyperthermia. Anesthesiology 53: S248, 1980
43. Fisher DM, Cronnelly R, Miller RD, et al: The neuromuscular pharmacology of neostigmine in infants and children. Anesthesiology 59:220–225, 1983
44. Fisher DM, Cronnelly R, Miller RD: Dose-response relationship for edrophonium in anesthetized children. Anesthesiology 59:A282, 1983
45. Meakin G, Sweet PT, Bevan JC, et al: Neostigmine and edrophonium as antagonists of pancuronium in infants and children. Anesthesiology 59:316–321, 1983

Jørgen Viby-Mogensen

15

Interaction of Other Drugs With Muscle Relaxants

Drugs that interfere with the action of muscle relaxants may exert their action proximal to the neuromuscular junction, at the neuromuscular junction, distal to the junction, or at two or all three of these sites, as is often the case.

An effect proximal to the neuromuscular junction may take place in the central nervous system or in the blood stream. Inhalational anesthetic agents probably owe at least a part of their influence on the effect of muscle relaxants to a reduced neural activity in the central nervous system. A classical example of an interaction taking place in the blood stream is the inhibition of plasma cholinesterase caused by echothiophate, preventing the normal metabolism of succinylcholine.

Interactions at the neuromuscular junction may in principle take place at three different sites: at the nerve terminal, at the postsynaptic membrane, or in the synaptic cleft. However, drugs often have an effect on more than one of these sites, and it may be impossible to decide which one is the more important; they may be equally important.

At the nerve terminal some drugs interfere with the propagation of the nerve terminal action potential (local anesthetic–like effect). Others modify calcium flow into the nerve terminal, either by blocking the calcium channels (like verapamil and nifedipine) or by interfering with one or more of the enzymes involved in the control of calcium flow into the nerve terminal and thus the quantal release of transmitter (theophylline and azathioprine; Fig 1). Certain antibiotics and lithium act presynaptically by inhibiting the synthesis of acetylcholine.

MUSCLE RELAXANTS
ISBN 0-8089-1784-6

Most drugs that have an effect on the postsynaptic membrane block the acetylcholine recognition sites of the receptor in a manner similar to the nondepolarizing muscle relaxants (some antibiotics and probably procainamide). However, certain drugs such as lidocaine, lincomycin, and clindamycin impair ion channel conductance by reducing open channel life time. Inhalation anesthetic agents also shorten the open channel life time. Recently it has been shown that some drugs may enter and occlude open ion channels. However, this action only occurs under certain conditions, and it is still not clear whether it has any clinical significance.

In the synaptic cleft any drug with anticholinesterase activity may interfere with the enzymatic hydrolysis of acetylcholine and, hence, with the effect of the nondepolarizing relaxants.

Among the drugs with an effect distal to the neuromuscular junction is dantrolene, used in the treatment of malignant hyperthermia. Dantrolene has no effect on the transmission of impulses from nerve to muscle but acts by blocking excitation-contraction coupling, thus preventing the normal mechanical performance of muscle. Tobramycin, lincomycin, and clindamycin also seem to have an effect on the muscle cell membrane.

In this paper, the drugs that might interfere with the action of muscle relaxants have been classified into two major groups: those that interfere with the effect of succinylcholine (Table 1) and those that interfere with the nondepolarizing relaxants (Table 2). With a few exceptions, only clinically relevant interactions are included.

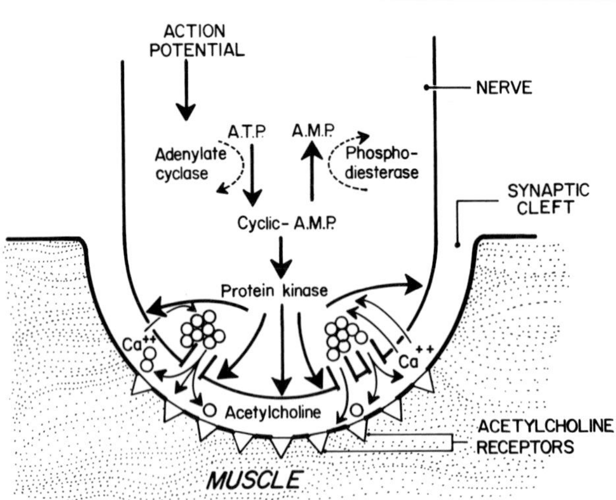

Figure 1. Diagrammatic representation of the enzyme cascade involved in the release of acetylcholine at the nerve terminal.

Table 1
Drugs That Might Interfere With the Effect of Succinylcholine.

Drug	Mechanism of Action	Effects and Comments
Antiarrhythmic drugs		
Beta-adrenergic blocking agents	Not known.	Propranolol potentiates the effect of succinylcholine in the cat.[1] It remains to be shown that this interaction also occurs in man.
Calcium channel blockers	Verapamil and nifedipine block conductance of the calcium channels prejunctionally as well as postjunctionally. Besides, verapamil has been shown to have local anesthetic-like effect on nerve conduction.	Whether calcium channel blockers in therapeutic doses can produce neuromuscular blockade is controversial.[2–4] However, in rabbits verapamil has been shown to potentiate the block produced by an infusion of succinylcholine.[5] Recently, respiratory failure has been reported following intravenous (IV) injection of verapamil in a patient with Duchenne's dystrophy.[6]
Procainamide	The main effect of procainamide is to decrease sensitivity of the postjunctional membrane.[7] However, it also decreases presynaptic transmitter release.	Procainamide potentiates the effect of succinylcholine in cats.[8] This interaction has not been shown in man.
Quinidine	Quinidine has both pre- and postjunctional actions. However, the exact mechanism is unknown.	In the cat, quinidine has been shown to augment the block caused by succinylcholine.[9] Prolonged neuromuscular blockade has been described following injection of quinidine to patients who have recently received succinylcholine.[10] Careful postoperative observation of respiration is mandatory.

Table 1
(Continued)

Drug	Mechanism of Action	Effects and Comments
Antibiotics Colistin Kanamycin Neomycin Streptomycin Polymyxin B	Not fully understood, but the antibiotics are known to have prejunctional as well as postjunctional effects.[11]	The effect of succinylcholine may be enhanced.[12]
Azothioprine	Unknown. Inhibition of phosphodiesterase at the motor nerve terminal? (Fig 1).	Azothioprine potentiates the block produced by succinylcholine in the cat.[13] So far, no such interaction has been reported in man.
Aprotinine Trasylol	Aprotinine is a weak inhibitor of plasma cholinesterase activity.[14]	Theoretically, a prolonged apnoea might occur following the injection of succinylcholine. However, unless plasma cholinesterase activity is already low from other causes, this is unlikely to occur.
Contraceptive pills	Contraceptive pills reduce plasma cholinesterase activity. This reduction most often only amounts to about 20% to 30%.[15]	Theoretically, a prolonged apnoea might occur following succinylcholine. However, unless plasma cholinesterase activity is already low from other causes, this is unlikely to occur.
Cyclophosphamide Endoxan	Endoxan causes long-lasting ("irreversible") inhibition of plasma cholinesterase activity. The inhibition is often 35% to 70%.	The duration of action of succinylcholine may be increased by 5 to 15 minutes.[15]

Table 1
(Continued)

Drug	Mechanism of Action	Effects and Comments
Digitalis	Digitalis seems to sensitize the myocardium to the effect of succinylcholine.[16] The exact mechanism is not clear. It has been hypothesized that the arrhythmias are caused by the sudden increase in plasma potassium often seen following the injection of succinylcholine.	Digitalized patients have been reported to be more prone to develop cardiac arrhythmias following succinylcholine than nondigitalized patients.[16]
Echothiophate	Echothiophate causes a long-lasting (irreversible) inhibition of plasma cholinesterase activity. One drop in each eye twice a day may reduce activity by 70% to 100%.[15]	The duration of action of succinylcholine is increased by 10 to 20 minutes. (Echothiophate eye drops are used in the treatment of glaucoma.)
Edrophonium	Like the other anticholinesterase drugs used for reversal of nondepolarizing neuromuscular blockade, edrophonium inhibits plasma cholinesterase.[17] The decrease in enzyme activity varies between little and 100%, depending on the dose of edrophonium.	So far, no prolonged neuromuscular blockade has been reported following injection of succinylcholine in patients given edrophonium for reversal of a nondepolarizing block.
Furosemide	The exact mechanism is not known. Tentatively, the mechanism has been explained on the basis of protein kinase inhibition (low doses) and phosphodiesterase inhibition (high doses), respectively, at the motor nerve terminal (Fig 1).	In cats, furosemide in low doses ($<10\ \mu g/kg$) intensifies the neuromuscular block produced by succinylcholine. In higher doses (1 to 4 mg/kg) it antagonizes the block.[18] Whether this interaction has any clinical significance remains to be shown.

Table 1
(Continued)

Drug	Mechanism of Action	Effects and Comments
Glucocorticoids	Long-lasting treatment with prednisone has been shown to reduce plasma cholinesterase activity by about 50%.[19]	Theoretically, a prolonged apnoea following succinylcholine might occur in patients on long-term steroid therapy. However, unless the plasma cholinesterase activity is already low from other causes, this is unlikely to occur.
Hexafluorenium	Hexafluorenium inhibits plasma cholinesterase activity and has a weak nondepolarizing neuromuscular blocking action.	Hexafluorenium has been used to potentiate and prolong the block produced by succinylcholine. Injection of hexafluorenium 0.5 mg/kg followed by succinylcholine 1 mg/kg causes an apnoea period of about 30 to 60 minutes. After the introduction of the new intermediate duration nondepolarizing relaxants there is hardly any indication for this drug combination. Simultaneous injection of succinylcholine and hexafluorenium may result in bronchospasm.
Inhalational anesthetic agents	The mechanism is multifactorial. Probably, the anesthetic agents exert their action on the central nervous system, at the postsynaptic membrane (by shortening open channel life time?), and at a point distal to the cholinergic receptor (the muscle cell membrane? The sarcoplasmatic reticulum?).	Halothane and enflurane have been shown to facilitate the occurrence of a phase 2 block and to potentiate the degree of its development. Halothane and enflurane also facilitate the development of tachyphylaxis to succinylcholine.[15]

Table 1
(Continued)

Drug	Mechanism of Action	Effects and Comments
Intravenous anesthetic agents		
Barbiturates	Barbiturates "stabilize" cell membranes, including the postsynaptic membrane. The mechanism is not fully understood.	Barbiturate induction decreases the outflow of potassium from the cells caused by injection of succinylcholine. Barbiturates are not normally considered to have any other clinically relevant effect on neuromuscular transmission.
Diazepam	Diazepam may act in the spinal cord to depress reflex activity evoked from muscle spindles, and it may suppress any repetitive firing in the motor nerve terminals (WC Bowman, personal communication).	Diazepam given IV before succinylcholine has been claimed to be more effective than d-tubocurarine in preventing the adverse effects of succinylcholine.[20,21] Others have found that diazepam has no effect on (1) frequency or intensity of succinylcholine fasciculations and, (2) the increase in serum potassium after succinylcholine.[22] Diazepam given IV seems to accelerate onset of succinylcholine block. The duration of block is not affected.[22]
Propanidid	Propanidid is broken down at least partly by plasma cholinesterase, and the enzyme activity is reduced after its administration. However, the exact mechanism of interaction with succinylcholine is not clear.[23]	The duration of action of succinylcholine may be prolonged by a few minutes.[24] This is normally without clinical significance.

Table 1
(Continued)

Drug	Mechanism of Action	Effects and Comments
Local anesthetics		
Lidocaine	Lidocaine is known to depress prejunctional as well as postjunctional functions. Whether this is the main mechanism or the interaction with succinylcholine is due to a competition between the two drugs for protein binding sites in plasma is not known. Lidocaine does inhibit plasma cholinesterase activity, but this is probably without clinical significance.	Lidocaine 50 to 100 mg IV may augment a phase 2 block caused by succinylcholine.[25]
Procaine	Like lidocaine, procaine has a weak anticholinesterase activity and competes with succinylcholine for the plasma protein binding sites. However, probably most significant is that succinylcholine and procaine both are metabolized by plasma cholinesterase, and large doses of the latter may therefore inhibit the hydrolysis of succinylcholine.[26]	The duration of action of succinylcholine may be (slightly) prolonged by the injection of procaine.[27] The hydrolysis of procaine is decreased in patients with a genetic defect in plasma cholinesterase. Accordingly, cardiovascular collapse has been described following injection of procaine in a patient with abnormal plasma cholinesterase activity.[28]
Magnesium	Magnesium decreases acetylcholine release prejunctionally, reduces the sensitivity of the postjunctional membrane to acetylcholine, and depresses the excitability of the muscle cell membrane.	In patients receiving magnesium sulphate (preeclamptic or eclamptic toxemia), the duration of action of succinylcholine may be prolonged. Calcium antagonizes the effects of magnesium.

Table 1
(Continued)

Drug	Mechanism of Action	Effects and Comments
Neostigmine	Neostigmine inhibits plasma cholinesterase. The decrease in enzyme activity may vary between little and 100%, depending on the dose of neostigmine. The inhibition of enzyme activity may last for hours.[29]	The duration of action of succinylcholine 1.0 to 1.5 mg/kg, when given within 1½ hours of the administration of neostigmine, may range from 35 to 180 minutes in normal patients. In patients with renal failure the enzyme activity may be reduced for several hours following injection of neostigmine.[30]
N′, N′′, N′′′, Triethylenthiophosphoramine Thiotepa	Thiotepa causes long-lasting (irreversible) inhibition of plasma cholinesterase activity. The activity may be reduced by 35% to 70%.[15]	The duration of action of succinylcholine is increased by 5 to 15 minutes. Thiotepa is a cytotoxic drug used in treatment of cancer.
Nondepolarizing relaxants (NDR) Pretreatment with NDR	The ultimate mechanism of action is not known. Presumably the NDR binds to a number of the cholinergic receptors, thus preventing the access of succinylcholine to these receptors. Besides, pancuronium (and to a lesser extent vecuronium) inhibits plasma cholinesterase.	The frequency and severity of succinylcholine side effects are reduced. D-tubocurarine and gallamine: The onset time and the duration of action of succinylcholine is slightly increased and decreased, respectively. Pancuronium: In patients with normal plasma cholinesterase genotype the duration of action of succinylcholine is increased by two to five minutes. Patients heterozygous for one of the abnormal cholinesterase genes and pretreated with pancuronium may develop a phase 2 block following an otherwise normal dose of succinylcholine (unpublished observation).

Table 1
(Continued)

Drug	Mechanism of Action	Effects and Comments
Prolonged relaxation with NDR	The mechanism is complicated and not fully understood.	The injection of succinylcholine to facilitate closure of peritoneum in a patient that has been relaxed with a NDR may increase the degree and duration of block, or counteract the block depending on (1) the amount of succinylcholine injected, (2) amount of residual block present, (3) the NDR in question, and (4) whether or not neostigmine has been given. The opinions differ as to whether or not it is advisable to inject succinylcholine to facilitate closure of peritoneum. Because of the many factors involved I normally prefer to deepen the anesthetic or to inject a small dose of a NDR in this situation.
Organophosphates		
Pesticides	Pesticides cause a long-lasting (irreversible) inhibition of plasma cholinesterase activity. The inhibition is often total, ie, 100%.[15]	The duration of action of succinylcholine may be increased by 20 to 30 minutes.
Psychotropic drugs		
Lithium carbonate	In vitro experiments indicate that lithium inhibits the synthesis and the release of acetylcholine at the nerve terminal.[31]	Onset time of succinylcholine may be prolonged.[32] The duration of action of succinylcholine may be prolonged, especially in patients with heterozygous occurrence of an abnormal cholinesterase gene.[33,34] Lithium may in its own right cause a myasthenic reaction.[35]

Table 1
(Continued)

Drug	Mechanism of Action	Effects and Comments
Phenelzine (a mono-amineoxidase inhibitor)	Long-lasting reduction in plasma cholinesterase activity has been reported,[36] but the reduction in enzyme activity is not consistent.	The duration of action of succinylcholine may be prolonged.
Physostigmine	Physostigmine inhibits plasma cholinesterase.	Respiratory insufficiency lasting more than one hour has been described following a normal dose of succinylcholine in a patient heterozygous for atypical plasma cholinesterase given physostigmine.[37]
Pyridostigmine	See neostigmine.	See neostigmine. The decrease in cholinesterase activity following pyridostigmine is longer lasting than that following neostigmine.[29] In patients with chronic renal failure, prolonged neuromuscular block following succinylcholine has occurred as long as six hours after the administration of pyridostigmine.[30]
Tetrahydroaminoacridine Tacrine	Inhibition of plasma cholinesterase activity.	Tacrine has been used to potentiate and prolong the effects of succinylcholine. The combination of tacrine 10 mg and succinylcholine 1 mg/kg causes an apnoea period of about 15 to 25 minutes. After the introduction of the new intermediate duration nondepolarizing relaxants there is hardly any indication for this drug combination.
Trimethapan Arfonad	Trimethapan does inhibit plasma cholinesterase activity.[38,39] However, the main effect is thought to be due to nondepolarizing postjunctional receptor blockade.[40]	The duration of action of succinylcholine may be prolonged.[38]

Table 2
Drugs That Might Interfere With Nondepolarizing Relaxants.

Drug	Mechanism of Action	Effects and Comments
Antiarrhythmic drugs		
Beta-adrenergic blocking agents	β-adrenergic blocking agents inhibit the normal sympathetic drive to the heart.	In patients receiving high doses of β-blockers, severe bradycardia have resulted from reversal of a nondepolarizing block with neostigmine, in spite of prior administration of an otherwise normal dose of atropine.[41,42] In a recent study in dogs, Wagner et al[43] found "that exaggerated heart rate slowing or other adverse effects do not follow the administration of anticholinesterase drugs in the presence of beta-adrenergic blockade." β-blockers have been shown to aggravate myasthenia gravis. Although animal experiments and a few case reports indicate prolongation of the action of d-tubocurarine, the evidence of interaction is inconclusive. It remains to be proven that an interaction occurs in man with the drug concentrations used clinically.
Bretylium	The exact mechanism is not known. Bretylium has been shown to inhibit acetylcholine synthesis.	In isolated muscle preparations, bretylium potentiates the effect of d-tubocurarine.[44] No case of clinically relevant interaction between bretylium and nondepolarizing relaxants has so far been reported. Careful postoperative observation is to be recommended in patients given bretylium during or after an operation.

Table 2
(Continued)

Drug	Mechanism of Action	Effects and Comments
Calcium channel blockers Verapamil Nifedipine	Verapamil and nifedipine block conductance of the calcium channels prejunctionally as well as postjunctionally. Besides, verapamil has been shown to have a local anesthetic-like effect on nerve conduction.	Whether calcium channel blockers in therapeutic doses can produce neuromuscular blockade is controversial.[2–4] However, in rabbits verapamil has been shown to potentiate the block produced by an infusion of pancuronium.[5] Recently, respiratory failure has been reported following IV injection of verapamil in a patient with Duchenne's dystrophy.[6] It is presumably only a matter of time before clinical studies in man confirm that calcium channel blockers may interact with other drugs with neuromuscular blocking actions. Meanwhile, caution should be exerted in the administration of verapamil and nifedipine in situations where the margin of safety of neuromuscular transmission is reduced.
Procainamide	The main effect of procainamide is to decrease sensitivity of the postjunctional membrane to acetylcholine.[7] However, it also decreases presynaptic transmitter release.	Procainamide has been shown to aggravate myasthenia gravis and to induce myasthenia-like weakness in normal subjects. In animal experiments it augments nondepolarizing neuromuscular blockade.
Quinidine	Quinidine has both pre- and postjunctional actions. The exact mechanism of interaction with nondepolarizing relaxants is not known.	Quinidine augments the block caused by nondepolarizing relaxants.[9] Patients have been "recurarized" after receiving quinidine postoperatively.[45] The block cannot be reversed by edrophonium.

Table 2
(Continued)

Drug	Mechanism of Action	Effects and Comments
Antibiotics[25,46–48]		
Aminoglycosides Amikain Dihydrostreptomycin Gentanmycin Kanamycin Streptomycin Tobramycin	The mechanism differs among agents. Generally speaking they all decrease acetylcholine release (Mg^{++}-like action) and lower postjunctional sensitivity to acetylcholine. Tobramycin has possibly an action directly on the muscle.	Several of the aminoglycosides can produce neuromuscular blockade in their own right, and numerous papers document the enhancement of nondepolarizing neuromuscular blockade by this type of antjbiotic. In clinical practice the reversal effect of cholinesterase inhibitors and of calcium is inconsistent. The beneficial role of 4-aminopyridine has not yet been fully elucidated.
Polypeptides Polymyxin A Polymyxin B Polymyxin E	The exact mechanism is not known. The polypeptides seem to have local anesthetic-like action. It is normally held that polymyxin B exerts its effects primarily by depressing the postjunctional action of acetylcholine. However, recently polymyxin B was found also to decrease acetylcholine release presynaptically.	These agents are very potent in producing neuromuscular blockade on their own. Intense blockade with respiratory insufficiency has been reported following the administration of polypeptides either as the sole agent or in combination with a nondepolarizing relaxant. The neuromuscular blockade is not reliably reversed by calcium or by 4-aminopyridine. Anticholinesterases enhance the block!
Tetracyclines Oxytetracycline Rolitetracycline Tetracycline	The exact mechanism is not known. The agents have been shown to have a prejunctional blocking action as well as an effect on muscle contractility. The tetracyclines chelate calcium. However, the action of the tetracyclines is not supposed to be the result of the resultant decrease in Ca^{++} at the region of the neuromuscular endplate.	These agents have been shown to depress neuromuscular function in vitro and in vivo. However, the clinical significance of these findings is not yet clear. Calcium is only partially effective in reversing the block. Anticholinesterases are without effect.

Table 2
(Continued)

Drug	Mechanism of Action	Effects and Comments
Miscellaneous Lincomycin Clindamycin	Both agents decrease acetylcholine release (prejunctional effect), impair ion channel conductance (postjunctional effect), and depress muscle contractility.	Lincomycin and clindamycin augment nondepolarizing neuromuscular blockade. Calcium and anticholinesterases are only partially effective in reversing the block. 4-Aminopyridine seems to be the drug of choice.
Metronidazol	The mechanism of action is unknown. It has been suggested that the effect is not at the neuromuscular junction. Rather, it may be secondary to an effect on the distribution or metabolism of the neuromuscular blocking drug.	In one study in cats, metronidazol was found to potentiate vecuronium but not pancuronium.[49] The clinical significance of this interaction is not yet clear.
Azathioprine	Unknown. Inhibition of phosphodiesterase at the motor nerve terminal is a possibility.	Azathioprine antagonizes nondepolarizing neuromuscular blockade.[13] However, it is not known whether this effect is clinically relevant.
Corticosteroids	Unknown. It has been suggested that the effect may be explained at least partly by a modulation of choline uptake presynaptically.[50]	Two clinical reports suggest that I.V. administration of corticosteroids may antagonize a pancuronium-induced neuromuscular blockade in patients on longterm steroid therapy.[51,52] Cat experiments have shown that the acute effect of corticosteroids is to decrease the sensitivity of the endplate, resulting in potentiation of pancuronium.[53] It has been suggested that the antagonism found in man might be related to the effect of chronic steroid therapy.

Table 2
(Continued)

Drug	Mechanism of Action	Effects and Comments
Dantrolene	Dantrolene has no neuromuscular blocking action. It does, however, block excitation-contraction coupling, thus preventing the normal mechanical performance of the muscle.	The combination of dantrolene and residual neuromuscular blockade may cause "muscle weakness" leading to respiratory insufficiency.
Digitalis	Pancuronium causes an increase in circulating catecholamine levels, which is known to cause cardiac dysrhythmias.	Digitalized patients have been reported to be more prone to develop cardiac arrhythmias following pancuronium than nondigitalized patients.[54]
Diuretics		
Diuretic-induced hypokalemia	Changes in transmembrane potential caused by low extra-cellular potassium concentration?	In cats, hypokalemia caused by diuretics decreases the dose of nondepolarizing relaxant required for neuromuscular blockade and anticholinesterase required for antagonism of the block.[55] So far, these findings have not been documented in man under prolonged treatment with diuretics.
Furosemide	The exact mechanism is not known. Tentatively, the mechanism has been explained on the basis of protein kinase inhibition (low doses) and phosphodiesterase inhibition (high doses), respectively, at the motor nerve terminal (Fig 1).	Furosemide has a biphasic effect on a nondepolarizing neuromuscular blockade; in low doses (<10 $\mu g/kg$) it augments, and in high doses (1 to 4 mg/kg) it antagonizes the block.[18,56]

Table 2
(Continued)

Drug	Mechanism of Action	Effects and Comments
Inhalational anesthetic agents Cyclopropane Diethyl ether Enflurane Fluroxene Halothane Isoflurane Methoxyflurane	The mechanism is multifactorial. Probably the anesthetic agents exert their action on the central nervous system, at the postsynaptic membrane (by shortening open channel life time?), and at a point distal to the cholinergic receptor (the muscle cell membrane? The sarcoplasmatic reticulum?).	All the listed inhalational anesthetic agents augment nondepolarizing neuromuscular blockade in a dose-dependent manner. Diethyl ether, enflurane, methoxyflurane, and isoflurane are more potent in this respect than halothane, which again is more potent than fluroxene and cyclopropane. A time-dependent increase in sensitivity to d-tubocurarine has been found during enflurane anesthesia. Nitrous oxide does not have any clinically significant influence on either the degree of block produced by relaxants or the rate of recovery. Adding a more potent inhalational anesthetic agent may decrease the dose of relaxant needed to 25% to 50% of that needed using nitrous oxide narcotic technique.
Intravenous anesthetic agents Althesin Diazepam Etomidate Droperidol Fentanyl Methohexitone Midazolam Morphine Pethidine Thiopentone	These agents have been shown (1) to increase the amount of acetylcholine released from the nerve terminal and (2) to decrease the sensitivity of the postsynaptic membrane to acetylcholine. These two opposite effects are normally balancing each other, preventing the interaction from becoming clinically significant.	In animal experiments, most IV anesthetic agents have been found to potentiate slightly the neuromuscular blockade produced by nondepolarizing relaxants. This potentiation is, however, not normally accompanied by an increase in recovery time. In man, these interactions are not normally of any clinical significance. Specifically, no clinically significant interaction has been found between nondepolarizing relaxants and diazepam, midazolam, thiopentone, morphine, fentanyl, or droperidol.

Table 2
(Continued)

Drug	Mechanism of Action	Effects and Comments
Ketamine	Ketamine, like the other IV anesthetics, decreases the sensitivity of the postsynaptic membrane to acetylcholine. However, at high doses it also decreases the amount of acetylcholine released from the nerve terminal.[23]	In man, ketamine has been found to potentiate d-tubocurarine but not pancuronium.[57]
Propanidid	This drug does not increase the acetylcholine release from the nerve terminal.[23]	Propanidid slightly potentiates nondepolarizing relaxants.
Local anesthetics Bupivacaine Lidocaine Mepivacaine Prilocaine Procaine	Local anesthetic drugs are "fast channel" blockers, thus depressing (1) the propagation of nerve terminal action potential, (2) the release of acetylcholine, (3) the sensitivity of the postsynaptic membrane to acetylcholine, and (4) the excitability of the muscle cell membrane.	Local anesthetic enhances the neuromuscular block from all nondepolarizing relaxants.[58] Caution should be exerted in the administration of these drugs when the margin of safety of neuromuscular transmission is otherwise reduced.
Magnesium sulphate	Magnesium decreases acetylcholine release prejunctionally, reduces the sensitivity of the postjunctional membrane, and depresses the excitability of the muscle cell membrane.	Magnesium enhances the neuromuscular block from all nondepolarizing relaxants. Several cases have been reported of prolonged neuromuscular blockade in patients with preechlamptic toxemia treated with magnesium sulphate. Recently it has been shown that the serum concentration of magnesium and the dose requirement of pancuronium is linearly and inversely related (cat experiments).[59]

Table 2
(Continued)

Drug	Mechanism of Action	Effects and Comments
Methylxanthines Aminophylline Theophylline	Inhibition of phosphodiesterase activity in the motor nerve terminal? Facilitation of Ca^{++} by a phosphodiesterase-independent action? (Fig 1) Aminophylline-stimulated catecholamine release from the adrenal medulla.	Methylxanthines in high concentrations antagonize nondepolarizing neuromuscular blockade.[60] Thus, patients on continuous infusion of theophylline may be resistant to the effect of a nondepolarizing relaxant. Simultaneous administration of pancuronium and aminophylline has caused cardiac arrhythmias.[61]
Nitroglycerine	Unknown.	In the cat, continuous IV infusion of nitroglycerine has been found to potentiate the neuromuscular blocking effect of pancuronium, provided (1) that the infusion is started before the injection of pancuronium and (2) that the dose exceeds 0.5–1.0 μg/kg (d-tubocurarine neuromuscular blockade was not affected).[62] So far, this effect has not been documented in man.
Nondepolarizing relaxants	The exact mechanism is not clear. A possible explanation is that the synergy is caused by simultaneous pre- and postjunctional receptor inhibition.	Recently it has been shown that simultaneous administration of a mixture of pancuronium and d-tubocurarine or pancuronium and metocurine results in a greater than additive neuromuscular blocking effect.[63–65] This interaction has been used clinically. The claimed advantages of this drug combination include (1) that lower total dose of each relaxant has to be given, (2) spontaneous recovery from equivalent degrees of blockade occurs more rapidly, and (3) greater cardiovascular stability is achieved.

Table 2
(Continued)

Drug	Mechanism of Action	Effects and Comments
Psychotropic drugs		
Lithium carbonate	In vitro experiments indicate that lithium inhibits the synthesis and the release of acetylcholine at the nerve terminal.[31]	In one case report lithium was found to potentiate the neuromuscular blockade produced by pancuronium.[66] No other evidence exists for clinical significant interaction between nondepolarizing relaxants and lithium. Several in vitro and in vivo experiments in animals indicate that lithium potentiates pancuronium. However, recently Waud et al published evidence that lithium has negligible effect on the block produced by pancuronium and d-tubocurarine.[67] Treatment with lithium may provoke a myasthenic reaction.[35]
Tricyclic antidepressants	Tricyclics, like halothane and pancuronium, stimulate the sympathetic nervous system.	Severe arrhythmias may occur in patients anesthetized with halothane and pancuronium while receiving tricyclic antidepressants.
Succinylcholine	The exact mechanism is not clear. One possibility is that the endplate receptors are "desensitized" by the injection of succinylcholine, making the endplates more susceptible to the effect of the nondepolarizing relaxant.	Recent investigations have shown that previous administration of succinylcholine augments both the degree and duration of the blockade induced by vecuronium.[68,69] This effect lasts at least 30 minutes after total clinical recovery from the neuromuscular block induced by succinylcholine.[70] Whether this interaction also applies to other nondepolarizing relaxants is controversial.

Table 2
(Continued)

Drug	Mechanism of Action	Effects and Comments
Trimethaphan Arfonad	Trimethaphan seems to cause nondepolarizing, junctional receptor blockade. Possibly it acts by occluding receptor-linked ion channels.	Two case reports have been published of prolonged neuromuscular blockade associated with trimethaphan.[71,72] The use of neostigmine to reverse the blockade is controversial. Augmentation as well as partial reversal have been reported following attempted reversal with neostigmine.

REFERENCES

1. Wislicki L, Rosenblum I: Effects of propranolol on the action of neuromuscular blocking drugs. Br J Anaesth 39:939–942, 1967
2. Kraynack BJ, Lawson NW, Gintautas J: Neuromuscular blocking action of verapamil in cats. Can Anaesth Soc J 30:242–247, 1983
3. Lawson NW, Kraynack BJ, Gintautas J: Neuromuscular and electrocardiographic responses to verapamil in dogs. Anesth Analg 62:50–54, 1983
4. Lehmann HD, Kretchmar R: Neuromuscular transmission and verapamil. Anesth Analg 62:1044–1052, 1983
5. Durant NN, Nguyen N, Katz RL: Potentiation of neuromuscular blockade by verapamil. Anesthesiology 60:298–303, 1984
6. Zalman F, Perloff JK, Durant NN, et al: Acute respiratory failure following intravenous verapamil in Duchenne's muscular dystrophy. Am Heart J 105:510–511, 1983
7. Lee DC, Liu HH, Johns TR: Presynaptic and postsynaptic actions of procainamide on neuromuscular transmission. Muscle Nerve 6:442–447, 1983
8. Cuthbert MF: The effects of quinidine and procainamide on the neuromuscular blocking action of suxamethonium. Br J Anaesth 38:775–779, 1966
9. Miller RD, Way WL, Katzung BG: The potentiation of neuromuscular blocking agents by quinidine. Anesthesiology 28:1036–1041, 1967
10. Grogono AW: Anaesthesia for atrial defibrillation. Effect of quinidine on muscular relaxation. Lancet 2:1039–1040, 1963
11. Singh YN, Marshall IG, Harvey AL: Pre- and post-junctional blocking effects of aminoglycoside, polymyxin, tetracycline and lincosamide antibiotics. Br J Anaesth 54:1295–1306, 1982
12. Griffin JP, D'Arcy PF: A manual of adverse drug interactions. Bristol, John Wright & Sons Ltd, 1979, pp 300–306
13. Dretchen KL, Morgenroth VH, Standaert FG, et al: Azathioprine: Effects on neuromuscular transmission. Anesthesiology 45:604–609, 1976
14. Doenicke A, Gesing H, Krumey I, et al: Influence of aprotinin (Trasylol) on the action of suxamethonium. Br J Anaesth 42:943–960, 1970
15. Viby-Mogensen J: Cholinesterase and succinylcholine. Dan Med Bull 30:129–150, 1983
16. Dowdy EG, Fabian LW: Ventricular arrhythmias induced by succinylcholine in digitalized patients. Anesth Analg 42:501–513, 1963
17. Barrow MEH, Johnson JK: A study of the anticholinesterase and anticurare effects of some cholinesterase inhibitors. Br J Anaesth 38:420–431, 1966
18. Scappaticci KA, Ham JA, Sohn YJ, et al: Effects of furosemide on the neuromuscular junction. Anesthesiology 57:381–388, 1982
19. Foldes FF, Arai T, Gentsch HH, et al: The influence of glucocorticoids on plasma cholinesterase (38219). Proc Soc Exp Biol Med 146:918–920, 1974
20. Eisenberg M, Balsley S, Katz RL: Effects of diazepam on succinylcholine-induced myalgia, potassium increase, creatine phosphokinase elevation, and relaxation. Anesth Analg 58:314–317, 1979
21. Fahmy NR, Malek NS, Lappas DG: Diazepam prevents some adverse effects of succinylcholine. Clin Pharmacol Ther 26:395–398, 1979
22. Erkola O, Salmenpera M, Tammisto T: Does diazepam pretreatment prevent succinylcholine-induced fasciculations? — A double-blind comparison of diazepam and tubocurarine pretreatments. Anesth Analg 59:932–934, 1980
23. Torda TA, Murphy EC: Presynaptic effect of i.v. anaesthetic agents at the neuromuscular junction. Br J Anaesth 51:353–357, 1979
24. Monks PS, Norman J: Prolongation of suxamethonium-induced paralysis by propanidid. Br J Anaesth 44:1303–1305, 1972

25. Miller RD: Neuromuscular blocking agents, in Smith NT, Miller RD, Corbascio AN (eds): Drug Interactions in Anesthesia. Philadelphia, Lea & Febiger, 1981
26. Foldes FF, McNall PG, Davis DL, et al: Substrate competition between procaine and succinylcholine diiodide for plasma cholinesterase. Science 117:383–386, 1953
27. Usubiaga JE, Wikinski JA, Morales RL, et al: Interaction of intravenously administered procaine, lidocaine and succinylcholine in anesthetized subjects. Anesth Analg 46:39–45, 1967
28. Zsigmond E, Eilderton TE: Abnormal reaction to procaine and succinylcholine in a patient with inherited atypical plasma cholinesterase. Case report. Can Anaesth Soc J 15:498–500, 1968
29. Mirakhur RK, Lavery TD, Briggs LP, et al: Effects of neostigmine and pyridostigmine on serum cholinesterase activity. Can Anaesth Soc J 29:55–58, 1982
30. Bishop MJ, Hornbein TF: Prolonged effect of succinylcholine after neostigmine and pyridostigmine administration in patients with renal failure. Anesthesiology 58:384–386, 1983
31. Vizi E, Illes P, Ronai A, et al: The effect of lithium on acetylcholine release and synthesis. Neuropharmacology 11:521–530, 1972
32. Hill GE, Wong KC, Hodges MR: Lithium carbonate and neuromuscular blocking agents. Anesthesiology 46:122–126, 1977
33. Hill GE, Wong KC, Hodges MR: Potentiation of succinylcholine neuromuscular blockade by lithium carbonate. Anesthesiology 44:439–442, 1976
34. Reimherr FW, Hodges MR, Hill GE, et al: Prolongation of muscle relaxant effects by lithium carbonate. Am J Psychiatry 134:205–207, 1977
35. Voetmann C, Jest P: A myasthenic reaction provoked by treatment with lithium carbonate. Ugeskr Laeger 140:2375– 2376, 1978
36. Bodley PO, Halwax K, Potts L: Low serum pseudocholinesterase levels complicating treatment with phenelzine. Br Med J 3:510–512, 1969
37. Kopman AAF, Strachovsky G, Lichtenstein L: Prolonged response to succinylcholine following physostigmine. Anesthesiology 49:142–143, 1978
38. Tewfik GI: Trimetaphan: Its effect on the pseudo-cholinesterase level in man. Anaesthesia 12:326–329, 1957
39. Sklar GS, Lanks KW: Effects of trimetaphan and sodium nitroprusside on hydrolysis of succinylcholine in vitro. Anesthesiology 17:31–33, 1977
40. Gergis SD, Sokoll MD, Rubbo JT: Effect of sodium nitroprusside and trimetaphan on neuromuscular transmission in the frog. Can Anaesth Soc J 24:220–227, 1977
41. Sprague DH: Severe bradycardia after neostigmine in a patient taking neostigmine to control paroxysmal atrial tachycardia. Anesthesiology 42:208–210, 1975
42. Prys-Roberts C: Hemodynamic effects of anesthesia and surgery in renal hypertensive patients receiving large doses of β-receptor antagonists. Anesthesiology 51:S122, 1979
43. Wagner DL, Moorthy SS, Stoelting RK: Administration of anticholinesterase drugs of beta-adrenergic blockade. Anesth Analg 61:153–154, 1982
44. Welch GW, Waud BE: Effect of bretylium on neuromuscular transmission. Anesth Analg 61:442–444, 1982
45. Way WL, Katzung BS, Larson CP: Recurarization with quinidine. JAMA 200:163–164, 1967
46. Sokoll MD, Gergis SD: Antibiotics and neuromuscular function. Anesthesiology 55:148–159, 1981
47. Argov Z, Mastaglia FF: Disorders of neuromuscular transmission caused by drugs. New Engl J Med 301:409–413, 1979
48. Bowman WC: Pharmacology of Neuromuscular Function, Bristol, John Wright & Son Ltd, 1980, pp 110–114
49. McIndewar IC, Marshall RJ: Interactions between the neuromuscular blocking drug ORG NC 45 and some anesthetic, analgesic and antimicrobial agents. Br J Anaesth 53:785–791, 1981
50. Leeuwin RS, Veldsema-Currie RD, Van Wilgenburg H, et al: Effects of corticosteroids on neuromuscular blocking actions of d-tubocurarine. Eur J Pharmacol 69:165–173, 1981

51. Meyers EF: Partial recovery from pancuronium neuromuscular blockade following hydrocortisone administration. Anesthesiology 46:148–150, 1977
52. Laflin MJ: Interaction of pancuronium and corticosteroids. Anesthesiology 47:471–472, 1977
53. Durant NN, Briscoe JR, Lee C, et al: The acute effects of hydrocortisone on neuromuscular transmission. Anesthesiology 57:A266, 1982
54. Bartolone RS, Rao TLK: Dysrhythmias following muscle relaxant administration in patients receiving digitalis. Anesthesiology 58:567–569, 1983
55. Miller RD, Roderick LL: Diuretic-induced hypokalaemia, pancuronium neuromuscular blockade and its antagonism by neostigmine. Br J Anaesth 50:541–544, 1978
56. Azar I, Cottrell J, Gupta B, et al: Furosemide facilitates recovery of evoked twitch response after pancuronium. Anesth Analg 59:55–57, 1980
57. Johnston RR, Miller RD, Way WL: The interaction of ketamine with d-tubocurarine, pancuronium and succinylcholine in man. Anesth Analg 53:496–501, 1974
58. Matsuo S, Rao DBS, Chaundry I, et al: Interaction of muscle relaxants and local anesthetics at the neuromuscular junction. Anesth Analg 57:580–587, 1978
59. Lee C, Nguyen BS, Tran BK, et al: Quantification of magnesium-pancuronium interaction in the diaphragm and the tibialis anterior. Anesthesiology 57:A392, 1982
60. Doll DC, Rosenberg H: Antagonism of neuromuscular blockade by theophylline. Anesth Analg 58:139–140, 1979
61. Belani KG, Anderson WW, Buckley JJ: Adverse drug interaction involving pancuronium and aminophylline. Anesth Analg 61:473–474, 1982
62. Glisson SN, Sanchez MM, El-Etr AA, et al: Nitroglycerin and the neuromuscular blockade produced by gallamine, succinylcholine, d-tubocurarine, and pancuronium. Anesth Analg 59:117–122, 1980
63. Lebowitz PW, Ramsey FM, Savarese JJ, et al: Potentiation of neuromuscular blockade in man produced by combinations of pancuronium and metocurine or pancuronium and d-tubocurarine. Anesth Analg 59:604–609, 1980
64. Lebowitz PW, Ramsey FM, Savarese JJ, et al: Combination of pancuronium and metocurine: Neuromuscular and hemodynamic advantages over pancuronium alone. Anesth Analg 60:12–17, 1981
65. Satwicz PR, Martyn JAJ, Szyfelbein SK, et al: Potentiation of neuromuscular blockade using a combination of pancuronium and dimethyltubocurarine. Studies in children following acute burn injury or during reconstructive surgery. Br J Anaesth 56:479–484, 1984
66. Borden H, Clarke MT, Katz H: The use of pancuronium in patients receiving lithium carbonate. Can Anaesth Soc J 21:79–82, 1974
67. Waud BE, Farrell L, Waud DR: Lithium and neuromuscular transmission. Anesth Analg 61:399–402, 1982
68. Krieg N, Crul JF, Booij LDH: Relative potency of Org NC 45, pancuronium, alcuronium and tubocurarine in anaesthetized man. Br J Anaesth 52:783–788, 1980
69. Krieg N, Hendrickx HHL, Crul JF: Influence of suxamethonium on the potency of ORG NC 45 in anaesthetized patients. Br J Anaesth 53:259–262, 1981
70. D'Hollander AA, Agoston S, DeVille A, et al: Clinical and pharmacological actions of a bolus injection of suxamethonium: Two phenomena of distinct duration. Br J Anaesth 55:131–134, 1983
71. Wilson SL, Miller RN, Wright C, et al: Prolonged neuromuscular blockade associated with trimetaphan. Anesth Analg 55:353–356, 1976
72. Nakamura K, Koide M, Imanaga T, et al: Prolonged neuromuscular blockade following trimetaphan. Anaesthesia 35:1202–1207, 1980

David R. Bevan
Francois Donati

16

Neuromuscular Relaxants: Complications

The recent release of two new neuromuscular relaxants in North America and the continued development of others indicates dissatisfaction with the available choice. This review will attempt to describe the complications associated with the established drugs, define the basic requirements of a neuromuscular blocker for use during anesthesia, and summarize the extent to which these criteria have been met by the introduction of atracurium and vecuronium. The established drugs will be discussed under the broad categories of depolarizing relaxants, of which only succinylcholine is used currently, and nondepolarizing relaxants (NDR) including D-tubocurarine, pancuronium, gallamine, atracurium, and vecuronium.

The complications associated with the neuromuscular relaxants may result from the normal action of the drug at the junction, activity at other sites, abnormal or idiosyncratic actions, or its use in abnormal situations.

SUCCINYLCHOLINE

The incidence and severity of complications following the use of succinylcholine probably exceeds that ascribed to all other relaxants combined. Nevertheless, it has been estimated that succinylcholine is used in about 75% of all anesthetics in North America. It retains its popularity because it is the only relaxant that will provide ideal intubating conditions within two minutes (Fig 1) and from which rapid recovery allows spontaneous respiration five to six minutes later.

MUSCLE RELAXANTS
ISBN 0-8089-1784-6

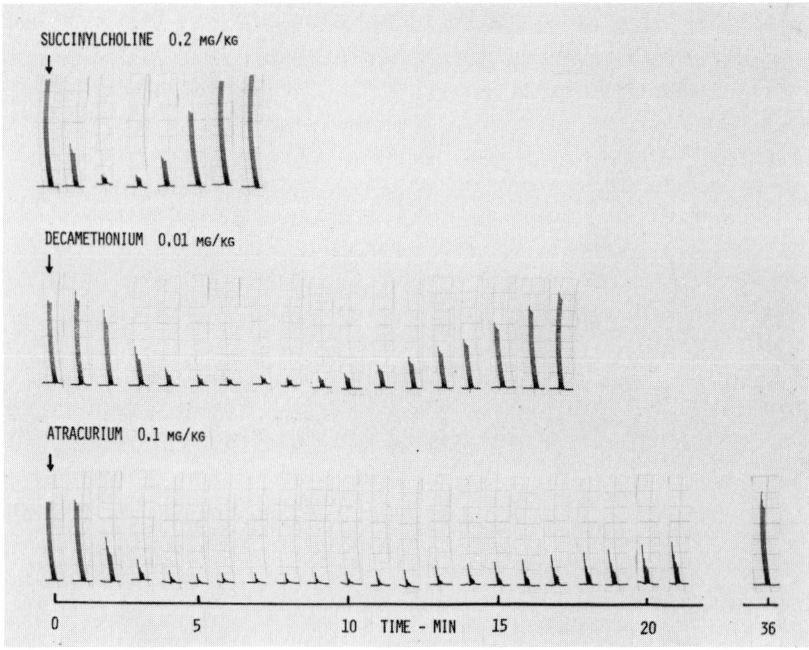

Figure 1. Comparison of speed of onset of neuromuscular blockade with equipotent doses of succinylcholine, decamethonium, and atracurium.

The onset of paralysis is preceded by depolarization and contraction of skeletal muscles. Its duration is determined by the rate of hydrolysis.

Complications of Initial Stimulation

Most patients exhibit generalized fasciculations after the rapid administration of succinylcholine. Some investigators, but not all, have found a relationship between the severity of the fasciculations and the intensity of postoperative muscle pains. The fasciculations are a nuisance and the pain may be distressing, particularly to patients after superficial surgery who expect to be mobile the next day. The pain associated with laparotomy incisions conceals that due to succinylcholine.

Generalized fasciculations and incoordinated contractions following depolarization may lead to the release of intracellular constituents including potassium, myoglobin, and creatine phosphokinase. In normal subjects the plasma potassium concentration increases by about 0.5 mEq/L, and a similar increase is observed in renal failure.[1] Far greater increases, sufficient to cause serious cardiac arrhythmias, have been observed after burns,[2] multiple trauma,[3] tetanus, radiation injury, and neurologic disease.[4] This exaggerated response is thought to result from multiplication of acetylcholine receptors. Their development takes several days, which explains why hyperkalemia after succinylcholine usually is not seen until 2 to 3 weeks after the injury. Hyperkalemia has also been observed in patients suffering from spinal cord transection, peripheral nerve injury, polyneuritis, Guillain-Barré syndrome, and Parkinson's disease.[5]

The initial stimulatory effect of succinylcholine is associated also with increases in intragastric[6] and intraocular pressures.

Several regimens have been advocated to avoid these problems. They include the administration of small doses of nondepolarizing relaxants, precurarization with D-tubocurarine 3 to 6 mg, pancuronium 0.5 to 1 mg, or gallamine 10 to 20 mg · 70 kg^{-1}, succinylcholine itself in a dose of 10 mg "self-taming", or pretreatment with xylocaine, diazepam, thiopental, fentanyl, calcium gluconate, and vitamin C. Several of these treatments, although successful in reducing the incidence of fasciculations and muscle pains, fail to modify the increases in serum potassium concentration or intraocular pressure.[7] Although intragastric pressure may increase after succinylcholine and the increase may be limited by precurarization, the risk of regurgitation and aspiration of stomach contents is dependent upon the integrity of the esophagogastric junction and this is preserved unless the normal oblique angle of entry of the esophagus into the stomach is altered.[6] Succinylcholine is unlikely to augment the risk of aspiration because it produces an increase in lower esophageal pressures that parallel the increase in intragastric pressure. It is our practice to administer prophylaxis to avoid muscle pains in those patients expecting to be ambulant the next day, and we give D-tubocurarine 3 mg or pancuronium 0.5 mg · 70 kg^{-1} three minutes before succinylcholine. If D-tubocurarine is used, the dose of succinylcholine is increased from 1 to 1.5 mg · kg^{-1}. Pretreatment is not innocuous. After even small doses of nondepolarizing relaxants most patients are aware of heavy eyelids and blurred vision, and some experience respiratory weakness.

Actions at Other Sites

Arrhythmias are common after succinylcholine, especially after repeated doses and particularly in children. These occur because succinylcholine stimulates nicotinic endings in sympathetic and parasympathetic ganglia and muscarinic receptors at the sinus node. In addition, the release of epinephrine and norepinephrine is increased. The arrhythmias vary from sinus bradycardia to junctional and ventricular arrhythmias. They occur frequently after intubation and are more common in the presence of hypoxia, hypercarbia, and hyperkalemia. The bradyarrhythmias can be prevented with atropine, which should be given before repeated administration of succinylcholine.

Idiosyncrasies of Succinylcholine Block

The characteristics of the neuromuscular block change after prolonged exposure to succinylcholine either by repeated bolus doses, prolonged infusion, or after impaired metabolism. This alteration is known as a change from phase I to phase II block. The response to nerve stimulation then resembles curare and demonstrates fade to tetanic or train-of-four stimulation, posttetanic facilitation, and reversibility with anticholinesterases.[8] If an attempt is made to maintain constant neuromuscular blockade with a continuous infusion of succinylcholine, the drug requirements are not constant. As phase II block develops (defined as a train-of-four ratio of less than 0.5), the requirement for succinylcholine increases (tachyphylaxis) by about 50% to 100%. Phase II block occurs earlier and after a lower dose in the presence of halothane, enflurane, and isoflurane. After about 90 minutes in adults, when the block is stable (train-of-four ratio = 0), the requirement decreases (bradyphylaxis) (Fig 2). Usually, it is possible to antagonize phase II block with small doses of neostigmine (1.2 to 2.5 mg · 70 kg^{-1}) and atropine except in the presence of atypical plasma cholinesterase. The cause of the alteration in the characteristics of the block remains uncertain.

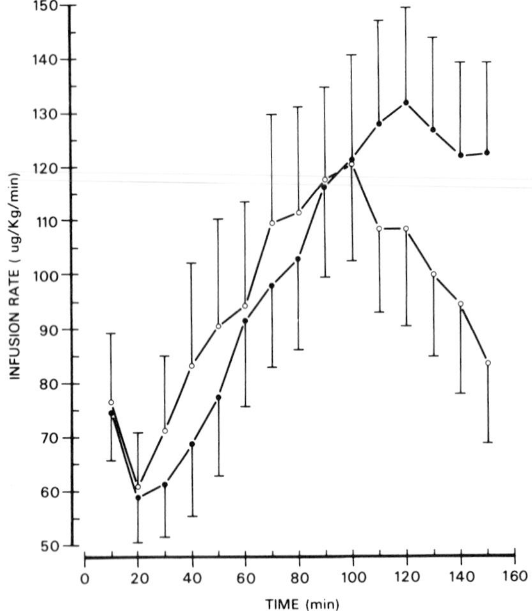

Figure 2. Infusion rates of succinylcholine required to maintain 85% to 90% twitch depression during halothane (○; n = 8) or fentanyl (●; n = 9) anesthesia. (Reproduced with permission from Fuller et al.[9])

Drug Interactions

The most important drug interactions with succinylcholine include those that inhibit plasma cholinesterase (see following text) and interactions with other neuromuscular blocking drugs. In general, depolarizing and nondepolarizing relaxants are antagonistic. Consequently, when small doses of NDRs are given for precurarization they decrease the potency and reduce the duration of action of succinylcholine. Thus, it is recommended that the dose of succinylcholine be increased. This is unnecessary after pancuronium, which is a weak inhibitor of plasma cholinesterase. When succinylcholine precedes NDRs their action is prolonged and potentiated. Finally, the anesthetist may be tempted to give succinylcholine to facilitate abdominal closure when NDRs have been used to provide relaxation. The effect will depend upon the degree of spontaneous recovery that has occured. If recovery is almost complete, succinylcholine will produce relaxation, but if the block is still intense, succinylcholine will antagonize the block and produce some recovery of neuromuscular activity. Anticholinesterases are powerful antagonists of plasma cholinesterase, so that if succinylcholine is given after neostigmine its action will be prolonged considerably.

Impaired Metabolism

The maximum rate of hydrolysis of succinylcholine, obtained from studies with continuous infusions, is about 100 $\mu g \cdot kg^{-1} \cdot min^{-1}$. When a bolus of 100 mg is given to an adult, it has been estimated that about 70% is metabolized within one minute. The biosynthesis of plasma cholinesterase in the liver is controlled by two allelic genes, E_1^a and E_1^u, and has a half-life of eight to 12 days. Thus, plasma cholinesterase activity may be reduced by physiologic variation, acquired or iatrogenic disease, and inherited abnormalities[10] (Table 1).

Physiological Variation

Plasma cholinesterase activity is greater in men than women. During pregnancy, plasma cholinesterase is reduced by 25%, and concentrations at birth are approximately half those of the adult. Normal values are not reached until 6 to 7 years.

Acquired Disease

Severe chronic illnesses are associated with decreased plasma cholinesterase activity and prolonged duration of action of succinylcholine. These diseases include collagen diseases, myocardial infarction, carcinoma, tuberculosis, and many chronic debilitating diseases.

Table 1
Decreased Plasma Cholinesterase Activity

Inherited	Cholinesterase variants
Physiologic	Pregnancy
	Neonates and infants
Acquired	Hepatic disease
	Uremia
	Malnutrition
	Carcinoma
	Acute infections
	Burns
Iatrogenic	Plasmapheresis
	Anticholinesterases
	Contraceptive pill
	Extracorporeal circulation
	Alkylating anticancer drugs
	Propranolol
	Pancuronium
	Echothiophate
	Monoamine oxidase inhibitors

Iatrogenic

Plasma cholinesterase activity may be reduced by many drugs and therapeutic procedures. Such interactions are not absolute contraindications to succinylcholine but require titration of the dose. With some drugs (eg, echothiophate) the requirement may be reduced by 75% to 80%, whereas with others, such as pancuronium pretreatment, the requirement is affected only slightly.

Inherited Disorders

The cholinesterase variants may be identified by their rates of hydrolysis of benzoylcholine and the distinct inhibition profiles with varying concentrations of the inhibitors dibucaine, fluoride, and choloride. At the present time, four allelic genes are recognized, although this list is not exhaustive: the normal gene E_1^u, the atypical gene E_1^a, the silent gene E_1^s, and the fluoride-resistant gene E_1^f. An abnormal gene is present in about 4% of the population.

The duration of neuromuscular block is prolonged to two to three hours in the patient homozygous for E_1^a or E_1^s whereas it is prolonged only slightly and in only half the heterozygotes.[11] When twitch activity begins to recover it has the appearance of phase II block, but it cannot be antagonized completely with neostigmine or edrophonium. Safe management includes respiratory support until spontaneous ventilation is restored. Plasma cholinesterase is stable so that stored whole blood or plasma are potential stores. However, the possible risks of transfusion may exceed those of ventilation for two to three hours.

Malignant Hyperthermia

The most dangerous complication after succinylcholine is the development of malignant hyperthermia.[12] It is a rare (1 in 50,000 in adults, 1 in 15,000 in children) disturbance of calcium movement within cells and has a multifactorial inheritance. The earlier catastrophic mortality of 70% has been reduced to 7% following the introduction of dantrolene treatment.

The syndrome may be triggered by exposure to halothane or succinylcholine and, theoretically, is recognized earliest by an increase in end-tidal CO_2 concentration. The first sign after succinylcholine may be ridigity, which makes intubation difficult. This is followed by other evidence of cellular hypermetabolism: tachycardia, hyperventilation, cyanosis, skin mottling, pyrexia, and unstable BP. Secondary changes including hyperkalemia, metabolic and respiratory acidosis, renal failure, and disseminated intravascular coagulation may follow without treatment.

Dantrolene, in an initial dose of 2 mg $\cdot$ kg^{-1} and repeated to a total of 10 mg $\cdot$ kg^{-1}, is the only effective drug remedy. General supportive methods such as removal of triggering agents, hyperventilation with oxygen, cooling, correction of acidosis and hyperkalemia should not be allowed to delay definitive therapy with dantrolene. Affected patients who recover, and their relatives, should be referred to the nearest center to confirm the diagnosis.

The provision of anesthesia in affected patients must avoid known triggering agents. Prophylaxis, if considered necessary, is achieved best with dantrolene 2 mg $\cdot$ kg^{-1} intravenously immediately before operation.

The relationship between malignant hyperthermia and other muscular diseases including Duchenne's muscular dystrophy, central core disease, and myotonia, remains unproven.

Miscellaneous

The responses to succinylcholine are modified in children. Neonates on a mg $\cdot$ kg^{-1} basis require two to four times the adult dose. The decrease in sensitivity probably results form an increased volume of distribution caused by an increase in extracellular fluid (ECF) volume. Attempts have been made to produce rapid paralysis by intramuscular injection in children whose venous access is difficult. Large doses (4 mg $\cdot$ kg^{-1}) are necessary, the onset is slow (three to four minutes), and three cases of pulmonary edema have been described using this technique. When succinylcholine is administered by continuous infusion, infants show a greater requirement than adults and phase II block occurs earlier, although this corresponds to a greater (5.3 mg · kg^{-1}) dose.[13]

Curiously, the duration of action of succinylcholine in adults appears to be shorter in New York than in London.

Acute sensitivity reactions to succinylcholine are rare. A recent study described 5 of 18 patients developing bronchospasm and cardiovascular collapse who had never had a general anesthetic previously.[14] Masseter spasm, often a harbinger of malignant hyperthermia, may also make intubation difficult or impossible in patients with myotonia congenita and dystophica, or polymyositis.

The sites of action of succinylcholine remain uncertain. Presynaptic actions have been inferred because they can (1) attenuate posttetanic repetitive activity, (2) cause repetitive firing, and (3) initiate an action potential in a motor nerve independent of external stimulation.

Present Position

Succinylcholine is an ''imperfect'' relaxant. It has several sites of action at the neuromuscular junction and elsewhere and is associated with a wide variety of complications that may be fatal. Nevertheless, it will remain a first-line agent until alternative means of producing intense, brief paralysis are available either with the development of new drugs or by altering the behavior of those currently available.

NONDEPOLARIZING RELAXANTS

The onset of neuromuscular blockade with the NDRs is slower than with succinylcholine (Fig 1). In part, this is because the rapid metabolism of succinylcholine allows flooding of the receptor with doses up to three to four timnes the ED_{95}. Increasing the dose of the NDR shortens the onset time but at the cost of prolonged block. Recent attempts to reduce the onset time with existing NDRs have included the administration of small ($0.1 \times ED_{95}$) doses three to five minutes before the main dose using either the same or different relaxants.

Repeated administration of most NDRs in clinical doses results in a progressive increase in the duration of action.[13] However, this cumulation is not a reflection of either increasing sensitivity of the neuromuscular junction or of decreased clearance but is a normal consequence of the pharmacokinetic behavior of the agent. The only exception is atracurium whose rapid metabolism ensures that each dose has the same duration.

Spontaneous recovery from the NDRs is slow; there is 95% recovery in about two hours after the ED_{95} dose of D-tubocurarine, pancuronium, metocurine, and gallamine, but this is reduced by two thirds with the newer agents atracurium and vecuronium. Recovery is accelerated with anticholinesterases so that rapid reversal can be anticipated as long as some neuromuscular activity is present before their administration. Reversal occurs more slowly with intense blocks, and very large doses may produce a block that is temporarily irreversible. It is disconcerting to realize that nearly half the patients given NDRs during anesthesia still demonstrate residual paralysis on arrival in the recovery room.[16]

Characteristically, all NDRs demonstrate fade in response to repeated nerve stimulation using either tetanic or train-of-four stimulation. The degree of fade is greater during recovery than onset of block, and it is greater with D-tubocurarine than pancuronium. It has been suggested that the fade represents a presynaptic site of action.[17] The irreversibility of profound blocks may be due to an additional action blocking the ionophore of the postjunctional receptor. Thus, all neuromuscular blocking drugs have actions at several sites around the neuromuscular junction.

Cardiovascular Effects

The most serious complications associated with the NDRs are the cardiovascular actions (Table 2). All are organic bases so that they may release histamine from mast cells. Also, they are related structurally to acetylcholine and they compete with and mimic its actions. Histamine release may produce urticaria, itching, and erythema at the injection site as well as hypotension and bronchospasm. Tubocurarine-induced histamine release is mainly responsible for the hypotension and tachycardia that follow its administration. In high doses ($3 \times ED_{95}$), metocurine and atracurium also release histamine (atracurium to a lesser extent). Rarely, D-tubocurarine may be associated with anaphylactoid reactions.

Table 2
Cardiovascular Effects of Nondepolarizing Muscle Relaxants

NDR	Histamine Release	Vagus	Ganglia	Sympathetic
D-Tubocurarine	Moderate	Block	Block	—
Metocurine	Slight	Slow block	Slow block	—
Gallamine	—	block + +	—	Stimulation
Pancuronium	—	Slow block	—	Stimulation
Atracurium	Slight	—	—	—
Vecuronium	—	—	—	—

Cardiovascular effects result from stimulation or inhibition of autonomic processes. The reduced clinical use of gallamine is a consequence of the unwanted tachycardia from vagal blockade, and a similar phenomenon prevented the release of fazadinium in North America. Conversely, the tachycardia and slight hypertension following sympathetic stimulation and weak vagal blockade after pancuronium are considered advantageous in opposing the bradycardia and hypotension that otherwise occurs when massive fentanyl doses are administered during cardiac surgery. In certain situations, the sympathetic stimulation is hazardous; the combination of pancuronium and halothane in a patient receiving tricyclic antidepressants may induce ventricular arrhythmias.[18]

Savarese[19] suggested that the extent of autonomic activity could be expressed by the autonomic margin of safety: the ED_{50} of autonomic effects (in cats) divided by the neuromuscular blocking effect (ED_{95}, in humans) (Table 3). The new NDRs, atracurium and vecuronium, are almost free of cardiovascular actions.

In a careful series of studies, Stoelting[20] has shown that during halothane anesthesia, equipotent doses of pancuronium, D-tubocurarine, and gallamine are associated with significant cardiovascular effects whereas metocurine and atracurium are innocent.

Pharmacokinetic Factors

Accurate assays of circulating concentrations of the NDRs have created a framework to predict their clinical behavior. All are ionized, water-soluble compounds that are distributed in volumes only slightly greater than the ECF. As the ECF volume is increased in infancy, greater dilution of the relaxants occurs. In general, the NDRs are poorly metabolized and are excreted unchanged by the kidney (gallamine), the liver (vecuronium), or both (D-tubocurarine, pancuronium). Obstruction to the routes of elimination leads to prolonged activity. Atracurium is different. It is metabolized nonenzymatically at body temperature and pH by a process known as Hofman elimination.

Table 3
Autonomic Margin of Safety

NDR	Vagus	Ganglia	Histamine
D-Tubocurarine	0.6	2.9	1.1
Metocurine	2.9	18.6	5.1
Gallamine	1	—	—
Pancuronium	2.9	329	—
Atracurium	23	55	3
Vecuronium	25	> 1,000	—

The decreased clearance of NDRs in the elderly is a consequence of impaired renal excretion and results in prolonged action. Also, the onset time is faster in the young than the old, a reflection of a shorter circulation time.

Drug Interaction

The effects of the mixed block associated with the combination of succinylcholine and the NDRs have been described previously. Mixtures of some NDRs have greater than additive effects, and this synergism has been described for mixtures of pancuronium, vecuronium, or atracurium with either metocurine or D-tubocurarine.[21] Such mixtures have been recommended to avoid the cardiovascular effects of each agent alone and to accelerate the onset on neuromuscular blockade. Blocks produced by the mixtures are antagonized easily with anticholinesterases.

Several groups of drugs potentiate the NDRs. In particular, the dose of relaxant can be reduced by about a third in the presence of halothane anesthesia and by about one half with enflurane or isoflurane if the vapors are given at 1-MAC concentrations.

Sensitivity to NDRs is increased in the presence of antibiotics (especially streptomycin, neomycin, polymyxin, colistin, and kanamycin), calcium (slow) channel blockers, ganglion-blocking drugs, magnesium, lithium, local anesthetic agents, and quinidine.[22] Conversely, the sensitivity is decreased by the phosphodiesterase inhibitors aminophylline and azathioprine.

Miscellaneous

The dose-response of neonates and small infants, on a $mg \cdot kg^{-1}$ basis, is similar to adults despite increased dilution of the relaxant in the larger ECF volume. Therefore, the sensitivity of the neuromuscular junction must be increased.[23]

In situations where spread of receptors causes hyperkalemia after succinylcholine, (burns, trauma, neurologic lesions), sensitivity to the NDRs is reduced. This may be confusing in the hemiplegic patient when neuromuscular monitoring of the affected side demonstrates resistance.

Transatlantic differences have been described so that D-tubocurarine seems to produce a greater block in patients in New York than in London.

RELAXANT REQUIREMENTS

Muscle relaxants are used during anesthesia for two purposes. First, they are needed to produce rapid, intense paralysis of short duration to facilitate endotracheal intubation. Second, they provide muscle relaxation for abdominal surgery and for the control of ventilation. For the latter, the paralysis need not be so intense, nor is the time scale so critical, although, for convenience, a duration of 30 to 40 minutes of near-complete paralysis would be appropriate for many procedures. It seems unlikely that one agent will perform both functions.

Other desirable properties include absence of side effects, particularly the cardiac action of the NDRs and the consequences of stimulation after succinylcholine. Control of the recovery of neuromuscular activity either with specific antagonists or by predictable metabolism would prevent the dangers associated with persistent postoperative paralysis.

WHAT IS AVAILABLE

The introduction of atracurium and vecuronium has provided drugs without significant side effects and with intermediate durations of action. Investigation in Europe of NDRs with more prolonged action but also devoid of cardiovascular effects (eg, pipecuronium) is promising. However, no rapidly acting agent is available at present. The obituary of succinylcholine has been written many times, but until a safe alternative appears, such essays are premature.

REFERENCES

1. Miller RD, Way WL, Hamilton WK, et al: Succinylcholine-induced hyperkalemia in patients with renal failure. Anesthesiology 36:138–141, 1972
2. Gronert GA, Theye RA: Pathophysiology of hyperkalemia induced by succinylcholine. Anesthesiology 43:89–97, 1975
3. Mazze RI, Escue HM, Houston JB: Hyperkalemia and cardiovascular collapse following administration of succinylcholine to the traumatized patient. Anesthesiology 31:540–545, 1969
4. Cooperman LH: Succinylcholine-induced hyperkalemia in neuromuscular disease. JAMA 213:1867–1871, 1970
5. John DA, Tobey RE, Homer LD, et al: Onset of succinylcholine-induced, hyperkalemia following denervation. Anesthesiology 45:294–298, 1976
6. Smith G, Dalling R, Williams TIR: Gastro-oesophageal pressure gradient changes produced by induction of anaesthesia and suxamethonium. Br J Anaesth 50:1137–1143, 1978
7. Cook JH: The effect of suxamethonium on intraocular pressure. Anaesthesia 36:359–365, 1981
8. Futter ME, Donati F, Bevan DR: Neostigmine antagonism of succinylcholine phase II block: A comparison with pancuronium. Can Anaesth Soc J 30:575–580, 1983
9. Futter ME, Donati F, Bevan DR: Prolonged suxamethonium infusion during nitrous oxide anaesthesia supplemented with halothane or fentanyl. Br J Anaesth 55:947–953, 1983
10. Whitaker M: Plasma cholinesterase variants and the anaesthetist. Anaesthesia 35:174–197, 1980
11. Viby-Mogensen J: Succinylcholine neuromuscular blockade in subjects heterozygous for abnormal plasma cholinesterase. Anesthesiology 55:231–235, 1981
12. Gronert GA: Malignant hyperthermia. Sem Anesthesia 2:197–204, 1983

13. Goudsouzian NG, Liu LMP: The neuromuscular response of infants to a continuous infusion of succinylcholine. Anesthesiology 60:97–101, 1984
14. Fisher MM, Munro I: Life-threatening anaphylactoid reaction to muscle relaxants. Anesth Analg 62:559–564, 1983
15. Fahey MR, Morris RB, Miller RD, et al: Clinical pharmacology of ORG NC45 (Norcuron™): A new nondepolarizing muscle relaxant. Anesthesiology 55:6–11, 1981
16. Viby-Mogensen J, Jorgensen BC, Ording H: Residual curarization in the recovery room. Anesthesiology 50:539–541, 1979
17. Bowman WC: Prejunctional and postjunctional cholinoceptors at the neuromuscular junction. Anesth Analg 59:935–943, 1980
18. Edwards RP, Miller RD, Roizen MF, et al: Cardiac responses to imipramine and pancuronium during anesthesia with halothane or enflurane. Anesthesiology 50:421–425, 1979
19. Savarese JJ: The autonomic margins of safety of metocurine and d-tubocurarine in the cat. Anesthesiology 50:40–46, 1979
20. Stoelting RK: The hemodynamic effects of pancuronium and d-tubocurarine in anesthetized patients. Anesthesiology 36:612–615, 1972
21. Lebowitz PW, Ramsey FM, Savarese JJ, et al: Potentiation of neuromuscular blockade in man produced by combinations of pancuronium and metocurine or pancuronium and d-tubocurarine. Anesth Analg 59:604–609, 1980
22. Ali HH, Savarese JJ: Monitoring of neuromuscular function. Anesthesiology 45:216–249, 1976
23. Fisher DM, O'Keefe C, Stanski DR, et al: Pharmacokinetics and pharmacodynamics of d-tubocurarine in infants, children and adults. Anesthesiology 57:203–208, 1982

Won W. Choi
Samir D. Gergis
Martin D. Sokoll

17

Controversies in Muscle Relaxants

In the past 20 years much knowledge has been acquired concerning the physiology of neuromuscular transmission and the pharmacology of neuromuscular blocking drugs. The knowledge acquired has made this area of anesthetic practice, to some extent, less controversial. However, a number of areas of controversy do remain. This section will be devoted to a discussion of some of these controversies, as listed below.

MUSCLE FASCICULATION

The origin of succinylcholine-induced fasciculation has been the source of considerable controversy. It was originally believed to be the result of asynchronous depolarization of the postsynaptic membrane of individual cells by succinylcholine. For several reasons this explanation appeared incomplete. First, the asynchronous depolarization of individual muscle cells would be imperceptible externally. Secondly, entire motor units appear to be activated almost simultaneously. Thirdly, repeated fasciculations occur in the same area of the muscle.

For many years there has been a slow accumulation of pharmacologic data suggesting that cholinergic agonists have actions not only postsynaptically at the neuromuscular junction but also prejunctionally on the nerve terminal. The recent demonstration of cholinergic receptor, both presynaptically and postsynaptically, along with the work of Riker[1] and of Standaert and Adams,[2] suggests that the origin of succinylcholine-induced fasciculations is

MUSCLE RELAXANTS
ISBN 0-8089-1784-6

due to the action of the drugs on the prejunctional receptor. The clinical significance of succinylcholine-induced fasciculations is their proposed relationship to increase in potassium efflux, intraocular and intragastric pressures (IOP and IGP, respectively), and postoperative muscle pain.[3] Though there is not a straightforward relationship between fasciculations and muscle pain, the abolition of fasciculations by the prior administration of a small dose of nondepolarizing neuromuscular blocking agent does decrease the incidence and severity of postoperative muscle pain. The efficacy of the nondepolarizing drug in blocking fasciculations is related to its ability to inhibit the presynaptic element of the action of succinylcholine. Pretreatment with a nondepolarizer does not greatly influence potassium efflux, intraocular pressure, or intragastric pressure.

INTRAOCULAR PRESSURE

The proper handling of the patient with an open eye injury presents a cluster of problems for the anesthesiologist. The patient must be anesthetized and the airway secured without elevation of intraocular pressure (IOP) and possible loss of vitreous humor. For many years this was frequently accomplished by a rapid induction-intubation sequence utilizing succinylcholine. This was done despite the knowledge that succinylcholine, because of its action on the extraocular and orbital muscles, perhaps as a result of fasciculations or production of contracture, increases IOP.[4] Following the observation that a small dose of nondepolarizing drug will prevent fasciculations, the efficacy of this maneuver in preventing succinylcholine-induced increased IOP was examined. Miller et al[5] observed that the prior administration of both gallamine and D-tubocurarine could prevent this increase in IOP. However, Meyers and associates[6] were unable to demonstrate the protective effect of the prior administration of D-tubocurarine or gallamine on IOP. The discrepancy between these two studies may be methodologic. Miller and colleagues used Schiotz tonometry, which is technically difficult to interpret. Meyers et al used applanation tonometry, a more recent technique for demonstrating IOP, which is more accurate than the former in determining IOP.*

Cook,[7] in a large series of patients in whom other factors that may cause an increase in IOP were kept constant, found that no regimen protected the patient from the development of increased IOP following succinylcholine.

---

*Editor's note: It is my belief that differences are due to the doses used. Nondepolarizing agents in sufficiently large doses will diminish or abolish the effect of succinylcholine on IOP. However, if the dose of succinylcholine is increased sufficiently this inhibition will be surmounted. Similarly, if the dose of nondepolarizer is increased, inhibition of the succinylcholine increase in IOP will again occur. It is simply a matter of size of dose of agonist and of antagonist.

SUCCINYLCHOLINE AND INTRAGASTRIC PRESSURE

It is a common practice to manage the patient with a full stomach by rapid induction of anesthesia with thiopental and succinylcholine, followed by tracheal intubation. There have been several studies of the effects of succinylcholine on IGP suggesting that the fasciculations produced by succinylcholine may raise the intragastric pressure (IGP)[8] sufficiently to overcome the opening pressure of the gastroesophageal junction and thereby produce regurgitation of gastric contents. In addition to skeletal muscle fasciculations mentioned previously, the ability of succinylcholine to produce contracture of slow muscle fiber may be a second mechanism for the observed increase in IGP. Unlike the rather consistent increase in IOP, the increase in IGP from succinylcholine is quite variable both in its occurrence and magnitude.

Miller and Way[8] found that 11 of 30 patients had essentially no increase in IGP. Salem et al,[9] in infants and children, found that succinylcholine does not appreciably increase IGP. Marchand[10] found that IGPs greater than 28 cm H_2O were frequently associated with incompetence of the cardioesophageal junction in cadavers. Miller and Way[8] reported that prior administration of a small dose of D-tubocurarine (3 mg) or gallamine (20 mg) and lidocaine (6 mg/kg) prevented succinylcholine-induced increase in IGP. LaCour (1969) recommends administration of 4 to 6 mg of D-tubocurarine prior to succinylcholine to prevent increase in IGP.

Does administration of succinylcholine increase IGP, and if so, is this increase in IGP enough to cause incompetence of the gastroesophageal junction resulting in regurgitation of gastric contents into oropharynx?

Contrary to the aforementioned reports, Smith et al[11] performed an in-depth study and reported that the difference betwen the IGP and the high-pressure zone (HPZ) of the lower eosphageal physiologic sphincter is more important than the absolute IGP in controlling the incidence of gastric regurgitation. When a modest increase in IGP was recorded during the fasciculations, there was always a corresponding increase in HPZ pressure. Indeed, the mean gradient between HPZ and IGP increased significantly during fasciculations. Thus they concluded that there is no increased risk of regurgitation when the gastric pressure increased in response to fasciculations induced by succinylcholine.

However, when the normal oblique angle of entry of the esophagus into the stomach is altered by increased intra-abdominal content, eg, pregnancy, ascites, bowel distension, or hiatal hernia, the IGP required to produce incompetence of the esophagogastric junction is frequently less than 15 cm H_2O. Thus, the risk of regurgitation and aspiration is greater in pregnancy. Precurarization prior to succinylcholine administration to prevent fasciculations has been advocated to prevent regurgitation and aspiration in obstetrical patients.

Marx et al[12] support this concept. This technique is supported on the grounds that succinylcholine-induced fasciculation increases IGP and also tends to increase oxygen consumption. Hence, prevention of succinylcholine-induced fasciculation may provide a greater margin of safety for both mother and baby. It has been argued that precurarization delays the onset, reduces the intensity, and shortens the duration of a succinylcholine-induced block. It also masks the end point for best intubating condition and may thus add to the risk of aspiration. Though rare, Engbek and Viby-Mogensen[13] reported unpleasant and serious reactions that may follow precurarization with small doses of nondepolarizing relaxants.

MUSCLE RELAXANTS AND INTRACRANIAL PRESSURE

Traditional practice cautions against the use of succinylcholine in patients with suspected intracranial hypertension. Cottrell et al demonstrated that a bolus injection of succinylcholine significantly increased intracranial pressure (ICP) in cats with normal or artificially elevated ICP and concluded that succinylcholine may be contraindicated in neurosurgical anesthesia.[14] However, Bormann et al[15] showed that in barbiturate-anesthetized dogs, succinylcholine does not increase ICP, even when it is acutely elevated or the intracranial compliance is decreased. One should always be careful in making inferences based on animal experiments. It is well known that species differences exist and that animal data may not be directly applicable to humans.

Stullken and Sokoll (1975) demonstrated in humans that neither succinylcholine nor D-tubocurarine have any significant effect on ICP in narcotic-barbiturate anesthesia.[16] Marsh et al[17] studied eight patients with elevated ICP and found that succinylcholine caused only a modest rise in ICP except one patient. The effects of positive pressure ventilation on central venous pressure (CVP) (therefore ICP) cannot be excluded as an explanation for this ICP increase. In acute neurosurgical patients who require rapid airway control, intubation can be facilitated by a thiopental-succinylcholine sequence with little expectation of a large, sustained ICP increase.

Lam et al,[18] in summarizing the available evidence, conclude that succinylcholine does not increase ICP in dogs, may increase ICP in cats, and in humans the response is variable with ICP increasing during intubation in the nonanesthetized or lightly anesthetized patient. Under adequate anesthesia and hypocapnia, the use of succinylcholine in neurosurgical anesthesia is compatible with safe practice.

SUCCINYLCHOLINE AND HYPERKALEMIA

A problem that has been of concern for some time is that of hyperkalemia following the administration of succinylcholine in patients with multiple trauma, burns, spinal cord transection, or demyelinating nervous disease. The magnitude of this serum potassium elevation can be clinically significant, and numerous cases of serious ventricular arrhythmia or cardiac arrest have been reported following the administration of succinylcholine to these patients. The mechanism by which this hyperkalemia occurs and the time frame of its occurrence are still not completely clear.

Carter et al[19] studied the effect of spinal cord transection in the rat and reported that, in control animals, the serum potassium was noted to rise approximately 0.5 mEq following the administration of succinylcholine. Following spinal cord transection, there was a progressive increase in the serum potassium following the administration of succinylcholine that peaked at ten days and by 60 days had returned toward normal. These data correspond well with the development of muscle contracture and increased acetylcholine sensitivity. From this work it was suggested that following a spinal cord transection injury there is a period of one to two days during which the administration of succinylcholine will cause no significant change in serum potassium level. By the third day, however, serum potassium may be expected to rise in response to succinylcholine and the drug should probably be avoided. Unfortunately, from these data they are unable to extract much information concerning when this hyperkalemic response may terminate since the response of the rat to spinal cord transection is in some ways dissimilar from that of the human. This dissimilarity is expressed by an initial atrophy of the muscle after spinal cord transection followed, in the rat, by a regaining of muscle bulk. In humans, spinal cord transection is followed by progressive atrophy with no recovery of muscle bulk. It is this difference, which begins to occur at about 2 weeks in the rat, that makes it difficult to extrapolate an end of the hyperkalemic response from the rat to the human. Carter et al concluded that the hyperkalemia originates from increased potassium efflux from the muscle in response to a cholinergic agonist from the cholinergic receptor that, following cord transection, spreads to involve practically the whole muscle membrane.

A hyperkalemic response can be seen in traumatized patients without muscle injury. Katz and Miledi reported that hypersensitivity of muscle to succinylcholine can occur following injury and does not require denervation.[20] Immobilization of an extremity, producing disuse atrophy, can result in hypersensitivity to succinylcholine.[21] Thus, succinylcholine-induced hyperkalemia is related to increased chemosensitivity of the membrane, as a result of the development of receptor sites in extrajunctional areas. Although succinylcholine induces a small release of potassium in normal muscle, it produces a potentially lethal efflux in the presence of increased sensitivity. The administration of nondepolarizing relaxants has been advocated to decrease succinylcholine potassium efflux in susceptible patients. However, the dose required approaches the full paralyzing dose of that agent. It is safest to avoid succinylcholine in these patients.

ANTAGONISM OF DESENSITIZATION BLOCK

The administration of succinylcholine by constant infusion frequently produces what has been called a desensitization or phase II block. Management of this type of block has been controversial.

Gissen et al[22] found that neostigmine antagonizes desensitization blockade only in the absence of succinylcholine in arterial blood. Although explanations for desensitization blockade by succinylcholine are numerous and controversial, certain observations indicate that neostigmine will antagonize a succinylcholine-induced phase II blockade.[23] Gissen et al concluded that without a method to determine the concentration of succinylcholine in blood, attempts to antagonize desensitization blockade by succinylcholine with acetylcholinesterase inhibitors should be avoided. Administration of edrophonium or neostigmine are indicated if the following criteria are met: (1) the infusion has been discontinued for ten to 15 minutes to allow for hydrolysis of circulating succinylcholine; (2) there is evidence of partial recovery of neuromuscular transmission; and (3) the nondepolarizing nature of the phase II block has been documented. Because of the unclear nature of the block, it is advisable to test the reversal with a small dose of edrophonium. If effective, the reversal can be completed with further doses of either edrophonium or neostigmine. Patients having either abnormal or deficient pseudocholinesterase almost always develop a phase II block and can be handled in the same manner. Monitoring neuromuscular function via peripheral nerve stimulation will help avoid succinylcholine overdose, detect development of phase II block, follow its rate of recovery, and assess the effect of reversal agents. In the event of inability to achieve complete recovery from a phase II block, ventilatory support is indicated.

MIXING OF RELAXANTS

In spite of the knowledge that nondepolarizing (D-tubocurarine, pancuronium, and gallamine) and depolarizing (succinylcholine and decamethonium) muscle relaxants may have antagonistic[24] or additive[25] actions, anesthesiologists often use depolarizing relaxants and nondepolarizing relaxants in the same patient. Both types of relaxants are administered concomitantly in the following possible situations.

Succinylcholine is commonly given to facilitate intubation of trachea, and then a longer-acting nondepolarizing relaxant such as D-tubocurarine or pancuronium is administered to provide prolonged relaxation for the surgical procedure. The use of succinylcholine to facilitate tracheal intubation prior to use of a nondepolarizing relaxant is open to the criticism that two antagonistic drugs have been used where one would suffice. Walts,[24] giving D-tubocurarine 4 mg/m^2 prior to full recovery from succinylcholine, decreased maximum intensity of D-tubocurarine–induced block when it was administered following succinylcholine. Katz[25] reported that prior administration of succinylcholine nearly doubled the depression of twitch height from the same dose of pancuronium. A comparable increase in duration of block occurred. Although succinylcholine and D-tubocurarine are supposedly antagonistic,[26] Katz[25] has speculated that perhaps the endplate is still desensitized from the first dose of succinylcholine.

Succinylcholine administration may result in increased IOP, increased IGP, fasciculation, muscle pain, or hyperkalemia. A small dose of nondepolarizing agent commonly is given prior to the administration of succinylcholine to attenuate some of these adverse effects. Despite its advantages, this technique has been questioned because a larger dose of succinylcholine is required, the possibility of producing a significant block with the small dose of nondepolarizing drug, and the loss of fasciculation as a sign of development of neuromuscular block. The advantages of this practice must be carefully weighed against the hazards of mixing different types of relaxants.

The third regimen of combined relaxant administration is to follow a nondepolarizing drug used for prolonged relaxation with succinylcholine to provide additional relaxation at the end of the procedure. The dose of succinylcholine required for adequate relaxation is directly dependent on the amount of residual neuromuscular blockade.[24] Foldes demonstrated that the efficacy of depolarizing drugs is reduced in the presence of residual curarization and that the dose required is likely to be excessive. Gray and Baraka[27] have demonstrated that a large dose of succinylcholine administered when the curarizing effect of a long-acting nondepolarizing relaxant is wearing off (1) reverses the residual action of that drug in a manner analogous to acetylcholine, and (2), would produce complete neuromuscular block provided the dose of succinylcholine was adequate.

The danger of administering succinylcholine in addition to a nondepolarizing drug to provide relaxation at the end of an operation lies in the possibility that its action may persist for a prolonged period, and that if neostigmine is subsequently administered it might cause a very prolonged and complex block. Despite the questionable pharmacologic reasoning, concomitant administration of an antagonist and an agonist in appropriate doses appears to be effective. Whether it is the best way to solve the problem is the subject of much debate. Many prefer to give an additional dose of nondepolarizing agent that can be easily antagonized at the end of the operation or to deepen the level of anesthesia.

The interaction between succinylcholine and cholinesterase inhibitors is very complex. Nastuk and Gissen[28] reported a marked reduction in the concentration of depolarizing drugs required to produce paralysis in presence of cholinesterase inhibitors, probably because acetylcholine and succinylcholine depolarize the postjunctional membrane in a similar and additive manner.

The need to provide additional relaxation following the reversal of a nondepolarizing block presents an even more difficult problem. In this circumstance the administration of further nondepolarizing drugs must be titrated to the minimum effective dose and even then may be difficult to reverse completely. The other alternative is to give a depolarizing agent. Sunew and Hicks[29] found a prolonged response to succinylcholine when administered following neostigmine under experimental conditions. All cholinesterase inhibitors appear to be similar in this regard. A similar but somewhat greater prolongation of action was found when succinylcholine was administered following reversal of a nondepolarizing block.

SINGLE LARGE OR SMALL DIVIDED DOSE

It has been proposed that antagonistic drugs, including all the nondepolarizing relaxants, achieve their effect by occupying a critical proportion of the receptor sites and rendering them unavailable to acetylcholine. In order to block transmission of normal motor nerve discharge (tetanic stimulus at 40 to 50 HZ), Waud and Waud (1970) suggest that in excess of 70% of the receptor sites must be occupied by curare or curare-like drug. It follows that once the concentration of drug in the synaptic cleft has been raised to a level that will produce occupancy of more than 80% of the receptors, twitch response will be reduced. Feldman[30] believes that a strong affinity between muscle relaxant and receptor, rather than blood flow, produces the rate-limiting step in recovery from paralysis. As the duration of paralysis will be the time required to reduce receptor occupancy below the critical paralytic threshold, the larger the dose, and the higher the initial receptor occupancy, the longer will be the duration of paralysis. In other words, a single large bolus of relaxant given at the start of anesthesia will produce prolonged adequate paralysis with a relatively low serum concentration of relaxant at the end of anesthesia. Because of this effect, Feldman suggested that frequently repeated small doses of relaxant that are just sufficient to produce adequate paralysis will result in higher blood level of drug at the end of operation. This is more likely to lead to difficulty with reversal and residual postoperative paralysis with its attendant potential for respiratory complications.

Certainly, initially administering large doses of muscle relaxant has its advantages. This technique will provide excellent surgical conditions and will mitigate the necessity of precisely regulating the anesthetic dose. However, the theory that neuromuscular blockade may be easier to antagonize if large doses of muscle relaxant were given initially rather than small repetitive doses was recently tested. Ham et al[31] found no difference in the pharmacokinetics and pharmacodynamics of D-tubocurarine when given as a single large bolus, repeated small doses, or a continuous infusion titrated to maintain a constant depression of twitch tension. Also, no difference in neostigmine antagonism between the three dosage schedules was found. These findings do not support Feldman's prediction of a lower serum muscle relaxant concentration with a large-dose technique. Despite the lack of difference between the three dosage schedules, the use of small frequent doses or of continuous infusion of muscle relaxant, while monitoring neuromuscular function with a peripheral nerve stimulator, may have advantages over the large-bolus technique.

MUSCLE RELAXANT AND TEMPERATURE

The problem of the effect of temperature on the action of neuromuscular blocking agents has been of concern for some time. In early studies Cannard and Zaimis[32] found that D-tubocurarine produced less neuromuscular blockade in a cold extremity or under the condition of hypothermia than it did at normal body temperature in humans. The extent of this change in potency appeared to be clinically significant. It was thought that the cause for this decrease in potency might be related to a temperature-induced decrease in the activity of acetylcholinesterase and hydrolysis of acetylcholine, resulting in an increased junctional acetylcholine and hence a decreased D-tubocurarine–induced blockade. In modern air-conditined operating rooms it is not uncommon for the patient to become moderately hypothermic. The clinical importance is the possible increased requirement for D-tubocurarine. This agrees with the original report of Bülbring[33] that moderate degrees of hypothermia lessened the onset and magnitude of a D-tubocurarine–induced block. Recently, Miller and colleagues[34] demonstrated that the infusion rate of D-tubocurarine necessary to maintain 90% depression of twitch tension is directly related to temperature. Thus, it would appear that in both the in vitro and in vivo preparations, neuromuscular block should be more effective at a low temperature.

Additionally, Ham et al[35] demonstrated the temperature dependence of the serum concentration of D-tubocurarine. They found that the serum D-tubocurarine concentration fell faster at 39 °C than it did at 28 °C, suggesting a prolonged excretion phase of the drug at lower temperature and hence a more prolonged effect on neuromuscular transmission. Because the decreased temperature inhibits the rate of hepatic metabolism and renal excretion of the neuromuscular blockers, the resultant higher blood concentration would impede drug redistribution from the endplate region.

Cannard and Zaimis' observations that cooling of the curarized preparation results in an increased twitch tension and rewarming increases the magnitude of the blockade is of clinical significance. One of the clinical implications of this controversy would be the possibility of recurarization on rewarming following adequate reversal of a neuromuscular block at a lower temperature. However, McKlveen et al[36] were unable to demonstrate this phenomenon in the experimental animal.

MUSCLE RELAXANTS AND ANTIBIOTICS

At approximately the same time that the neuromuscular blocking agents were being developed, antibiotics were also coming into clinical use. Though the sulfonamides and penicillin had no significant effect on neuromuscular transmission, the aminoglycoside antibiotics did prove to have neuromuscular blocking properties. The first clinical cases of antibiotic-induced neuromuscular block reported are apparently those of Pridgen[37] in 1956. Since then a large number of antibiotics, principally those of the aminoglycoside group, but also including clindamycin, lincomycin, and polymyxins, which are non-aminoglycoside antibiotics, have been demonstrated to have neuromuscular blocking properties.

The mechanism by which antibiotics induce blockade at the neuromuscular junction may be rather complex. There are four possible sites of action: (1) the nerve terminal, (2) the postsynaptic cholinergic receptors, (3) the extrajunctional muscle membrane, and (4) the contractile mechanism in the muscle.[38,39] For example, the available information implies the existence of three possible modes of action of streptomycin: (1) a postsynaptic receptor blockade, (2) inhibition of acetylcholine release from the nerve terminal, and (3) a minor nonspecific local anesthetic type of action.

Other information concerning the mode of action of antibiotics as neuromuscular blockers can be obtained from observing the ability of calcium or neostigmine to reverse the antibiotic-induced neuromuscular block. Reversal of a magnesium-induced block by calcium suggests that the block is presynaptic in origin and may involve inhibition of transmitter release. Likewise, reversal of a neuromuscular block by neostigmine has been interpreted to indicate a primary site of action at the postjunctional cholinergic receptor. Many of the antibiotics probably induce their neuromuscular effect by a combination of presynaptic and postsynaptic activity, as is suggested by the fact that, for example, a gentamycin-induced block is reasonably well reversed by both calcium and neostigmine. Conversely, drugs such as polymyxin, colistin, clindamycin, and erythromycin show no reversal of neuromuscular block by either calcium or neostigmine. The assumption here would be that neuromuscular block induced by these agents does not involve transmitter release from the nerve terminal or the action of this transmitter with the cholinergic receptor. The actual mechanism of neuromuscular block produced by these agents has, to a great extent, not been elucidated beyond the fact that the blockers are not completely reversed by either calcium or neostigmine.

The postoperative management of patients with an antibiotic- or combined neuromuscular blocking agent-antibiotic–induced neuromuscular block can be difficult. The degree of difficulty in reversing the block depends on its depth and the drugs that have produced it. In the case of a combined block it is almost impossible to tell what percentage of the block is due to the neuromuscular blocking agent and what percentage is due to the antibiotic. Reversal of a combined neuromuscular blockade may be attempted by the administration of a total of 0.07 mg/kg neostigmine (5 mg/70 kg) preceded by 0.017 mg/kg atropine. If this does not produce adequate reversal, then calcium chloride can be administered gradually to a total dose of 30 mg/kg over a ten-minute period while the ECG is constantly monitored. However, use of calcium for reversal of antibiotic-induced neuromuscular block is no longer recommended by some groups[40] for two reasons. First, the antagonism calcium produces usually is not sustained, and second, calcium may antagonize the antibacterial effect of the antibiotics. If these drugs have not produced reversal of the blockade, then the patient should be artificially ventilated and the block permitted to wear off spontaneously.

REFERENCES

1. Riker WF: Prejunctional effects of neuromuscular blocking and facilitatory drugs, in Katz RL (ed): Muscle Relaxants. Amsterdam, North Holland Publishing Co, 1975, pp 59–102
2. Standaert FG, Adams JE: The action of succinylcholine on the mammarian motor nerve terminal. J Pharmacol Exp Ther 149:113–123, 1965
3. Dottori O, Loff BA, Ygge H: Muscle pains after suxamethonium. Acta Anaesth Scand 9:247–256, 1965
4. Katz RL, Eakins KE: Mode of action of succinylcholine on intraocular pressure. J Pharmacol Exp Ther 162:1, 1968
5. Miller RD, Way WL: Inhibition of succinylcholine induced increased intraocular pressure by non-depolarizing muscle relaxant. Anesthesiology 29:123–126, 1968
6. Meyers EF, Krupin T, Johnson M, et al: Failure of non-depolarizing neuromuscular blockers to inhibit succinylcholine induced increased intraocular pressure, a controlled study. Anesthesiology 48:149–151, 1978
7. Cook JH: The effect of suxamethonium on intraocular pressure. Anaesthesia 36:359–365, 1981
8. Miller RD, Way WL: Inhibition of succinylcholine-induced increased intragastric pressure by non-depolarizing relaxant and lidocaine. Anesthesiology 34:185–188, 1971

9. Salem MR, Wong AY, Lin YH: The effect of suxamethonium on the intragastric pressure in infants and children. Br J Anaesth 44:166, 1972
10. Marchand P: A study of the forces productive of gastroesophageal regurgitation and herniation through the diaphragmatic hiatus. Thorax 12:189, 1957
11. Smith G, Dalling R, Williams TIR: Gastro-esophageal pressure gradient changes produced by induction of anaesthesia and suxamethonium. Br J Anaesth 50:1137–1143, 1978
12. Marx GF: In defense of the use of D-tubocurarine prior to succinylcholine in obstetrics. Anesthesiology 59:157, 1983
13. Engbek J, Viby-Mogensen J: Precurarization—A hazard to the patient? Acta Anaesth Scand 28:61–62, 1984
14. Cottrell JE, Hartung J, Giffin JP, et al: Intracranial and hemodynamic changes after succinylcholine administration in cats. Anesth Analg 62:1006–1009, 1983
15. Bormann BE, Smith RB, Bunegin L, et al: Does succinylcholine raise intracranial pressure? Anesthesiology 53:S262, 1980
16. Stullken EH Jr, Sokoll MD: Anesthesia and subarachnoid intracranial pressure. Anesth Analg 54:494–498, 1975
17. Marsh ML, Dunlop BJ, Shapiro HM, et al: Succinylcholine—Intracranial pressure effects in neurosurgical patients. Anesth & Analg 59:550–551, 1980
18. Lam AM, Gelb AW: Succinylcholine and intracranial pressure—A cause for ''pause.'' Anesth Analg 63:619–625, 1984
19. Carter JG, Sokoll MD, Gergis SD: Effect of spinal cord transection on neuromuscular function in the rat. Anesthesiology 55:542–546, 1981
20. Katz B, Miledi R: Development of acetylcholine sensitivity in nerve-free segments of skeletal muscle. J Physiol 170:389, 1964
21. Solandt DY, Partridge RC, Hunter J: The effect of skeletal fixation on skeletal muscle. J Neurophysiol 6:17, 1943
22. Gissen AJ, Katz RL, Karis JH, et al: Neuromuscular block in man during prolonged arterial infusion with succinylcholine. Anesthesiology 27:242–249, 1966
23. Miller RD: Antagonism of neuromuscular blockade. Anesthesiology 44:318–329, 1976
24. Walts LF, Dillon JB: Clinical studies of the interaction between D-tubocurarine and succinylcholine. Anesthesiology 31:39, 1969
25. Katz RL: Modification of the action of pancuronium by succinylcholine and halothane. Anesthesiology 35:602, 1971
26. Jenkinson DH: The antagonism between tubocurarine and substances which depolarize the motor endplate. J Physiol 152:309, 1960
27. Gray TC, Baraka A: Progress in anesthesiology. Proceedings of the 4th World Congress of Anesthesiologists, London, Excerptamesica, 1968
28. Nastuk WL, Gissen AJ: Acetion of acetylcholine and other quaternary ammonium compounds at the muscle post-junctional membrane, in Paul WM, Daniel EE (eds): Muscle. Oxford, Pergamon Press, p 389, 1965
29. Sunew KY, Hicks RG: Effects of neostigmine and pyridostigmine on duration of succinylcholine action and pseudocholinesterase activity. Anesthesiology 49:188, 1978
30. Feldman SA: The rational use of muscle relaxants, in: Muscle Relaxants. London, WB Saunders, 1973, pp 149–155
31. Ham J, Miller RD, Sheiner LB, et al: Dosage schedule independence of D-tubocurarine pharmacokinetics and pharmacodynamics and recovery of neuromuscular function. Anesthesiology 50:528, 1979
32. Cannard TH, Zaimis E: The effect of lowered muscle temperature on the action of neuromuscular blocking drugs in man. Physiol 149:112–119, 1959
33. Bülbring E: Observations on isolated phrenic nerve diaphragm preparation of rat. Br J Pharmacol 1:38, 1946

34. Miller RD, Van NyHuis LS, Eger EI II: The effect of temperature on a D-tubocurarine neuromuscular blockade and its antagonism by neostigmine. J Pharmacol Exp Ther 195:237–241, 1975
35. Ham J, Miller RD, Benet LZ, et al: The pharmacokinetics and pharmacodynamics of D-tubocurarine during hypothermia in the cat. Anesthesiology 49:324, 1978
36. McKlveen JR, Sokoll MD, Gergis SD, et al: Absence of recurarization upon rewarming. Anesthesiology 38:153–156, 1973
37. Pridgen JE: Respiratory arrest thought to be on the action of intraperitoneal neomycin. Surgery 40:571–574, 1956
38. Sokoll MD, Gergis SD: Antibiotics and neuromuscular function. Anesthesiology 55:148–159, 1981
39. Singh YN, Marshall IG, Harvey AL: The mechanism of the muscle paralyzing action of antibiotics and their interaction with neuromuscular blocking agents. Review on Drug Metabolism and Drug Interaction, London, Freund Publishing, 3:129, 1980
40. Miller RD, Savarese JJ: Pharmacology of muscle relaxants, in Miller RD (ed): Anesthesia, vol 1. New York, Churchill Livingstone, 1981, pp 523–524

Sandor Agoston
Dieter Langrehr
Douglas E.F. Newton

18

Pharmacology and Possible Clinical Applications of 4-Aminopyridine

Chemical work with pyridine started as early as 1846 and resulted in the synthesis of the first heterocyclic compound, methylpyridine, by Klaus in 1862. Further development was marked by the synthesis of three isomeric aminopyridines in 1894 and that of 2-aminopyridine in 1915. The first pharmacologic studies with aminopyridines were initiated by Dohrn in 1924, and, thereafter, much experimental work has been done in order to clarify the pharmacologic profile and define the potential clinical usefulness of aminopyridines. Although a great number of compounds has been tested under various experimental conditions in the course of subsequent decades, Lemeignan and Lechat (1967) were the first to notice the ability of 4-aminopyridine to reverse neuromuscular block induced by d-tubocurarine. After investigating these effects in detail, Bulgarian scientists, Paskov and Stojanov, in 1973 introduced 4-aminopyridine hydrochloride as an anticurare agent into anesthetic practice. For this purpose it has been used clinically in Bulgaria under the trade name Pymadin for the last 10 years. The first clinical reports of Stojanov and co-workers were followed by more extensive clinical investigations in The Netherlands that have triggered a wide and rapidly growing interest in aminopyridines and similarly acting drugs. For references, a comprehensive review of Bowman and Savage[1] and the proceedings of an international symposium devoted to aminopyridines, edited by Lechat et al, may be consulted. (The structural formula of 4-aminopyridine is shown in Fig 1).

MUSCLE RELAXANTS
ISBN 0-8089-1784-6

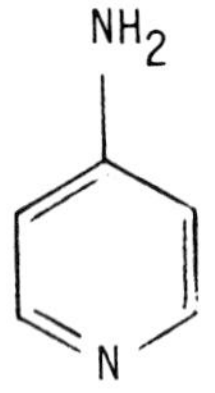

NH_2

N

4-AMINOPYRIDINE

Figure 1. Structural formula of 4-aminopyridine.

PHARMACOLOGIC ACTIONS OF 4-AMINOPYRIDINE

Presynaptic Effects at the Nerve Terminal

It is a generally accepted view that, when an action potential invades the nerve terminal, the large change in membrane potential causes a transient increase in membrane permeability to Na^+ and K^+ resulting in a transmembrane movement of these cations in accordance with their concentration gradients. Although most of the current (nerve action potential) is carried by Na^+ and K^+, at this stage the membrane becomes also permeable to calcium. It is well known that voltage-sensitive calcium channels exist in the presynaptic membrane of the motor nerve terminals and that calcium current through these channels mediates evoked transmitter release.[3] Therefore, small changes in the amplitude or in duration of the nerve action potential will in turn determine the size and duration of the ionic fluxes and also the inward flux of calcium ions that activate the transmitter release mechanism. The main action of 4-aminopyridine at the motor nerve terminal is to decrease membrane potassium conductance. Such an inhibitory action results in slowing of the action potential during its repolarization phase. The prolongation of the duration of the nerve action potential results in a greater influx of calcium into the nerve terminal and, thus, increased release of acetylcholine.

Actions on Muscle Contractility

Calcium ions play an essential role not only in acetylcholine release from motor nerve ending but also in the contractile mechanism of skeletal, smooth, and heart muscle. There is accumulating experimental evidence that 4-aminopyridine, either by prolongation of the muscle action potentials or by direct action on the membrane calcium channels at the sarcoplasmatic reticulum, makes more calcium available to the processes that couple excitation to contraction, which ultimately will result in increase of muscle contractility.[1,4]

Central Nervous System Effects

There is also animal experimental and clinical evidence indicating some analeptic actions of 4-aminopyridine. The central actions are thought to be mediated by a similar presynaptic mechanism to that seen in the periphery and are not necessarily restricted to effects upon any particular type of synapse or transmitter; although it is probable that central cholinoceptive sites are most sensitive to the actions of this compound. 4-Aminopyridine has been shown to facilitate transmission in the excitatory and inhibitory pathways in the spinal cord and to stimulate respiratory drive in the cat. In man the central stimulant action of 4-aminopyridine convincingly shortened recovery to full consciousness from ketamine-diazepam anesthesia or reversed respiratory depression induced by narcotics.[1,2]

Many of the various actions of 4-aminopyridine could be potentially useful in clinical practice. The accumulated clinical experience with this compound so far includes its therapeutic application in anethesia for reversal of residual neuromuscular blockade resulting from nondepolarizing neuromuscular blocking agents and certain antibiotics, but it might also be extended to treatment of patients with Botulinus intoxication or myoneural disorders, such as myasthenia gravis and Eaton-Lambert syndrome.[2]

Further discussion in this review will, therefore, be focused on the possible clinical application of 4-aminopyridine in anesthesiology and in other clinical disciplines. Its pharmacokinetics in man and toxic effects will be discussed as well.

Use of 4-Aminopyridine in Anesthesiology

In our hands, when given alone, 4-aminopyridine showed only a modest anticurare effect. Such a case is shown in Fig 2.

In this case, following intubation with succinylcholine (SCh), a constant 90% depression of the twitch tension was maintained with pancuronium bromide administered by intravenous (IV) infusion. After stopping the infusion when the twitch tension returned to 20% of its control value, 230 μg/kg 4-aminopyridine was injected. Thereafter the recovery rate visibly increased; however, there was less than 80% recovery by 15 minutes, and, therefore, neostigmine 12 μg/kg was given with atropine, which resulted in complete reversal of the twitch tension within a few minutes.

Also in subsequent Western European studies, using the dose of 4-aminopyridine suggested by the Bulgarian authors (0.3 mg/kg IV), a complete reversal of pancuronium-induced neuromuscular blockade required 20 to 25

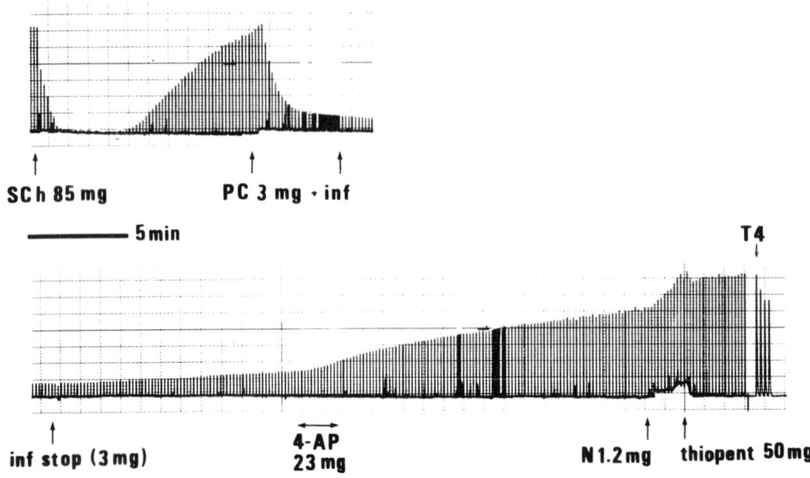

Figure 2. Reversal of pancuronium (Pc) induced neuromuscular blockade by 4-amino-pyridine (4-AP) and neostigmine (N). (Reprinted with permission[5].)

minutes. Under similar conditions neostigmine usually produced complete reversal in less than ten minutes. In order to shorten the reversal time, the use of larger doses (up to 0.5 mg/kg of 4-aminopyridine) was investigated. These larger doses, however, were frequently associated with central nervous system stimulation, resulting in postoperative restlessness and confusion.

Since 4-aminopyridine increases acetylcholine release, whereas cholinesterase inhibitors delay acetylcholine breakdown, it can be expected that when administered together they will mutually potentiate the antagonistic effects of each other. This possibility has been extensively studied by Miller et al[6] who showed that in the presence of small, by itself inactive, doses of 4-aminopyridine the antagonistic doses of neostigmine or pyridostigmine could be reduced by 70% and 80%, respectively, due to the apparent synergism between these drugs. Therefore, the dose of one or both drugs in such a combination can be reduced, yet still provide increased antagonistic activity with, at the same time, a decreased risk of side effects. Drugs used in fixed-dose combinations should have similar pharmacokinetic profiles. For this reason, pyridostigmine is the drug of choice when 4-aminopyridine is to be used together with an anticholinesterase drug for the reversal of the effects of neuromuscular blocking agents. The prejunctional effects of this compound, resulting in an increase of acetylcholine release, have been successfully utilized to reverse the neuromuscular effects of certain antibiotics. Neomycin and streptomycin appeared to be more effectively reversed than polymixin B, which suggests that the affinity of these polypeptide antibiotics for sites of acetylcholine release may be greater than that of aminoglycosides.

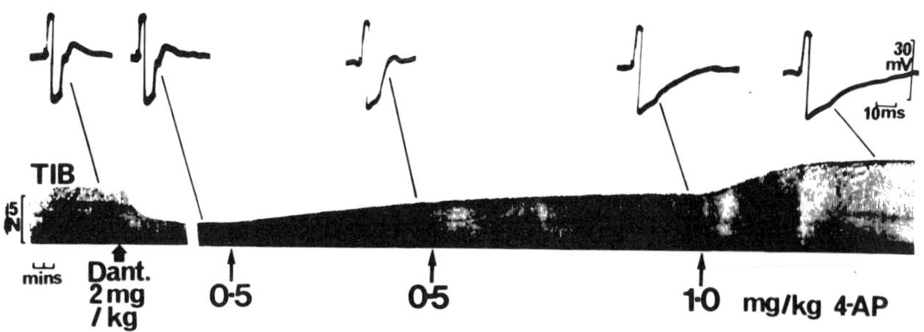

Figure 3. Maximal twitches and gross muscle action potentials of the tibialis anterior muscle of the cat. The oblique lines indicate the twitches with which the representative action potentials are associated. At D and at the remaining arrows, dantrolene sodium and 4-aminopyridine were injected IV, respectively. (Reprinted with permission[4].)

Besides its facilitatory effects at the neuromuscular junction, 4-aminopyridine also exerts a direct effect on skeletal muscle that is reflected in its ability to reverse muscle paralysis induced by dantrolene sodium.

Dantrolene is known to inhibit the release of calcium from the sarcoplasmatic reticulum; therefore, the 4-aminopyridine–induced reversal of dantrolene effects indicates that this compound also facilitates the excitation-contraction coupling processes in skeletal muscle. This effect of 4-aminopyridine is entirely different from and complementary to its presynaptic actions by which the curare-like agents are antagonized. Note that the muscle action potentials (Fig 3) simultaneously recorded with the twitch response remained unchanged, even after the development of the maximum twitch depression by dantrolene. In contrast, the administration of incremental doses of 4-aminopyridine reversed the twitch height depression and prolonged the duration of the action potentials in a dose-dependent fashion. This is in agreement with the proposed mechanism of action of 4-aminopyridine (Lechat, et al[2]).

Central analeptic effects of 4-aminopyridine were described by the Bulgarian investigators and confirmed later in western European studies. In cats, Folgering et al[7] demonstrated the ability of 4-aminopyridine to increase central respiratory drive using the quantified phrenic nerve activity as an indication of the activity of the respiratory center. This effect could be abolished by high doses of atropine, suggesting the involvement of cholinergic mechanisms. In human volunteers[8] 4-aminopyridine was shown to shorten significantly the recovery time from diazepam-ketamine anesthesia. Both ketamine and benzodiazepines have been reported to interfere with central cholinergic pathways, although this is probably not their main mechanism of action. 4-Aminopyridine is known to facilitate cholinergic transmission in both central and peripheral nervous system as described above, and so it might reverse the inhibitory effects of the above anesthetics at cholinergic synapses in the brain.

The possibility that a relatively specific interaction occurs between diazepam (and other benzodiazepines) and 4-aminopyridine is supported by a recent case history[9] of a nurse who, after taking an overdose of flunitrazepam preoperatively (without informing the anesthesiologist), underwent general anesthesia for a minor surgical intervention after which she remained in a naloxone- and physostigmine-resistent deep coma for five hours. This state was promptly terminated by the injection of 0.15 mg/kg 4-aminopyridine. In the serum samples, obtained from the patient just before the administration of 4-aminopyridine, extremely high concentrations (118 μg/mL of flunitrazepam, normal values 5 to 20 μg/mL) were found by the hospital pharmacist. The postoperative course after this episode was uneventful.

Although the facilitation of cholinergic transmission both in peripheral and central nervous system seems to be an important feature of 4-aminopyridine, other pathways might also be affected as is demonstrated by the ability of this compound to reverse opiate-induced respiratory depression.[10] This effect of 4-aminopyridine would by no means justify its use as an opiate antagonist. However, the antagonism of opiate-induced respiratory depression together with its anticurare effects could be beneficial at the end of anesthesia.

Other Clinical Disciplines

Besides its application as a curare antagonist and its other possible uses in clinical anesthesia, 4-aminopyridine has been shown to exert beneficial effects in a number of clinical conditions, particularly in certain neuromuscular diseases. Marked therapeutic effects were observed after 4-aminopyridine was electrophoretically applied in patients with traumatic nervus recurrent injuries after partial thyroidectomy and also in patients with nervus facialis injuries. Therapeutic efficacy appeared to be dependent on the duration of the disease and on the functional state of the muscles involved at the time when therapy was started. In patients with Eaton-Lambert syndrome (characterized by muscular weakness due to prejunctional lesion), 4-aminopyridine has been shown to be effective; therefore this might be another indication for the therapeutic use of this compound. Also there have been sporadic reports on the ability of 4-aminopyridine to improve neuromuscular transmission in patients with myasthenia gravis.[1]

The first reports on the usefulness of 4-aminopyridine in experimental botulism[11] and later in human botulism[12] evoked considerable interest in the therapeutic potential of this compound. In patients with severe paralytic botulism, 4-aminopyridine 0.35 to 0.5 mg/kg IV produced marked progressive improvement in peripheral muscle power persisting for two to four hours. However, these beneficial effects were pronounced in the extrinsic ocular and limb muscles and only to a lesser extent in the respiratory muscles, as judged by clinical observations. Nevertheless, the authors concluded that at present the benefits of 4-aminopyridine therapy are outweighed by its potential toxicity in the treatment of human botulism.

A recent report of Wesseling et al[13] on the effects of 4-aminopyridine in Alzheimer's disease might further stimulate the research focused on the central nervous system effects of this compound. The available experimental evidence indicates that in Alzheimer's type senile dementia choline-acetyltransferase deficiency reflected in reduced acetylcholine turnover is the underlying cause of the disease. However, all neurones are not impaired to the same extent; therefore it is conceivable that a compound that promotes the release of acetylcholine from those neuronal terminals that are still functional may have beneficial effects. The study of Wesseling and co-workers[13] revealed that 4-aminopyridine (20 mg per day) significantly improved recent memory and other related functions like daily activity and recognition in demented elderly residents of a nursing home. The results of this study support the contention that aminopyridines, either alone or in combination with centrally acting cholinesterase inhibitors, might open new perspectives in the treatment of Alzheimer's senile dementia.

Another area of potential clinical application of 4-aminopyridine is in cases of intoxication with verapamil. In animal experiments, Agoston et al[14] demonstrated the ability of 4-aminopyridine to reverse completely profound cardiovascular depression and also partial neuromuscular block induced by toxic doses of verapamil (4 to 25 mg/kg IV) in the cat. A typical experiment is shown in Fig 4.

More importantly, the six animals that received 4-aminopyridine survived the verapamil intoxication, whereas four animals in the control group died. Considering the results of the above study and the wide spectrum of pharmacologic actions of 4-aminopyridine on calcium-dependent biologic functions, this compound deserves a trial in the treatment of massive verapamil intoxication also in man, particularly in cases where conventional measures have failed.

Human Pharmacokinetics

The pharmacokinetic profile of 4-aminopyridine after both oral and IV administration has been extensively studied in human volunteers by Uges et al.[15] The kinetic analysis of the serum concentrations following IV administration of a bolus injection of 20 mg 4-aminopyridine revealed a long elimination half-life of 3.6 hours, large distribution volume of 2.6 L/kg, and a high total plasma clearance of 0.6 L/kg/hr. Most of the drug (approximately 90% of the administered dose) appears unchanged in the urine within 24 hours. Elimination appears, therefore, to occur almost exclusively in the kidney, with an average renal clearance of 670 mL/min. As the normal glomerular filtration

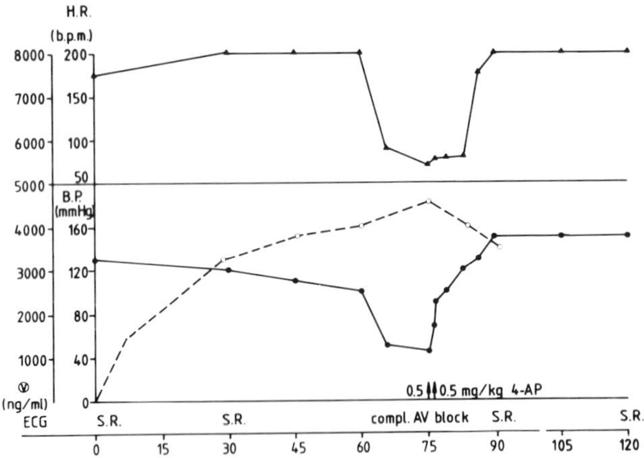

Figure 4. The effects of 4-aminopyridine on the verapamil-induced heart rate and blood pressure change in the cat. Outer scale along ordinate: serum concentrations of verapamil (nanograms per milliliter) (-------). Inner scale along ordinate: (▲) heart rate (HR; beats per minute). Inner scale along ordinate: (●) mean arterial blood pressure (BP; mm Hg). Abscissa: time (minutes). Arrows indicate time at which 4-aminopyridine (4-AP) was given (SR, sinus rhythm).

rate is approximately 130 mL/min, it is deduced that active tubular secretion plays an important role in the elimination of 4-aminopyridine in man.

SIDE EFFECTS

Following the administration of moderate clinical doses (0.15 to 0.3 mg/kg) of 4-aminopyridine, apart from a slight increase in systolic blood pressure and heart rate no other side effects were seen in any of the patients receiving this compound. However, one of the most important shortcomings of 4-aminopyridine is its narrow therapeutic index; in man doses greater than 0.5 mg/kg are likely to produce toxic effects, including restlessness, confusion, nausea, weakness, and generalized tonic-clonic seizures. High doses of diazepam (up to 80 mg IV) might be necessary to counteract such effects of 4-aminopyridine overdose.

CONCLUSIONS

The multitude of pharmacologic actions of 4-aminopyridine at various sites may complicate and limit its clinical use by increased risks of dangerous side effects and unpredictable interactions. At present its clinical use (either alone or in combination with cholinesterase inhibitors) is best restricted to the treatment of some relatively uncommon clinical conditions in which there is either a known failure of prejunctional transmission or where there are theoretical grounds to believe that the compound might be effective where routine measures have failed. Such conditions include the Eaton-Lambert syndrome, myasthenia gravis, and neuromuscular blockade complicated by concomitant use of certain antibiotics. Another area of potential clinical application is in cases of intoxication with benzodiazepines, botulinus toxin, or verapamil.

At present 4-aminopyridine cannot be considered to be a drug for routine clinical use. The synthesis and pharmacologic testing of new, more selectively acting derivatives are continuing in order to develop new drugs with improved therapeutic index and 'clean' pharmacologic profile.

REFERENCES

1. Bowman WC, Savage AO: Pharmacological actions of aminopyridines and related compounds. Rev Pure Appl Pharmacol Sci 2:317–371, 1981
2. Aminopyridines and similarly acting drugs: Effects on nerves, muscles and synapases, in Lechat P, Thesleff S, Bowman WC (eds): Advance in the Biosciences, vol 35. Oxford-New York-Toronto-Sydney-Paris-Frankfurt, Pergamon Press, 1982
3. Katz R, Miledi R: Spontaneous and evoked activity of motor nerve endings in calcium Ringer. J Physiol 203:689–706, 1969
4. Agoston S, Bowman WC, Houwertjes MC, et al: Direct action of 4-aminopyridine on the contractility of a fast contracting muscle in the cat. Clin Exp Pharmacol Physiol 9:21–34, 1982
5. Sohn YJ, Uges DRA: Pharmacokinetics and side-effects of 4-aminopyridine. Anesthesiology—Int Congress Series no. 538, Proceedings of the 7th World Congress of Anaesthesiologists. Amsterdam-Oxford-Princeton, Excerpta Medica, 1980
6. Miller RD, Booij LHDJ, Agoston S, et al: 4-Aminopyridine potentiates neostigmine and pyridostigmine in man. Anesthesiology 50:416–420, 1979
7. Folgering H, Rutten J, Agoston S: Stimulation of phrenic nerve activity by an acetylcholine releasing drug: 4-Aminopyridine. Pflügers Arch 379:181–185, 1979
8. Agoston S, Salt PJ, Erdmann W, et al: Antagonism of ketamine and diazepam anaesthesia by 4-aminopyridine in human volunteers. Br J Anaesth 52:367–370, 1980
9. Schmutzler S, Uges D, Agoston S, et al: Rohypnol-Intoxikation als Ursache eines postanaesthetischen Komas und Behandlungserfolg mit 4-aminopyridine. Anaesthesist 33: 294– 295, 1984
10. Sia RL, Zandstra DF: Use of 4-aminopyridine to reverse morphine induced respiratory depression in man. Br J Anaesth 53:865–868, 1981
11. Lundh H, Leander S, Thesleff S: Antagonism of the paralysis produced by botulinum toxin in the rat. The effects of tetraethylammonium, guanidine and 4-aminopyridine. J Neurol Sci 32:29–43, 1977
12. Ball AP, Hopkinson RB, Farrel ID, et al: Human botulism caused by Clostridium botulinum type E: The Birmingham outbreak. Q J Med New Series XLVIII 191:473–491, 1979
13. Wesseling H, Agoston S, van Dam GBP, et al: Effects of 4-aminopyridine in elderly patients with Alzheimer's disease. N Engl J Med 310:988–989, 1984
14. Agoston S, Maestrone E, van Hezik EJ, et al: Effective treatment of verapamil intoxication with 4-aminopyridine in the cat. J Clin Invest 73:1291–1296, 1984
15. Uges DRA, Sohn YJ, Greijdanus B, et al: 4-aminopyridine kinetics. Clin Pharmacol Ther 31:587–593, 1982

INDEX